Pass Finals: A Companion to Kumar and Clark

Commissioning Editor: Ellen Green
Project Development Manager: Siân Jarman
Project Manager: Frances Affleck
Designer: Sarah Russell
Cartoons: Roger Penwill
Illustrations: Cactus Illustration

Pass Finals

A Companion to Kumar and Clark

GEOFF SMITH
Specialist Registrar in Gastroenterology, University
College London Hospitals; Honorary Research Fellow,
Digestive Diseases Research Centre, St Bartholomew's
and the London School of Medicine, Queen Mary's
University of London

ELIZABETH CARTY
Consultant Physician and Gastroenterologist, Whipps
Cross University Hospital, London

LOUISE LANGMEAD
Specialist Registrar in Gastroenterology and Medicine,
St Bartholomew's and the London NHS Trust

WB 18
SMITH
HO4 050 95

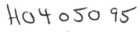

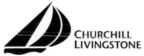

CHURCHILL
LIVINGSTONE

EDINBURGH   LONDON   NEW YORK   OXFORD   PHILADELPHIA   ST LOUIS
SYDNEY   TORONTO   2004

SAUNDERS
An imprint of Elsevier Science Limited

First published 2004

ISBN 0-7020-2653-0

British Library Cataloguing in Publication Data
A catalogue record for this book is available from the British Library

Library of Congress Cataloging in Publication Data
A catalog record for this book is available from the Library of Congress

Notice
Medical knowledge is constantly changing. Standard safety precautions must
be followed, but as new research and clinical experience broaden our
knowledge, changes in treatment and drug therapy may become necessary
or appropriate. Readers are advised to check the most current product
information provided by the manufacturer of each drug to be administered
to verify the recommended dose, the method and duration of
administration, and contraindications. It is the responsibility of the
practitioner, relying on experience and knowledge of the patient, to
determine dosages and the best treatment for each individual patient.
Neither the Publisher nor the authors assumes any liability for any injury
and/or damage to persons or property arising from this publication.

ELSEVIER
SCIENCE

your source for books,
journals and multimedia
in the health sciences

www.elsevierhealth.com

Printed in China

The
publisher's
policy is to use
paper manufactured
from sustainable forests

Preface

The range and depth of knowledge that medical students seem to be expected to retain grows continuously. This is despite the stated policy of many medical schools that the 'information load' should be reduced in undergraduate teaching. Over the last decade many traditional styles of examination have become less common, replaced by multiple-choice style examinations based on clinical scenarios and OSCE examinations in place of long and short cases.

The advance of molecular medicine and the increasing links between basic sciences and clinical medicine have led us to include these topics in the text. Common radiological investigations are also included as they are becoming a key part of many examinations. The use of evidence-based medicine demands an understanding of statistics and trial design and these topics are, as a result, also included.

In this book we have tried to distil a core dataset in general and speciality medicine. The information is provided as bulleted lists and is supported by diagrams and self-assessment questions. By its nature, therefore, this is not a definitive textbook of clinical medicine and the page references to the 5th edition of Kumar and Clark's *Clinical Medicine* are designed to point the reader towards a more in-depth explanation of the subject. We hope, however, that it will act as a source of rapid access information for the important disease processes and thereby act as a useful revision aid.

Finally we would like to thank those individuals that have supported our efforts — notably Ellen Green and Siân Jarman at Elsevier for their efforts and Sarah Russell for the design work. Also to Parveen Kumar and Michael Clark for their critique of the text and for writing *Clinical Medicine* in the first place and to our families for support and coffee during the writing. Finally we should thank the Good Samaritan for ongoing inspiration.

Good Luck!
London   G.S.
                                                          E.C.
                                                          L.L

Acknowledgements

Our thanks go to Nick Reading (Consultant Radiologist, Whipps Cross University Hospital) for supplying images for the radiology chapter.

Contents

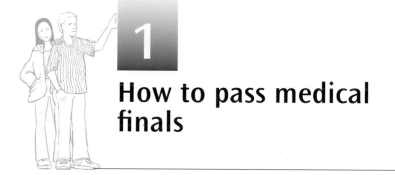

How to pass medical finals

There are, and always have been, several truisms about sitting final exams in medicine. At the end of the day, the vast majority of students pass their final exams and earn the right to call themselves 'Doctor'. There are, however, tactics and techniques that you can use to make the process less painful.

Written exams

Much of this sounds obvious, but 'schoolboy errors' are commonly made in the stress of final exams.

Be prepared
- Exam technique is a learned skill
- Know the distribution of marks for the paper
- Make sure you know the format of the exam
- Practise questions from past papers
- Practise keeping to time

Directed learning
- The vast majority of questions are about common and important areas of medicine
- Rare syndromes are very unlikely to come up
- Medical emergencies are often asked about

Read the instructions
- Make sure you are quite clear on how many questions you have to answer and how much time you have for each one
- If need be, write the start and finish times for each section on the top of the paper and stick to them

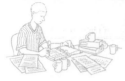

Answer the question asked	▌ Read the question carefully – preferably twice ▌ Answer the question asked, not the one you want to answer
Answer all the questions	▌ Attempt the correct number of questions ▌ If you are running out of time, try to put something down on paper, even if it is only an essay plan – you may get some credit
Presentation	▌ Clear, neat handwriting is easier to mark ▌ Headings and subheadings speed up marking ▌ Spell accurately
Anonymous papers	▌ Many exams require you to put a name or candidate number on each page – make sure you do

Clinical exams

Clinical exams can be more nerve-racking than written papers. The 'performance' in front of examiners is stressful. Again, basic tactics will help you out.

Dress code	▌ Go for smart, conservative and comfortable dress. Loud waistcoats and cartoon ties will not help
Equipment	▌ The vast majority of the equipment you will need for a clinical examination will be provided ▌ You will need: — A stethoscope – make sure it is clean and working — A pen – most important for long cases! ▌ Ophthalmoscopes should be provided, but if you have your own and are comfortable using it, take it with you. Make sure the batteries are fresh ▌ Everything else is a luxury. Pockets bulging with equipment are uncomfortable and heavy

Three key aims

I Make the diagnosis
I Ensure the examiner sees you carry out all parts of the examination competently
I Do not hurt or embarrass the patient

The order of importance of the above depends upon the examiner and the case. If the diagnosis is straightforward, the examiner will want you to reach it without too much of a performance. If the diagnosis is difficult, he or she will want you to demonstrate your ability to elicit clinical signs, even if the underlying cause escapes you.

Examination technique

I Make sure that your examination technique is swift and professional
I Do what you are asked
— 'Examine the cardiovascular system' means a full examination starting with the hands
— 'Listen to the heart' means just auscultation
— Examiners should make it clear what they want

Dignity

I *NEVER* hurt or embarrass the patient
I *ALWAYS* introduce yourself
I *ALWAYS* ask permission to examine
I *ALWAYS* ask whether the area you are going to examine is painful or tender
I *THANK* the patient at the end of the exam

Scoring points

I A professional introduction, followed by an examination technique that is fluent and clearly well practised, is as important as reaching a diagnosis
I Even if the diagnosis eludes you, describe your findings
I Outline the positive findings at examination and the important negatives
I If you can, come up with a diagnosis and differential
I The longer you can talk, the fewer questions can be asked (although talking rubbish does not help)

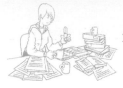

Viva voce exams

Vivas or oral examinations still make up a part of final examinations in some medical schools. They may be routine for all candidates or used specifically to re-examine a borderline candidate. If you are called for a viva in the latter situation, remember that honours students may be examined as well and that a selection of candidates across the whole range of marks will be examined to provide a standard range of scores.
In general it is difficult to fail the whole exam because of a poor performance in a viva.

Dress
I Be smart and conservative

Format
I There are usually two examiners – one may be external
I You may be:

Asked questions
I e.g. What classes of drug are useful in the management of hypertension?

Given a case scenario
I e.g. Outline the management options for a 74-year-old woman who comes to see you with rheumatoid arthritis

Asked about medical emergencies
I e.g. A 55-year-old man is admitted with haematemesis and a blood pressure of 90/50. What would you do?

Asked to report the results of an investigation
I e.g. A chest X-ray or ECG

Tactics
I 'Engage your brain before your mouth'
I Structure your answer (Tables 1.1 and 1.2)
I Do not dig holes; if you realize that you are completely wrong, apologize and start again – the examiners expect you to be nervous
I When giving lists of causes, start with the commonest first

Table 1.1   The structured answer

For any disease, outline:

Incidence – common → rare
Age
Sex
Geographical   } distribution
Racial
Pathology
Aetiology
Clinical features
Investigations
Therapeutic options
Outcome
Complications

▌ When giving lists of investigations, start with the least invasive and explain how they help with the diagnosis

▌ Make sure the tests are appropriate; if you are going to mention a blood count, chest X-ray and so on, make sure you state why you are discussing them

Table 1.2   Disease aetiology

For any clinical symptom or sign (e.g. diarrhoea*), classify the causes into:

Infective	**Metabolic**
Viruses	Hypercalcaemia
Rotavirus	
Adenovirus	**Endocrine**
Bacteria	Thyrotoxicosis
Staphylococcus aureus	
Salmonella	**Neurological**
Cholera	Autonomic neuropathy
Inflammatory	**Trauma/surgery**
Inflammatory bowel disease	Post-gastrectomy
Malignant	**Iatrogenic**
Colorectal cancer	Drugs, e.g. laxatives
Autoimmune	
Coeliac disease	**Idiopathic**

* List is not complete.

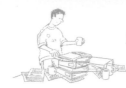

Last-minute revision

What to revise
I Revising facts you already know is easier than learning new information in the weeks prior to the exam. Consistent learning throughout the course is the best preparation

I Target the revision to the exam. Base revision around past papers and the type of exam you are sitting

I In the last week, go over notes and take timed practice exams rather than trying to learn new data

How to revise
I Practise MCQs in a group. It is more fun and you will remember more

I Outline essay plans and fill in the essential facts. You do not need to write out complete essays except to check timings

I If your university offers mock or prize exams, sit them. They are good practice and will highlight weak areas

I Use tools such as mind maps and revision aids. The more senses you use, the better the chance of the information sinking in. Jotting down lists and notes will help you absorb what you read

I Remember to give yourself time to relax. Play sport, go out or meet your friends rather than burning the midnight oil. Learning when you are half-comatose is ineffective

I Sleep and eat properly and avoid stimulants such as caffeine tablets

I The night before the exam, do as little as possible. Find a way of relaxing and get a good (and sober) night's sleep

I And finally, do you really learn anything by frantically flicking through a book as you walk into the exam?

2

Question types in medical finals

The ideal exam question, from the examiners' point of view, is one that discriminates between different levels of knowledge or ability. A question that everybody gets right says little about an individual and is therefore a poor discriminator.

Question types in written exams

MULTIPLE CHOICE QUESTIONS (Table 2.1)

▌ Questions usually comprise a stem that introduces the question, and five branches or options

Best answer questions

▌ Choose the branch that provides the correct or best answer

Example Which *one* of the following is a cause of liver cirrhosis?
A. Cigarette smoking
B. Alcohol
C. Heroin
D. Cannabis
E. Methadone

Answer: B

True or false?

▌ For each branch, decide whether the statement is true or false

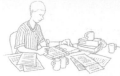

Table 2.1   MCQ styles

1. Which of the following are true of aspirin?
   A. It may cause gastric ulceration
   B. It is associated with an increased risk of transient ischaemic attacks
   C. It is associated with renal dysfunction
   D. Its use is never indicated in acute myocardial infarction
   E. It may exacerbate inflammatory bowel disease

2. Which of the following are not true of paracetamol?
   A. It is an anti-inflammatory drug
   B. It results in hepatic necrosis in severe overdose
   C. It is metabolized in the liver
   D. It is often given intravenously
   E. It is a non-steroidal anti-inflammatory drug

3. The following drugs are associated with the stated complication:
   A. Flucloxacillin: jaundice
   B. Loperamide: diarrhoea
   C. Enalapril: cough
   D. Prednisolone: weight loss
   E. Metronidazole: nausea

1. A, C, E
2. A, D, E
3. T, F, T, F, T

Example   The following are recognized causes of cirrhosis:
A. Alcohol
B. Autoimmune hepatitis
C. Hepatitis C
D. Haemochromatosis
E. Cystic fibrosis

Answer: All are true

Negative marking   ❙ A point is given for each correct answer, but a point is deducted for an incorrect answer. This system is designed to discourage blind guessing

Tips and tactics   ❙ Always ensure that you know how to complete the question paper – read the instructions carefully
❙ For computer-scored papers, make sure that the marks you make on the paper are clear and confined to the correct part of the paper. Always

use the pencil provided. Pens may not be detected properly by the computerized reader

I Keep an eye on the time. You may only have 2–3 minutes per question

I Going through the whole paper once, answering the questions you are sure of, then going back to those that need more time may ensure that you don't miss any easy points

I Look for obvious incorrect answers. *Always* and *never* are rarely correct. Read the stem very carefully.

I Check for negatives in the stem: e.g. Which of the following are *not* causes of abdominal pain? Getting this wrong could cost you five marks

I 'Educated guesses' are usually correct; however, 'blind guesses' are risky if the paper is negatively marked

I Even if you have no idea about the subject of a question, read the possible answers – there may be sections for which no specialist knowledge is required

EXTENDED MATCHING QUESTIONS

I For a small set of questions, a common list of 15–30 options provides the list of possible answers

Example Question 1 *Theme: jaundice*

A. Alcohol-related cirrhosis
B. Carcinoma of the pancreas
C. Hepatitis A
D. Hepatitis B
E. Hepatitis C
F. Haemochromatosis
G. Wilson's disease
H. Acute haemolysis
I. Gilbert's syndrome
J. Primary sclerosing cholangitis
K. Primary biliary cirrhosis
L. Autoimmune hepatitis
M. Budd–Chiari syndrome
N. Cystic fibrosis
O. Gallstone in the common bile duct

For each of the following questions, select the best answer from the list above.

I. A 28-year-old man notices that his eyes have a yellow tinge following a bad cough and cold. His liver function tests are normal apart from a bilirubin of 78 μmol/L.

II. A 76-year-old woman presents with jaundice and weight loss. She denies any abdominal pain. Her bilirubin is 280 μmol/L and the alkaline phosphatase 590 IU. The alanine

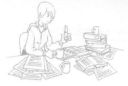
aminotransferase is 87 IU. She has a family history of ischaemic heart disease. An ultrasound of her abdomen reveals a dilated common bile duct (Table 2.2).

III. A 45-year-old man with known diabetes presents

with jaundice. He is noted to have a deep tan and hepatomegaly. His ferritin is 1201 μg/L.

Answers:
1. I.   I
   II. B
   III. F

Table 2.2   Picking out key facts

'A 76-year-old woman presents with *jaundice* and *weight loss*. *She denies any abdominal pain*. Her bilirubin is 280 μmol/L and the alkaline phosphatase 590 IU. The alanine aminotansferase is 87 IU. She has a family history of ischaemic heart disease. An ultrasound of her abdomen reveals a *dilated common bile duct*.'

Here, the classical combination of painless jaundice and weight loss gives you the diagnosis of carcinoma of the pancreas

---

Example   Question 2

A. Haemoglobin
B. Myoglobin
C. Albumin
D. Ferritin
E. Transferrin
F. Alanine transaminase
G. Collagen
H. Fibrinogen
I. Factor VIII
J. Immunoglobulin
K. Serotonin (5-hydroxytryptamine, 5HT)
L. Tryptophan
M. Intrinsic factor
N. Glucose-6-phosphatase
O. Lactate dehydrogenase

For each of the following questions, select the best answer from the list above:

I.   A peptide important in the absorption of vitamin B_{12} *(M)*

II. An iron-containing protein derived from muscle   *(B)*

III. A neurotransmitter released by carcinoid tumours   *(K)*

IV. A helical structural connective tissue protein   *(G)*

V.   A protein to which bilirubin is bound in the blood   *(C)*

VI. A protein capable of carrying oxygen in the circulation   *(A)*

VII. A substance the deficiency of which results in pellagra   *(L)*

VIII. A protein precursor of bilirubin   *(A)*

IX. A protein released by injured hepatocytes   *(F)*

X.   A protein that exists in five subclasses   *(J)*

> **I** Note that any answer from the list may be appropriate for more than one question

A second type of EMQ   ▌ This asks for more than one answer for each question

Example

XI. State two molecules capable of carrying oxygen   *(A, B)*

XII. State two proteins secreted into the intestine   *(J, M)*

XIII. State three proteins found in erythrocytes or leucocytes   *(A, N, O)*

Tips and tactics   ▌ The examiner is usually looking for the best answer to the question; however, there may be other possible answers that will gain some marks
▌ Make an attempt at each part if you can, for the reasons given above. For each part of the question, underline the key facts and investigation results that may help you reach the correct answer
▌ Don't be put off by diseases on the list of options that you know little about. They may well not be the answer to any of the questions posed

SHORT ANSWERS

▌ These questions ask you to write notes or a short summary on three or four related topics

Example   1. Write short notes on each of the following:
   A. Thrombolysis in myocardial infarction
   B. Risk factors for ischaemic heart disease
   C. Aspirin in ischaemic heart disease

Tips and tactics   ▌ These require short, structured answers
▌ If time is short, consider bulleted points or headings and lists
▌ Do not attempt to put down everything you know about the subject – stick to answering the question being asked
▌ Keep a close eye on the time – it is easy to get carried away and spend far too much time on a single part of a question
▌ There are only a limited number of marks. Writing excessive amounts will not get you extra points

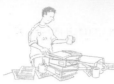
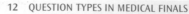

PATIENT MANAGEMENT PROBLEMS

❚ A description of a patient history and examination is given, followed by two or three questions. For each question there is a list of options and you are asked to grade the correctness of each option

Example   A 55-year-old man, who works for a building company, is referred complaining of a cough. The cough has been present for 3 months and on four occasions he has coughed up some blood. He now feels breathless after mild exertion. His wife has rheumatoid arthritis and he is her main carer. He has had a previous admission for angina and attends a diabetes clinic at his local GP's. He is a smoker who drinks about 40 units of alcohol a week as beer.

He is 180 cm tall and weighs 70 kg. He has some crackles at left midzone of his lungs but no other findings on examination.

Which four of the following would be most useful in making an immediate diagnosis?

1. ECG
2. Exercise ECG
3. CT of the chest
4. MRI of the lungs
5. Peak flow measurements
6. Lung function tests
7. Full blood count
8. Blood cultures
9. Arterial blood gases
10. Chest X-ray

Answer: 1, 5, 8, 10

A chest X-ray reveals calcified pleural lesions and increased lung markings, most notably in the bases. Based on this, what is the most likely diagnosis?

A. Carcinoma of the bronchus
B. Chronic congestive cardiac failure
C. Streptococcal pneumonia
D. Asbestosis

E. Rheumatoid lung disease

Answer: D

I The second variation of this question type asks for one-line answers to a series of questions about a case

Example A 66-year-old man presents with chest pain. This started suddenly 2 hours ago. The pain is central and radiates to both shoulders. He is sweaty and feels very unwell. On examination he is apyrexial and tachycardic with a blood pressure of 110/60.

1. What is the most likely diagnosis?

Answer: Acute myocardial infarction

2. What two investigations would be of immediate use?

Answer: ECG and troponin

3. State four immediate therapeutic steps you would institute.

Answer: High-flow oxygen, i.v. diamorphine, aspirin and consider thrombolysis

4. Suggest three possible complications of the therapies you suggest.

Answer: Haemorrhage, gastrointestinal ulceration, respiratory depression

ESSAY QUESTIONS

I These provide a title and sometimes some specific requirements for an essay

Example Outline the important considerations in palliation of a patient with an inoperable lung carcinoma. In your answer outline the important therapies you would consider using.

Tips and tactics I Read the question carefully and underline any 'riders' or specific instructions

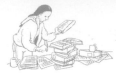

I Spend a minute or so sketching an essay plan with section headings. This allows you to order your thoughts before committing them to paper
I Headings help the examiner as they speed up marking
I Answer the specific questions being asked; do not write a general essay on the subject in the hope of getting credit
I Time the paper carefully. Writing two 30-minute essays instead of three 20-minute essays makes passing much harder
I Read through your answer
— Does it all make sense?
— Does it answer the question?
— Is the spelling correct?
— Is it structured and easy to read?
I If you are running out of time, write out a structured essay plan with key facts about the subject. Most marking schemes will give you some credit for this
I If the examiners cannot read your writing, they cannot mark the essay!

Clinical exams

SHORT CASES

I A series of patients are seen with the examiners who give you specific instructions
— 'Look at this patient – what is the diagnosis?'
— 'Examine this man's chest'
— 'Listen to this woman's heart'
I You will then be expected to:
— Introduce yourself
— Carry out the appropriate examination
— Present your findings and give a diagnosis, differential and management plan

Tips and tactics
I Be professional
I Do not embarrass or hurt the patient
I Follow the instructions you are given
I Answer the questions you are asked

▌ Remember, very unwell patients are unlikely to be in a clinical exam. Chronic conditions are more common. You may be given tips or a brief introduction
  — 'This gentleman gets breathless on exertion – examine the heart'
  — Think about heart valve murmurs and cardiac failure

Common topics for short cases

Cardiac
▌ Heart sounds and murmurs
▌ Cardiomegaly
▌ Dextrocardia (rare)
▌ Hypertensive retinopathy

Respiratory
▌ Chronic obstructive pulmonary disease
▌ Surgery for tuberculosis
▌ Pulmonary fibrosis
▌ Pleural effusions
▌ Chest infections
▌ Cystic fibrosis

Gastrointestinal
▌ Chronic liver disease
▌ Ileostomy/colostomy
▌ Fistulating Crohn's disease
▌ Hepatosplenomegaly

Urinary
▌ Transplanted kidney (right iliac fossa)
▌ Arteriovenous shunt for dialysis (left arm)
▌ Ileal urinary conduit (urine in the bag)
▌ Palpable kidneys (often polycystic kidney)

Neurological
▌ Multiple sclerosis
▌ Ophthalmoplegia
▌ Facial palsy
▌ Brachial plexus injury
▌ Ulnar or radial nerve damage
▌ Carpal tunnel syndrome
▌ Hemiparesis or paraparesis
▌ Charcot–Marie–Tooth
▌ Friedreich's ataxia (check speech)
▌ Parkinson's disease
▌ Cerebellar ataxia

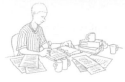

Table 2.3   'Examine this patient and assess her thyroid gland'

Hypothyroidism
Thick, rough, dry skin
Obesity
Bradycardia
Slow relaxing reflexes

Hyperthyroidism
Thin patient
Sweaty
Tachycardia ± atrial fibrillation
Exophthalmos with lid lag
Tremor

Endocrine   I Thyroid status (Table 2.3)
I Acromegaly
I Diabetic retinopathy
I Diabetic sensory loss
I Hypopituitarism
I Cushing's syndrome

Rheumatological   I Systemic sclerosis
I Rheumatoid arthritis
I Osteoarthritis
I Ankylosing spondylitis
I Paget's disease of bone

LONG CASES

I A prolonged period with a patient prior to presenting the case to an examiner. You may be taken back to the patient in order to assess a specific part of the examination technique
I Take a detailed history
I With chronic disabling conditions, the social history is very important
I Perform a thorough clinical examination
I Keep an eye on the time and make legible notes. Divide the time into:
— History-taking

— Examination
— Reviewing your findings
— Going back to ask further questions
I When presenting, adhere to the preferred format for your medical school
I Give the positive and important negative findings
I Outline a diagnosis and a differential
I Outline the investigations that are appropriate
I Outline treatment options, including long-term care needs if appropriate

OBJECTIVE STRUCTURED CLINICAL EXAMINATION (OSCE)

I This is a 'round robin' of test stations
I The examiner stays at the station
I Each station lasts 4–5 minutes
I Stations may be paired, e.g. a clinical examination at one station and questions about the examination and diagnosis at the next
I As every student does the same OSCE, the results are fairer to the individual

Types of station

General
I Taking a history
I Examining a patient
I Patient photographs
I X-rays
I ECGs
I Laboratory test interpretation

Practical skills
I Measuring blood pressure
I Inserting a cannula
I Taking blood
I Checking a blood transfusion
I Cardiopulmonary resuscitation

Management questions
I Medical emergencies
I Writing a fluid chart
I Writing a prescription
I Reviewing a drug chart

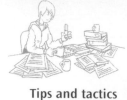

Tips and tactics I Make sure you are comfortable with the common procedures that crop up in OSCEs
I Practise the commonly needed practical skills in a clinical skills lab if possible. These are easy marks to get

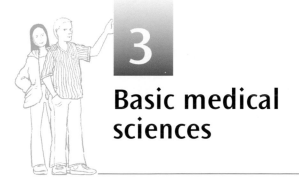

3

Basic medical sciences

Cell biology

CELL STRUCTURE (Figs 3.1 and 3.2) *(K&C, p. 153)*

Cell membrane
- Outer phospholipid bilayer
- Allows specialization:
  - — e.g. microvilli/cilia
  - — Receptors recognize extracellular signals
  - — Ion channels and active uptake systems
  - — G proteins activate intracellular signals

Cytoskeleton
- Determines structure and shape of cell
- Microtubules ($\alpha + \beta$ tubulin)
- Intermediate filaments
- Microfilaments (actin)

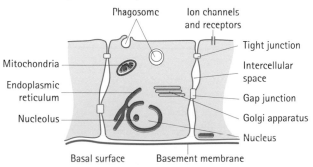

Apical surface – specialized for cell function

Phagosome   Ion channels and receptors

Mitochondria

Endoplasmic reticulum

Nucleolus

Tight junction

Intercellular space

Gap junction

Golgi apparatus

Nucleus

Basal surface   Basement membrane

Fig. 3.1   Overview of cell structure.

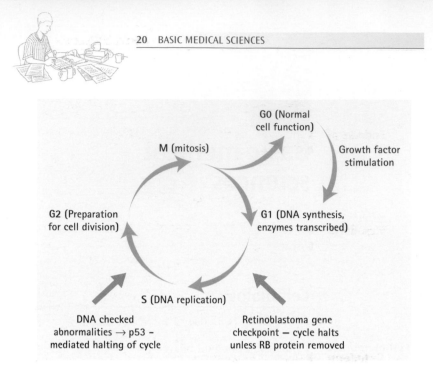

Fig. 3.2 The cell cycle. (*K&C*, p. 162)

Nucleus	▌ Contains genomic DNA (chromosomes) ▌ Apparatus for mRNA transcription
Endoplasmic reticulum (ER)	▌ Nuclear membrane ▌ Rough ER: protein synthesis ▌ Smooth ER: storage and secretion
Golgi apparatus	▌ Protein processing
Mitochondria	▌ Oxidative phosphorylation ▌ Have own DNA genome
Lysosomes	▌ Digestive vesicle

Intercellular junctions

Tight junctions	▌ Apical margin of epithelial cells ▌ Block movement of ions and solutes
Gap junctions	▌ Protein channels between cells ▌ Allow direct passage of substances

CELL TYPES

Endoderm
- Innermost of the three germ cell layers
- Gives rise to
  - Gut, liver and pancreas
  - Urinary tract
  - Bronchial tree and alveoli

Mesoderm
- Middle layer of germ cells
- Gives rise to
  - Skeleton
  - Musculature
  - Vascular tree
  - Kidneys
  - Gonads

Ectoderm
- Outer layer of germ cells
- Gives rise to
  - Nervous system
  - Sensory organs
  - Skin

Epithelium
- Cells lining luminal spaces and body surfaces
- Squamous cells
  - Skin
  - Oesophagus
- Columnar cells
  - Gastrointestinal system
  - Bronchial tree
- Transitional cells
  - Bladder

Endothelium
- Primary layer lining vascular lumens
  - e.g. Arteries

Molecular biology

DNA AND CHROMOSOMES (K&C, p. 163)

DNA structure
(Fig. 3.3)
- Double-stranded
- Two intertwined helices

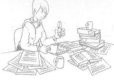

Fig. 3.3
DNA and
chromosome
structure.

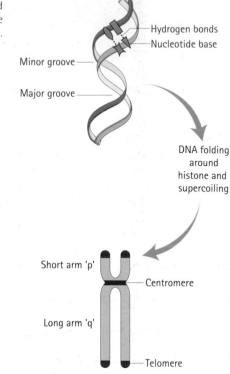

- four nucleotide bases
  — Adenine (A)
  — Cytosine (C)
  — Thymine (T)
  — Guanine (G)
- Hydrogen bonds between strands
- A–T and G–C pairings only
- Nucleotide triplets encode specific amino acids

Chromosomes
(Fig. 3.3)
(*K&C*, p. 170)

- DNA coiled around histone proteins
- Then supercoiled into nucleosomes
- Further folding and coiling → chromosome
- Each
  — Has a short arm (p)
  — Has a long arm (q)
  — Is joined at the centromere

- 22 pairs of autosomes
- Two sex chromosomes: ♀ XX ♂ XY
- Contain 6×10^9 base pairs
- Classified by size (chromosome 1 largest)
- When condensed in metaphase staining → visible bands
- Each band is numbered, e.g. 7q21 = band 21 long arm chromosome 7

Gene structure
- Genes code for proteins
- Expression controlled by binding of proteins to
  — Promoter regions: binding sites for RNA polymerase
  — Operator regions: modify promoter binding
  — Enhancer regions: distant sites that increase transcription

Exons
- Coding section of gene

Introns
- 'Junk' DNA – does not code for protein

RNA AND PROTEIN SYNTHESIS (K&C, p. 164)

Structure of RNA (Fig. 3.4)
- Single nucleotide chain
- Uracil (U) replaces thymine
- Can hybridize with complementary DNA chains

Messenger RNA (mRNA)
- Formed by transcription of DNA
- Carries information from nucleus to cytoplasm

Ribosomal RNA (rRNA)
- Combines with protein to form ribosomes
- Attaches to mRNA
- Exposes base triplets (codons)
- Catalyses translation from 5′ → 3′

Transfer RNA (tRNA)
- Each displays specific nucleotide triplet
- Carries a specific amino acid
- Hybridizes with exposed mRNA codon
- Amino acid is then added to polypeptide chain

Proteins
- Chains of amino acids
- Nine essential amino acids

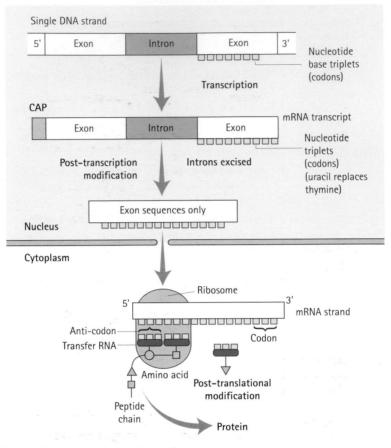

Fig. 3.4 DNA transcription and translation.

I Basic α-helix and β-pleated sheet structure
I Folding → functional structure

ANALYTICAL METHODS IN MOLECULAR BIOLOGY
(*K&C*, p. 168)

DNA

Restriction enzymes
(Fig. 3.5)

I Cut DNA at specific base sequences
I → Thousands of fragments
I → Electrophoresis by size and charge
I → Stained → all fragments visible
I Pattern of bands = DNA fingerprint

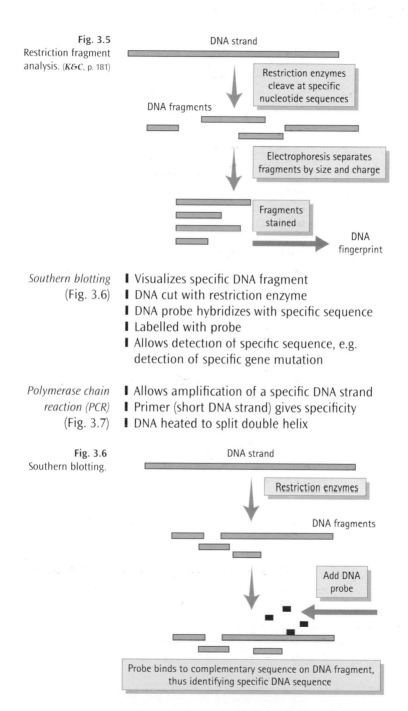

Fig. 3.5
Restriction fragment
analysis. (*K&C*, p. 181)

Southern blotting
(Fig. 3.6)

I Visualizes specific DNA fragment
I DNA cut with restriction enzyme
I DNA probe hybridizes with specific sequence
I Labelled with probe
I Allows detection of specific sequence, e.g.
detection of specific gene mutation

Polymerase chain
reaction (PCR)
(Fig. 3.7)

I Allows amplification of a specific DNA strand
I Primer (short DNA strand) gives specificity
I DNA heated to split double helix

Fig. 3.6
Southern blotting.

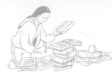

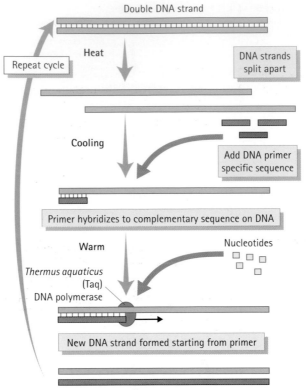

Double DNA strand

Heat

Repeat cycle

DNA strands
split apart

Cooling

Add DNA primer
specific sequence

Primer hybridizes to complementary sequence on DNA

Warm

Nucleotides

Thermus aquaticus
(Taq)
DNA polymerase

New DNA strand formed starting from primer

New double-stranded DNA

Fig. 3.7   Polymerase chain reaction mechanism of amplifying specific DNA sequence.

I Primer attaches to specific DNA sequence
I Polymerase synthesizes new DNA chain
I System cycled to amplify the DNA chain
I Depends on heat-stable bacterial polymerase
I Once amplified, DNA chain can be detected

Sequencing   I Uses radio-labelled nucleotides
I DNA chain produced using labelled nucleotide
I Reveals nucleotide sequence of a DNA strand

RNA
Northern blotting   I Same technique as Southern blotting
I Allows detection of specific mRNA sequence

Reverse transcriptase	❙ mRNA converted into DNA
PCR	❙ PCR then carried out on DNA as above

Proteins

Western blotting (Fig. 3.8)	❙ Proteins electrophoresed ❙ Antibody against specific protein introduced ❙ Desired protein is bound by antibody ❙ Antibody conjugated to a signalling substance ❙ Allows detection of specific protein
Enzyme-linked *immunosorbent* *assay (ELISA)* (Fig. 3.9)	❙ Detects protein (e.g. antibody or cytokine) ❙ Utilizes antibody specificity for target ❙ Detecting antibody conjugated to an enzyme ❙ Enzyme → colour change ∝ amount of target

Fig. 3.8
Western blotting.

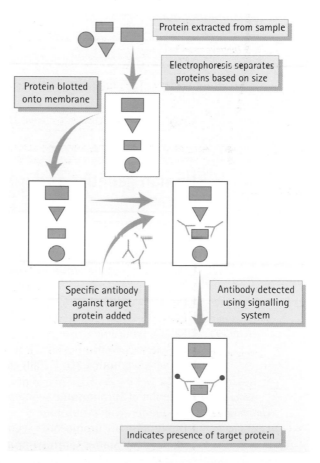

Protein extracted from sample

Electrophoresis separates proteins based on size

Protein blotted onto membrane

Specific antibody against target protein added

Antibody detected using signalling system

Indicates presence of target protein

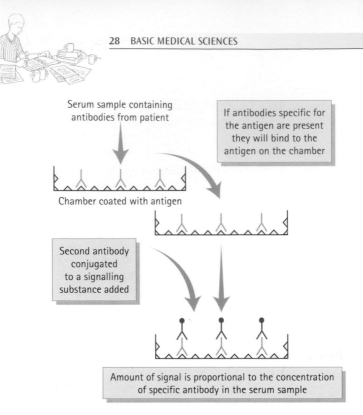

Serum sample containing antibodies from patient

If antibodies specific for the antigen are present they will bind to the antigen on the chamber

Chamber coated with antigen

Second antibody conjugated to a signalling substance added

Amount of signal is proportional to the concentration of specific antibody in the serum sample

Fig. 3.9   Enzyme-linked immunosorbent assay (ELISA).

Human genetics and inherited disease

HUMAN GENETICS (K&C, p. 172)

Chromosomal disorders

I Majority → spontaneous abortion

Abnormal chromosome numbers
I Down's syndrome: trisomy 21,1:650 live births
I Edward's syndrome: trisomy 18,1:3000
I Pataú's syndrome: trisomy 13,1:5000
I Klinefelter's syndrome: XXY, 1:1000 males
I Turner's syndrome: XO, 1:2500 girls

Abnormal chromosome structure
I Deletion of chromosome segment,
  — Prader–Willi syndrome
I Duplication of chromosome segment,
  — Charcot–Marie–Tooth syndrome

Table 3.1   Autosomal dominant, autosomal recessive and X-linked recessive disorders

Autosomal dominant	β-thalassaemia
Achondroplasia	Friedreich's ataxia
Adult polycystic kidney disease	Haemochromatosis
Familial Alzheimer's disease	Phenylketonuria
Familial	Sickle cell disease
hypercholesterolaemia	Wilson's disease
Huntington's chorea	**X-linked recessive**
Marfan's syndrome	Duchenne muscular
Neurofibromatosis type I	dystrophy
Von Willebrand's disease	Haemophilia A
Autosomal recessive	Haemophilia B
Albinism	Red-green colour blindness
Cystic fibrosis	Wiskott–Aldrich syndrome

Mitochondrial DNA abnormalities *(K&C, p. 173)*

- Inherited mitochondrial DNA mutations
- Passed via maternal line (sperm do not donate mitochondria)
- → Myopathies and neuropathies

Gene defects
(Table 3.1)
(K&C, p. 176)

- Result in abnormal protein being synthesized
- Homozygous: both gene copies abnormal
- Heterozygous: one gene copy abnormal

Autosomal dominant disorders (Fig. 3.10)

- One of the two gene copies is mutated
- Normal gene not sufficient to compensate
- Or mutated protein is toxic
- Effect may vary in each generation
- Varying penetrance

Fig. 3.10
Autosomal dominant inheritance.

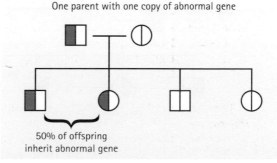

One parent with one copy of abnormal gene

50% of offspring inherit abnormal gene

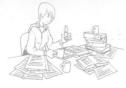

I → Disease skipping generations
I New cases arise due to germ-line mutations

Autosomal recessive
disorders (Fig. 3.11)

I Both gene copies have mutation (homozygous)
I No functioning protein synthesized
I Carrier state exists if only one copy affected
I → Inborn errors of metabolism

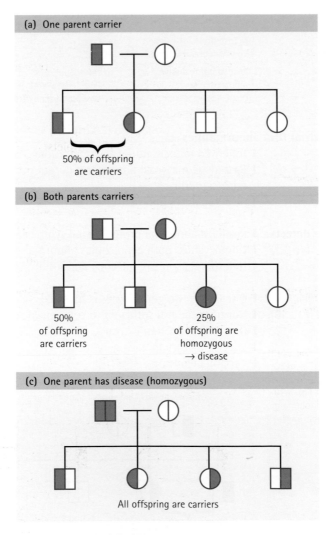

Fig. 3.11   Autosomal recessive inheritance.

Sex-linked inheritance
I Mutations of genes on the X chromosome
I Vast majority are recessive (Fig. 3.12), but
— Males only have one X chromosome, therefore are affected by mutation
— Females act as carriers if heterozygotes

X-linked dominant
I Heterozygote ♀ has the disease
I Rare
I e.g. Vitamin D-resistant rickets

Trinucleotide repeats
I Multiple repeats of three nucleotides
I Severity of the disease ∝ number of repeats
I Number of repeats increases with each generation
I Therefore severity increases with each generation = genetic anticipation
— Myotonic dystrophy (CTG triplets)
— Huntington's chorea (CAG triplets)

Genetic imprinting
I Disease phenotype varies
I Depends on origin of mutant gene
I e.g. Deletion of long arm of chromosome 15
— If inherited from mother → Prader–Willi syndrome
— If inherited from father → Angelman syndrome

Multifactorial inheritance
(*K&C*, p. 179)
I Encoded for by multiple genetic loci (polygenic)
— Height
— Hair colour

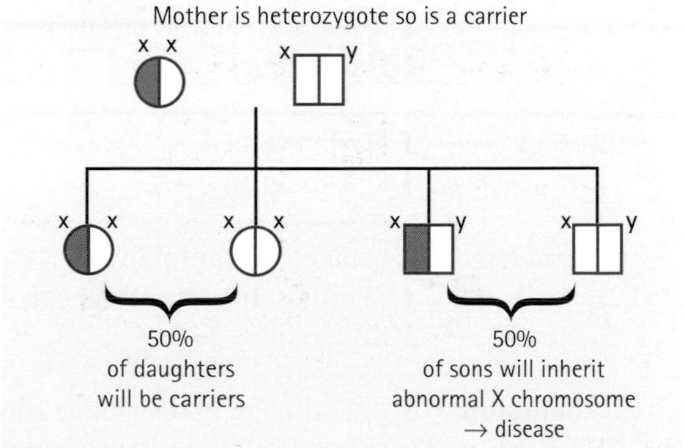

Fig. 3.12
X-linked recessive inheritance.

Mother is heterozygote so is a carrier

50% of daughters will be carriers

50% of sons will inherit abnormal X chromosome → disease

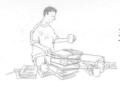
— Hypertension
— Pyloric stenosis
— Ankylosing spondylitis

GENETIC SCREENING AND COUNSELLING (K&C, p. 180)

Provision of information to prospective parents who are carriers of an inherited disease is vital for informed decisions to be made. Determination of these risks is important and requires screening.

Screening ▌ Detection of carrier of a mutation, e.g.
— Thalassaemia
— Sickle cell disease
— Tay–Sachs disease
— Haemophilia
— Cystic fibrosis

Prenatal diagnosis

Maternal serum ▌ Maternal α-fetoprotein – neural tube defects
▌ Bart's triple test on maternal serum assesses risk of fetal trisomy 21
— α-fetoprotein (low)
— β-human chorionic gonadotrophin (high)
— Unconjugated oestriol (low)

Imaging ▌ Ultrasound for anatomical abnormalities
▌ Nuchal fold translucency for Down's syndrome

Amniocentesis ▌ Sampling amniotic fluid for fetal cells
▌ α-fetoprotein and biochemical analysis
▌ Risk to fetus < 1%

Chorionic villus sampling ▌ Chromosome/DNA analysis
▌ Risk to fetus 1–2%

Cordocentesis ▌ Fetal blood sampling
▌ Chromosome and DNA analysis
▌ Risk to fetus 1–2%

Counselling ▌ Risk of passing on genetic abnormality to child depends on inheritance and parental genome

Medical immunology (K&C, p. 191)

STRUCTURE

Cellular immunity
I T cells – antigen-presenting cells
I → Cell-mediated defence

Humoral immunity
I B cells → antibody production
I With complement → activation
I → Organism lysis, phagocytosis

Innate immunity
I Non-specific defence

ANATOMY

Innate immunity
Physical barriers
I Skin
I Gut wall

Chemical barriers
I Gastric acid
I Lysozyme in tears

Removal
I Sneezing/coughing
I Urinary washing
I Bronchial cilia

Non-specific
I Phagocytes
I Natural killer cells
I Complement
I Defensins

Lymphoid organs
Primary
I Bone marrow
I Thymus

Secondary
I Lymph nodes
I Tonsils
I Spleen
I Mucosa-associated lymphoid tissue (MALT)

CELLS OF THE IMMUNE SYSTEM (K&C, pp. 192–201)

Neutrophils
I Phagocytes
I Complement C5a/C3a attracts cell to site

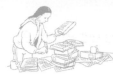

I Cell adheres to endothelium
I Diapedesis → extracellular matrix
I Target organism/substance is coated with complement and antibodies
I Phagocyte internalizes the antigen

Eosinophils
I 5% of leucocytes
I Surface IgE receptors
I Active against parasitic infections
I Involved in hypersensitivity reactions

Basophils
I Histamine granules
I IgE receptors
I Involved in hypersensitivity reactions

Mast cells
I Histamine-releasing cells
I IgE receptors
I Release of histamine in allergy

B lymphocytes
(Fig. 3.13)
I 25% of lymphocytes
I Produce antibody
I Once activated proliferates →
— Plasma cells (antibody production)
— Memory cells (memory for the antigen)

T lymphocytes
(Fig. 3.13)
I CD3 surface marker
I T cell receptor for antigen processing
I Interact with antigen-presenting cells
I → Cytokine response

Helper cells
I Enhance the immune response
I CD4 positive

Th1 cells
I Produce Interleukin-2 (IL-2), IL-3 and γ-interferon
I Promote cell-mediated immunity

Th2 cells
I Produce IL-4, IL-5, IL-10
I Promote antibody-mediated immunity
I Drive IgE responses

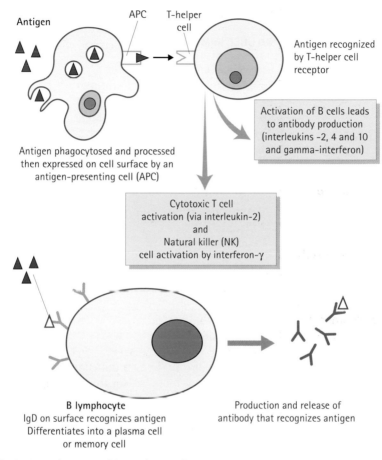

Fig. 3.13 Antigen recognition and processing.

Antigen-presenting cells	❙ Process foreign material
	❙ Express antigen fragments on surface
	❙ Interact with T cell receptor
Types	❙ Phagocytes
	❙ Follicular dendritic cells (lymph nodes)
	❙ Langerhans' cells (skin)
	❙ Dendritic cells (blood)
	❙ Kupffer cells (liver)

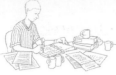

Natural killer cells ▌ Kill tumour and virally infected cells

SOLUBLE IMMUNE FACTORS

Complement
(Fig. 3.14)
(K&C, p. 195)

▌ Cascade of serum glycoprotein
▌ Results in membrane attack complex
▌ → Osmotic lysis of bacteria
▌ Recruits cells to inflammatory site
▌ Opsonizes bacteria → phagocytosis
▌ Modulates B cell responses

Classical pathway:
Ca^{2+}/Mg^{2+}-
dependent

▌ Initiated by
— IgM
— Antibody–antigen complex
— Apoptotic cells
— Some bacteria

Alternative pathway

▌ Initiated by
— Yeast cells
— IgA
— Bacterial endotoxin
— C3 nephritic factor
— Viruses
— Tumour cells

Activators
IgM
Antibody–antigen
complex

Activators
IgA
Endotoxin
Yeasts
C3 nephritic factor

Classical pathway
(calcium and
magnesium-
dependent)

C3

Alternative
pathway

MBL
pathway

Final common pathway

Mannose binding
lectin binds to
mannose on bacterial
surface

C3b

Membrane
attack complex

Fig. 3.14 The complement cascade.

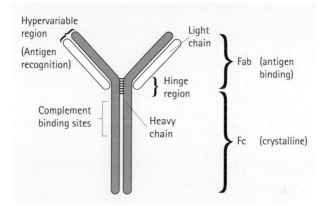

Fig. 3.15 Antibody structure.

Antibodies (Fig 3.15) (K&C, p. 199)	I Glycoproteins I Two antigen-binding sites I Specific for single antigen I → Antigen recognition I Complement binding site I → Complement activation I Stops adhesion of organism to cell I Aids opsonization → organism lysis I Blocks toxin activity I B cell receptor function
IgM	I Pentamer I Earliest antibody response
IgG	I Monomer I Most abundant type I Second response to antigen
IgD	I B cell surface I Immunoregulatory role
IgE	I Mast cell receptor I Anti-nematode function I Important in allergy
IgA	I Secretory I Found at mucous membranes I Usually a dimer in secretions

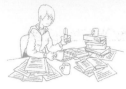

IMMUNE RECOGNITION

Human leucocyte antigen (HLA) system (Table 3.2) (*K&C*, p. 202)

- Genes on chromosome 6 (= major histocompatibility complex)
- Genes encode cell surface proteins
- Denotes 'self'
- Thus allows identification of 'non-self'
- Presents antigens to T lymphocytes

Class I: A/B/C
- Expressed on all cell types except erythrocytes and trophoblasts
- Present antigen to T-helper (CD4) cells

Class II: DP/DQ/DR
- Expressed on
  — B lymphocytes
  — Monocytes
  — Dendrocytes
  — Activated T lymphocytes
  — Antigen-presenting cells
- Present antigen to cytotoxic (CD8) cells

Antigen recognition
- Differentiation of 'self' and 'non-self'
- Antigen presented by HLA I and II
- T cells recognize the antigen
- If 'self' → no response
- If 'non-self' → immune activation occurs

Table 3.2   HLA disease associations

Disease	HLA
Polycystic kidney disease	B5
Addison's disease	B8/DR3
Graves' disease	B8/DR3
Coeliac disease	B8/DR3/DR7/DQ2
Ankylosing spondylitis	B27
Type I diabetes mellitus	DR4/DR3
Rheumatoid arthritis	DR4

IMMUNE DEFICIENCY SYNDROMES

Phagocyte abnormalities (K&C, p. 208)

Neutropenia –
reduced numbers
of neutrophils

I Congenital (rare)
I Racial (Afro-Caribbean)
I Drugs
  — Chemotherapeutics
  — Immunosuppressants
  — Carbimazole
I Hypersplenism
I Myeloid leukaemia

Abnormal function

I Leucocyte adhesion defects
I Hyper-IgE syndrome
I Drugs: steroids
I Diabetes mellitus

Symptoms of
phagocyte
abnormalities

I Bacterial and fungal infections
I Often benign

Complement deficiencies (K&C, p. 210)

C3/C1q

I Infections with capsulated organisms, e.g. pneumococcus/*Haemophilus*
I Systemic lupus erythematosus (SLE)-like disorders C5–C9
I → *Neisseria* infections, e.g. meningococcus/gonococcus

C1 esterase inhibitor
deficiency

I → Hereditary angio-oedema
I → Airway or gastrointestinal obstruction

Antibody deficiencies (K&C, p. 210)

X-linked
hypogamma-
globulinaemia

I Failure of B cell maturation
I Mutation of Xq21–22
I → *Mycoplasma*/meningococcus infections
I Treatment: i.v. immunoglobulin

Common variable
deficiency

I Late-onset antibody deficiency
I Notably IgG deficiency
I → Bacterial infection

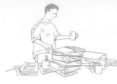

IgA deficiency ▋ Common (1:600)
▋ Often asymptomatic

T cell deficiencies (*K&C*, p. 211)
▋ Congenital: DiGeorge syndrome
▋ → *Candida/Pneumocystis*
▋ Acquired: HIV → decreased CD4 T lymphocytes

Combined immunodeficiencies (*K&C*, p. 212)
Severe combined ▋ Absent lymphoid tissue
immunodeficiency ▋ Hypogammaglobulinaemia
(SCID) ▋ Lymphopenia
▋ → Severe infections from birth
▋ X-linked or autosomal recessive
▋ Poor prognosis

HYPERSENSITIVITY DISEASES (*K&C*, p. 213)

Type I ▋ Immediate type
▋ Occur within minutes of exposure
▋ IgE-mediated mast cell activation, e.g.
— Pollens
— Food allergens
— Drugs
— Dust mite
▋ → Allergic reaction/atopy
▋ Oedema
▋ Bronchospasm
▋ Atopic eczema
▋ Anaphylaxis

Type II ▋ Cytotoxic
▋ IgG/IgM/complement-mediated
▋ → Damage to targeted cell, e.g.
— Transfusion reactions
— Autoimmune haemolytic anaemia
— Myasthenia gravis

Type III ▋ Immune complex deposition
▋ Antibody-mediated
▋ → Antibody–antigen complex deposition

▌ → Inflammation and vasculitis, e.g.
— Glomerulonephritis
— Rheumatoid arthritis
— SLE
— Farmer's lung

Type IV   ▌ Delayed type
▌ Macrophages and T lymphocytes
▌ → Granulomas and caseation, e.g.
— Tuberculosis
— Leprosy

Type V   ▌ Stimulating/blocking
▌ Antibodies → altering cell function
▌ Usually IgG, e.g. Graves' disease

MANAGEMENT OF ACUTE ANAPHYLAXIS

Clinical features
Shock – hypotension and tachycardia
Oedema – periorbital/laryngeal swelling → stridor
Skin rash – local or generalized erythematous rash
Bronchospasm → wheezing

First-line
Ensure airway is secure
Ensure patient is breathing
Ensure that there is a circulation
Ask for senior help in management

Give
Adrenaline (epinephrine) 500 µg i.m.; repeat this every
    5 minutes
High-flow oxygen (> 60% or 10 L/minute)
Antihistamine, e.g. chlorphenamine (chlorpheniramine) 10 mg
    i.v.
Reassess the patient

Consider
Hydrocortisone 200 mg i.v. (N.B. This provides a delayed
    response)
Salbutamol nebulizers for bronchospasm
Salbutamol i.v. for continued anaphylaxis
Nursing in a high-dependency area

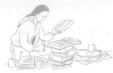

Self-assessment questions

Multiple choice questions

1. The following are correct:
   A. Translation is the production of a messenger RNA strand from DNA
   B. Exons are DNA sequences that code for peptides
   C. Restriction enzymes cut DNA at specific nucleotide sequences
   D. Northern blotting is the detection of specific DNA sequences
   E. Polymerase chain reactions amplify DNA sequences

2. The following are correct nucleotide base pairs:
   A. Thymine–guanine
   B. Uracil–adenine
   C. Cytosine–guanine
   D. Uracil–thymine
   E. Adenine–cytosine

3. The following are correct:
   A. There are 23 pairs of autosomes in the human
   B. Chromosome 1 is the smallest of the chromosomes
   C. The two chromosomes in a pair have identical base pair sequences
   D. q denotes the long arm of a chromosome
   E. DNA is coiled around histones

4. The following are autosomal dominant:
   A. Haemophilia A
   B. Achondroplasia
   C. Haemochromatosis
   D. Red–green colour blindness
   E. Leprosy

5. The following genetic abnormalities result in the named condition:
   A. Trisomy 19 — Down's syndrome
   B. XO — Turner's syndrome
   C. XXY — Klinefelter's syndrome
   D. Trisomy 21 — Patau's syndrome
   E. XXO — Smith's syndrome

6. The following are inherited in an X-linked recessive manner:
   A. Down's syndrome
   B. Polycystic kidney disease
   C. Wiskott–Aldrich syndrome
   D. Haemophilia A
   E. Acute intermittent porphyria

7. The following are antigen-presenting cells:
   A. Dendritic cells
   B. Hepatocytes
   C. Erythrocytes
   D. Kupffer cells
   E. Phagocytes

8. The following are functions of T lymphocytes:
   A. Phagocytosis
   B. Antigen recognition
   C. Cytokine production
   D. Killing of virally infected cells
   E. Antibody production

9. The following are useful in the immediate relief of anaphylactic shock:
   A. Adrenaline (epinephrine)
   B. Hydrocortisone
   C. Oxygen at 2 litres per minute (24%)

D. Chlorphenamine
(chlorpheniramine)

E. Atropine

10. The following are features of type I hypersensitivity:
   A. Immune complex deposition
   B. Mast cell degranulation
   C. Granuloma formation
   D. Bronchospasm
   E. Rapid onset after exposure to an allergen

Short answer questions

1. Write short notes on the following:
   A. Polymerase chain reaction
   B. Transcription
   C. Chromosome structure

2. Outline the role of the following:
   A. Messenger RNA
   B. Ribosomal RNA
   C. Transfer RNA

3. Write short notes on the following:
   A. Trinucleotide repeats
   B. Genetic anticipation
   C. Autosomal dominant inheritance
   D. Multifactorial inheritance

4. Outline the role of the following in the immune response to an antigen:

A. Complement
B. Antibodies
C. T-helper lymphocytes
D. Phagocytes

5. Write short notes on the following:
   A. Delayed (type IV) hypersensitivity
   B. Atopy
   C. Autoimmune disease

Essay questions

1. What is prenatal screening? Outline the techniques commonly used.

2. With reference to a specific inherited disease, discuss its mode of inheritance and its diagnosis and management.

3. A 55-year-old woman is seen in casualty following a wasp sting. She is unresponsive and there is audible wheeze. Her blood pressure is 80/50. Outline your initial management.

4. Discuss the roles of antibodies in the immune response.

5. What is innate immunity? Outline the different mechanisms of innate immunity giving specific examples of each.

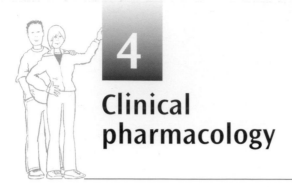

4
Clinical pharmacology

I The study of chemicals or drugs that interact with the human body

Principles of drug action (K&C, p. 957)

Pharmacodynamics

I The study of biochemical and physiological effects of drugs and their mechanism of action

Pharmacokinetics I The study of the way the body handles a drug

PHARMACODYNAMICS (K&C, p. 959)

Non-specific drug action
I Drugs act by virtue of their physicochemical properties
— Osmotic diuretic (mannitol)
— Antacids (sodium bicarbonate)

Inhibition of transport systems
I Drugs act by blocking or facilitating transport mechanisms in tissue or cells
— Calcium channel blockers (nifedipine)
— Na/K-ATPase inhibitor (digoxin)
— Neurotransmitter reuptake inhibitors (imipramine)

Enzyme inhibitors
I Drugs act by competitively or irreversibly altering enzyme function

— Angiotensin-converting enzyme (ACE) inhibitor (captopril)
— Cyclo-oxygenase (COX) inhibitor (aspirin)
— Phosphodiesterase inhibitor (sildenafil)

Hormones ▌ Drugs may act by inhibiting or enhancing hormone production and/or release
— Oral contraceptive pill (inhibits FSH/LH production)
— Sulphonylureas (enhance insulin secretion)

▌ Or hormone may be replaced if production is deficient
— Insulin in type 1 diabetes mellitus
— Thyroxine in primary hypothyroidism

Receptor agonists and antagonists ▌ The majority of drugs act by interacting with target receptors either to activate them (agonists) or to inactivate and block them (antagonists)
— β_2-adrenergic agonists (salbutamol)
— H_2-receptor antagonists (ranitidine)

DRUG–RECEPTOR INTERACTIONS

The biological effects of a drug which acts via a receptor will depend on several factors. Important terms and their definitions are listed below.

Affinity ▌ Capacity of drug to bind to receptor

Efficacy ▌ Pharmacological response resulting from drug–receptor interaction

Potency ▌ Dose of drug required to produce a given effect

Dose-response ▌ Biological response measured with increasing doses of a drug

LD_{50} ▌ Lethal dose of a drug in 50% of population

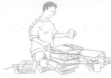

ED_{50} | Effective dose of a drug in 50% of population

Therapeutic index | LD_{50}/ED_{50}

Agonists | Drugs that bind to receptors to elicit a dose-response effect, e.g. salbutamol is a β_2-agonist

Partial agonists | Drugs that competitively bind and activate receptor, but cannot elicit same maximal response as full agonist
| Antagonize effects of full agonist
— buprenorphine is an opiate receptor partial agonist

Antagonists | Drugs that bind to receptors but do not activate them; they may be competitive or irreversible

Competitive antagonists | Drugs that compete with agonist for receptor-binding
| Effect can be reversed by agonist in adequate concentration
— propranolol is a competitive β-antagonist

Irreversible antagonists | Drugs that bind irreversibly with receptors so that any amount of agonist cannot reverse effect
— phenoxybenzamine is an irreversible antagonist

PHARMACOKINETICS *(K&C, p. 957)*

Routes of administration

Oral | Drug enters body by gastrointestinal absorption via the portal venous system, before entering systemic circulation

Intravenous | Drug enters directly into systemic bloodstream

Intramuscular or subcutaneous injection | Drug enters systemic circulation rapidly via absorption through muscle or subcutaneous capillaries

Topical | Drug acts locally to application
— ointments, eye drops
— usually minimally absorbed into circulation

Inhalation | Drug may be absorbed or act locally
— volatile anaesthetics
— asthma drugs

Sublingual and rectal | Drug is absorbed directly into systemic circulation, bypassing portal system

Absorption | The mechanism by which a drug enters the systemic circulation from the site of administration

Dependent on | Route of administration
| Lipid solubility of drug
| Stability in acid and digestive enzymes
| Food in the stomach
| Gut motility
| Degree of first-pass metabolism (see below)

Distribution | Distribution of a drug around the body tissues after it has reached the circulation

Dependent on | Lipid solubility
| Plasma protein-binding

Volume of distribution (V_D) | The apparent volume into which a drug is distributed

Low V_D (< 5 L) | Drug is retained in vascular compartment

Medium V_D (< 15 L) | Drug is restricted to extracellular space

High V_D (> 15 L) | Drug is distributed throughout total body water

$t_{1/2}$ (half-life) | Time taken for the concentration of drug in the blood to fall by half its original value

Dependent on | Elimination in urine
| Elimination in bile
| Metabolism (usually by the liver)

Elimination kinetics | The fall in plasma concentration of drug with time

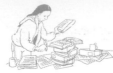

First-order kinetics
(K&C, p. 959)
- Most drugs
- Exponential fall in plasma concentration
- Elimination is dependent on drug concentration

Zero-order kinetics
- Rate of elimination is constant and not affected by increased concentration of drug
- Usually due to saturation of enzyme responsible for metabolism
  — phenytoin

Excretion
- Most drugs/metabolites are excreted by the kidneys

Renal excretion dependent on
- Glomerular filtration rate
- Lipid solubility
- Reabsorption in renal tubules

Biliary excretion
- Some drugs are concentrated in the bile
- May be reabsorbed from the intestine (enterohepatic circulation)

DRUG METABOLISM

- Drug is made more hydrophilic, therefore is more rapidly excreted by the kidney
- Metabolites are usually less active than the parent drug

Phase I
- Transformation of drug into more polar metabolite

Oxidation
- Most common
- Cytochrome P450-dependent mixed function oxidases
  — Warfarin

Reduction
— Methadone

Hydrolysis
— Aspirin

Phase II
- Drugs or phase I metabolites that are not sufficiently polar to be excreted by the kidneys are

conjugated with endogenous compounds to facilitate renal elimination

Types of conjugation
- Acetylation
- Glucuronidation
- Methylation
- Sulphation
- Glutathione
- Glycine

ENZYME INDUCTION/INHIBITION

- Some drugs increase or inhibit cytochrome P450 activity. This may affect their own and other drug metabolism

Inducers
- **P**henytoin
- **C**arbamazepine
- **B**arbiturates
- **R**ifampicin
- **A**lcohol
- **G**riseofulvin

Inhibitors
- **O**meprazole
- **D**iltiazem
- **E**rythromycin
- **V**alproate and verapamil
- **I**soniazid
- **C**imetidine and ciprofloxacin
- **E**rythromycin
- **S**ulphonamides

PHARMACOGENETICS

- How genetic determinants affect drug metabolism

Slow acetylation
- Half the population acetylate isoniazid slowly due to autosomal recessive gene
- Causes accumulation of drug and adverse reactions
- Similar polymorphisms exist for other drug acetylation

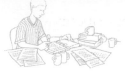

Plasma pseudocholinesterase

I 1:2500 have inactive enzyme
I Causes grossly prolonged action of suxamethonium

Adverse drug reactions (K&C, p. 960)

Types   I Dose-dependent
I Often result from known pharmacological effects of drugs
— gout and thiazide diuretics
I Dose-independent (idiosyncratic)

TYPE I HYPERSENSITIVITY (ANAPHYLACTIC REACTION)

I Common in atopic individuals
I Occurs on second or third exposure to drug

Pathology   I IgE-mediated mast cell degranulation with release of histamine and other inflammatory mediators

Clinical features   I See page 41
— Penicillin

TYPE II HYPERSENSITIVITY

Pathology   I Humoral type response
I Production of antibody to drug protein complex, causing complement activation
— Coombs' positive haemolytic anaemia with methyldopa

TYPE III HYPERSENSITIVITY

Pathology   I Formation of antigen–antibody complex, which lodge in small vessels
I Eosinophilia
— Lupus-type reaction with hydralazine

TYPE IV HYPERSENSITIVITY

Pathology   ▌ Cell-mediated response to antigen
— Contact dermatitis to topical antibiotic

LONG-TERM ADVERSE EFFECTS

▌ Occur after long-standing exposure to a drug
— Osteoporosis with corticosteroids
— Pulmonary fibrosis with amiodarone

REPORTING ADVERSE EVENTS

Doctors and pharmacists are urged to report adverse
drug reactions to the appropriate control agency

United Kingdom   ▌ Prepaid yellow cards for reporting adverse events
yellow cards   are available at the back of the British National
Formulary (BNF) and from the Medicines and
Healthcare Regulatory Authority (MHRA)

Drug interactions

Types   ▌ Pharmacokinetic
▌ Pharmacodynamic

EXAMPLES OF PHARMACOKINETIC INTERACTIONS

Absorption   ▌ Impaired absorption of iron with coadministration
of calcium salts

Distribution   ▌ Displacement from plasma proteins and tissue-
binding sites of digoxin by quinidine

Metabolism   ▌ Induction of P450 enzymes (see above)
▌ Inhibition of an enzyme used to metabolize
another drug
— Allopurinol (xanthine oxidase inhibitor)
— Azathioprine (metabolized via xanthine oxidase)

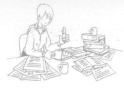

Table 4.1   Common important drug interactions

Drug	Interacting drugs	Effect
Warfarin	P450 inhibitors	Increased INR Bleeding
Theophylline	P450 inhibitors	Arrhythmias
Digoxin	Amiodarone Verapamil Quinidine Diuretics	Arrhythmias Heart block
β-blockers	Verapamil Diltiazem	Bradycardia Asystole
Lithium	Thiazides	Ataxia Fits
Oral contraceptive pill	Antibiotics	Failure of contraception
Azathioprine	Allopurinol	Bone marrow failure

Elimination   ❙ Impaired excretion of lithium by thiazide diuretics

EXAMPLES OF PHARMACODYNAMIC INTERACTIONS

❙ ACE inhibitors and loop diuretics cause hypotension
❙ Verapamil and β-blockers cause bradycardia
❙ Digoxin toxicity in hypokalaemia caused by thiazide diuretics

COMMON IMPORTANT DRUG INTERACTIONS

See Table 4.1.

Poisoning (K&C, p. 973)

Causes   ❙ Deliberate self-harm
❙ Substance abuse
❙ Accidental
❙ Criminal
❙ Iatrogenic

Table 4.2   Antidotes of common poisons

Poison	Antidote	Mechanism
Iron	Desferrioxamine	Formation of inert complex
Paracetamol	N-acetylcysteine	Accelerates detoxification
Methanol	Ethanol	Competes with metabolic enzymes
Organophosphates	Atropine	Blocks receptors which mediate toxic effect
Opiates	Naloxone	Drug receptor antagonist

General management

▌ Decrease drug absorption (within 4 hours of ingestion)
— Gastric lavage
— Absorbent, e.g. activated charcoal
— Induced vomiting (in children)
— Whole bowel lavage
▌ Antagonize effects of poisoning (Table 4.2)

ASPIRIN POISONING (K&C, p. 979)

Pathology

▌ Salicylate stimulates respiratory centre → Hyperventilation → respiratory alkalosis → Renal compensation
▌ Salicylate
▌ Lactate, ketones and pyruvate
} Metabolic acidosis

Clinical features

▌ Tinnitus
▌ Nausea and vomiting
▌ Hyperventilation
▌ Hyperpyrexia
▌ Sweating
▌ Tachycardia
▌ Confusion
▌ Fits
▌ Coma
▌ Cerebral oedema
▌ Pulmonary oedema

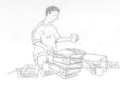

Management
I Gastric lavage (up to 12 hours due to delayed gastric emptying)
I Activated charcoal

Salicylate levels > 500 mg/L
I Forced alkaline diuresis (use with care)

Salicylate levels > 700 mg/L
I Haemodialysis

PARACETAMOL POISONING (*K&C*, p. 985)

I Most common form of poisoning; 45% of cases in UK

Pathology
(see Fig. 10.9)
I Paracetamol converted to toxic metabolite
I Metabolite is normally inactivated by reduction glutathione
I Glutathione reduced by large doses of paracetamol
I Toxic metabolites
I Hepatic necrosis

Clinical features
I Malaise
I Nausea and vomiting
I Abdominal pain
I Jaundice
I Bleeding
I Delirium

Management
(Fig. 4.1)
I Blood for paracetamol level
I Gastric lavage (for large amounts)
I Activated charcoal (within 4 hours of ingestion)
I N-acetylcysteine (Table 4.3)
I Treatment is given if plasma paracetamol concentration is on or above the treatment line

High-risk groups
I Malnourishment
I Concomitant or chronic alcohol ingestion

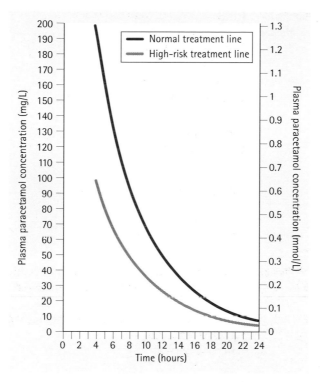

Fig. 4.1 Normogram for the treatment of paracetamol overdose. From: *British National Formulary* (1988) with permission.

▮ Use of P450 enzyme-inducing drugs
▮ AIDS

Treatment is given stat if a potentially toxic dose is known to have been taken – no need to wait 4 hours for levels (Table 4.3)
▮ Treatment is continued while paracetamol level > 10 mg/L or patient symptomatic

Table 4.3   N-acetylcysteine (NAC) treatment regime

150 mg/kg NAC in 200 mL 5% dextrose over 15 minutes

50 mg/kg NAC in 500 mL 5% dextrose over 4 hours

100 mg/kg NAC in 1000 mL 5% dextrose over 16 hours

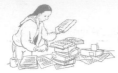

Monitoring for　❚ INR
liver damage　❚ Creatinine
　　　　　　　❚ Arterial pH

Refer to specialist　❚ INR > 3
liver unit　❚ Creatinine > normal (or rising)
　　　　　❚ pH < 7.3
　　　　　❚ Encephalopathy

BENZODIAZEPINES *(K&C*, p. 980)

❚ 40% of drug overdoses

Clinical features　❚ Drowsiness
　　　　　　❚ Ataxia
　　　　　　❚ Dysarthria
　　　　　　❚ Nystagmus
　　　　　　❚ Coma

Management　❚ Supportive
　　　　　❚ Ventilate if necessary

TRICYCLIC ANTIDEPRESSANTS *(K&C*, p. 988)

Clinical features　❚ Reduced level of consciousness
　　　　　　❚ Fits
　　　　　　❚ Increased muscle tone
　　　　　　❚ Hyperreflexia
　　　　　　❚ Fixed dilated pupils
　　　　　　❚ Urine retention
　　　　　　❚ Hypotension
　　　　　　❚ Sinus tachycardia
　　　　　　❚ Ventricular arrhythmias
　　　　　　❚ Electromechanical dissociation

Management	**I** Gastric lavage **I** Activated charcoal **I** ITU with assisted ventilation if necessary **I** Correct acid–base disturbances **I** Cardiac monitoring

ETHANOL POISONING

Clinical features	**I** Depression of conscious level **I** Vomiting **I** Fits **I** Hypoglycaemia **I** Respiratory depression **I** Aspiration of stomach contents
Management	**I** Gastric lavage **I** Respiratory support

Common drug groups

The following section lists the important features of many commonly used drugs.

British National Formulary (BNF)
There are many preparations and formulations of most of the commonly used drugs. The BNF lists all prescribable and over-the-counter medications licensed for use in the UK.

It also has sections on prescribing in liver disease, renal failure and pregnancy and a comprehensive list of drug–drug interactions. It is an invaluable reference for both revision and prescribing.

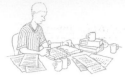

GASTROENTEROLOGY (Tables 4.4 and 4.5)

Table 4.4 H_2-receptor antagonists

Examples
Cimetidine
Ranitidine

Indications
Dyspepsia
Reflux oesophagitis

Mechanism of action
Reduce gastric acid secretion by blocking H_2-receptors

Side-effects
Diarrhoea
Abnormal LFTs
Headache
Rash
Confusion in elderly
Gynaecomastia (cimetidine)

Cautions/contraindications
Renal failure

Interactions
Warfarin
Phenytoin   } Cimetidine
Theophylline

Table 4.5   Proton pump inhibitors

Examples
Omeprazole
Lansoprazole

Indications
Peptic ulcer healing
Reflux oesophagitis
H. pylori eradication

Mechanism of action
Reduce gastric acid secretion
   by blocking proton pumps

Side-effects
Diarrhoea
Headache
Rash
Nausea

Cautions/contraindications
Liver disease

Interactions
Omeprazole – Warfarin

DIURETICS (Tables 4.6–4.8)

Table 4.6   Thiazide diuretics

Examples	**Side-effects**
Bendroflumethiazide (bendrofluazide)	Postural hypotension
Metolazone	Hypokalaemia
	Hyponatraemia
Indications	Impotence
Hypertension	Gout
Chronic heart failure	Rash
	Nausea
Mechanism of action	**Cautions/contraindications**
Inhibit sodium reabsorption in proximal tubule	Severe renal impairment
	Hypokalaemia
	Hyponatraemia
	Addison's disease

Table 4.7   Loop diuretics

Examples
Furosemide (frusemide)
Bumetanide

Indications
Pulmonary oedema
Chronic heart failure
Oliguria due to renal failure

Mechanism of action
Inhibit reabsorption in ascending limb of loop of Henle

Side-effects
Postural hypotension
Hypokalaemia
Hyponatraemia
Gout
Tinnitus and deafness

Cautions/contraindications
Anuric renal failure
Liver failure

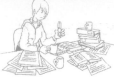

Table 4.8   Potassium-sparing diuretics

Examples
Amiloride
Spironolactone

Indications
In addition to potassium-
  wasting diuretics
Chronic heart failure
  (spironolactone)
Ascites due to liver disease

Mechanism of action
Spironolactone inhibits
  aldosterone
Amiloride blocks renal
  sodium uptake

Side-effects
GI disturbance
Hyperkalaemia
Hyponatraemia
Impotence
Gynaecomastia
  (spironolactone)
Rash

Cautions/contraindications
Severe renal impairment
Hyperkalaemia
Hyponatraemia

CARDIAC DRUGS (Tables 4.9–4.14)

Table 4.9   Cardiac glycosides

Examples
Digoxin

Indications
Heart failure
Supraventricular
  arrhythmias, particularly
  atrial fibrillation

Mechanism of action
Increase contractility of heart
  and reduce conductivity

Side-effects
Associated with toxicity
Anorexia
Nausea and vomiting

Diarrhoea
Headache
Drowsiness
Confusion
Arrhythmias
Heart block

Cautions/contraindications
Hypokalaemia
Renal impairment
Complete heart block
Wolff–Parkinson–White
  syndrome

Interactions
Potassium-wasting diuretics

Table 4.10   β-blockers

Examples
Propranolol (non-selective)
Atenolol (cardioselective)
Metoprolol (cardioselective)
Acebutolol (partial agonist)

Indications
Hypertension
Angina
Myocardial infarction
Arrhythmias
Thyrotoxicosis
Chronic heart failure

Mechanism of action
Block β-adrenergic receptors

Side-effects
Hypotension
Bradycardia
Bronchospasm
Peripheral vasoconstriction
Fatigue
Sleep disturbance
Impotence
Rash

Cautions/contraindications
Asthma
Obstructive airways
   disease
Uncontrolled heart failure
Heart block
Cardiogenic shock

Interactions
Calcium channel blockers

Table 4.11   Angiotensin-converting enzyme (ACE) inhibitors

Examples
Captopril
Enalapril
Lisinopril

Indications
Hypertension
Diabetic nephropathy
Myocardial infarction
Chronic heart failure

Mechanism of action
Block conversion of
   angiotensin I to
   angiotensin II

Side-effects
Profound hypotension
Renal impairment
Hyperkalaemia
Dry cough
Tachycardia
Fatigue
Impotence
Rash

Cautions/contraindications
Renovascular disease
Aortic stenosis

Interactions
Diuretics (hypotension)
Potassium salts

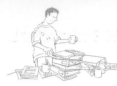

Table 4.12 Angiotensin II receptor antagonists

Examples
Losartan
Valsartan

Indications
Hypertension

Mechanism of action
Block angiotensin II receptors
(do not effect breakdown
of bradykinin)

Side-effects
Hypotension
Hyperkalaemia
Cough

Cautions/contraindications
Renovascular disease
Pregnancy

Interactions
Diuretics (hypotension)
Potassium salts

Table 4.13 Nitrates

Examples
Glyceryl trinitrate (GTN)
Isosorbide mononitrate

Indications
Acute angina (GTN)
Angina prophylaxis

Mechanism of action
Vasodilatation
Reduced cardiac preload
Coronary artery dilators

Side-effects
Throbbing headache
Postural hypotension
Tachycardia

Cautions/contraindications
Severe renal impairment
Severe liver disease
Hypotension
Aortic stenosis
Closed angle glaucoma

Table 4.14 Calcium channel blockers

Examples
Verapamil
Nifedipine
Amlodipine
Diltiazem

Indications
Hypertension
Angina prophylaxis
Supraventricular tachycardia
(verapamil)

Mechanism of action
Smooth muscle relaxation
Peripheral vasodilatation
Reduce myocardial
contractility
Coronary artery dilatation

Slow heart rate (verapamil,
diltiazem)

Side-effects
Headache
Oedema hypotension
Worsen heart failure
Atrioventricular block
(verapamil, diltiazem)

Cautions/contraindications
Severe renal impairment
Severe liver disease
Hypotension
Left ventricular failure

Interactions
β-blockers

ANTICOAGULANTS (Tables 4.15 and 4.16)

Table 4.15   Heparin

Examples
Unfractionated heparin
Low molecular weight heparin (LMWH) (enoxaparin, tinzaparin)

Indications
Unstable angina
Myocardial infarction
Deep venous thrombosis (DVT)/Pulmonary embolism (PE)
DVT prophylaxis

Side-effects
Bleeding
Thrombocytopenia

Cautions/contraindications
Severe liver disease

Monitoring
Requires monitoring of activated partial thromboplastin time
(not for LMWH)

Table 4.16   Warfarin

Indications
DVT/PE
Prophylaxis of thromboembolism
Prosthetic heart valves
Previous PE
Arrhythmias (especially atrial fibrillation)

Mechanism of action
Antagonizes vitamin K

Side-effects
Bleeding
Teratogenic

Cautions/contraindications
Severe renal impairment
Severe liver disease
Pregnancy

Monitoring
Requires monitoring of INR (prothrombin ratio)

Interactions
P450 inhibitors

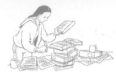

LIPID-MODULATING DRUGS (Tables 4.17–4.19)

Table 4.17   Anion exchange resins

Examples
Cholestyramine

Indications
Hyperlipidaemia

Mechanism of action
Prevents bile acid
   reabsorption and alters
     hepatic lipid metabolism

Side-effects
GI disturbance
Constipation

Cautions/contraindications
Severe renal impairment
Liver disease
Pregnancy
Breast-feeding

Table 4.18   Fibrates

Examples
Bezafibrate

Indications
Hyperlipidaemia

Mechanism of action
Unknown

Side-effects
Gallstones
Pruritus
Impotence

Cautions/contraindications
Severe renal impairment
Liver disease
Pregnancy
Breast-feeding

Table 4.19   Statins

Examples
Simvastatin
Atorvastatin

Indications
Hypercholesterolaemia

Mechanism of action
HMG CoA reductase inhibitors

Side-effects
Myositis
Headache
Abnormal LFTs

Cautions/contraindications
Severe renal impairment
Liver disease
Pregnancy
Breast-feeding

OTHERS (Tables 4.20–4.22)

Table 4.20   Benzodiazepines

Examples	**Side-effects**
Diazepam	Drowsiness
Nitrazepam	Dependence
Temazepam	Withdrawal syndrome
Indications	**Cautions/contraindications**
Insomnia	Respiratory disease
Anxiety	Pregnancy
Mechanism of action	Severe liver disease
Potentiate action of GABA	

Table 4.21   Non-steroidal anti-inflammatory drugs (NSAIDs)

Examples	**Side-effects**
Non-selective COX inhibitors	Dyspepsia
Ibuprofen	GI ulceration and bleeding
Indometacin	Hypersensitivity reactions
Naproxen	Renal impairment
Diclofenac	**Cautions/contraindications**
COX-2 inhibitors (fewer GI	Elderly
side-effects)	Peptic ulcer disease
Rofecoxib	Renal impairment
Indications	Asthma
Inflammatory joint disease	Pregnancy
Pain associated with	**Interactions**
inflammation (e.g. post-	Warfarin (enhance
operative)	anticoagulant effect)
Musculoskeletal pain	Diuretics (increase risk of
Mechanism of action	renal toxicity)
Cyclo-oxygenase inhibitors	

Table 4.22   Oxygen

Indications
Acute hypoxaemia (e.g. asthma)
  High-flow 60–100%
Chronic respiratory failure
  Low concentration 24–28%

Side-effects
Hypercapnia due to loss of hypoxic respiratory drive

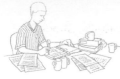

Prescriptions

Writing prescriptions
- Write in ink/biro
- State full name and address or hospital number of patient
- State date of birth of patient
- State dose and frequency of drug
- State number of days drug is prescribed for
- Use generic name of drug
- Do not use abbreviations
- Sign and date prescription

Controlled drug prescriptions
- Must be written in prescriber's own handwriting
- State name and address of patient
- Name, preparation and strength of drug
- Total quantity of drug in words and figures
- Dose and frequency
- Repeat prescriptions are not permitted

Name: John Smith
Address: St Elsewhere's
London
AB1 2CD

Date of birth: 13.9.40

1 **Prescription**
Morphine sulphate tablets (MST Continus)
20 mg three times daily to be taken orally
5 days' supply

Total = 300 mg, three hundred milligrams

Signature: **Date:** 01.01.01
Name of prescriber: Dr I Hope
The Surgery
West Street
London
AB2 3EF

Self-assessment questions

Multiple choice questions

1. The following drugs exert their effect by binding to receptors:
   A. Aspirin
   B. Propranolol
   C. Nifedipine
   D. Cimetidine
   E. Omeprazole

2. The following drugs are receptor agonists:
   A. Salbutamol
   B. Atenolol
   C. Pilocarpine
   D. Phenylephrine
   E. Captopril

3. The following drugs undergo extensive first-pass metabolism:
   A. Glyceryl trinitrate
   B. Lidocaine (lignocaine)
   C. Insulin
   D. Benzylpenicillin
   E. Probenecid

4. The following drugs induce P450 enzymes:
   A. Phenobarbital
   B. Rifampicin
   C. Cimetidine
   D. Omeprazole
   E. Carbamazepine

5. In paracetamol overdose:
   A. Paracetamol levels are essential in planning treatment
   B. Hepatic necrosis can occur up to 48 hours after ingestion
   C. N-acetylcysteine prevents paracetamol absorption from the stomach
   D. Rising INR is a poor prognostic indicator
   E. Coingestion of alcohol enhances paracetamol toxicity

6. In salicylate overdose:
   A. Aspirin delays gastric emptying
   B. Respiratory alkalosis occurs in conjunction with metabolic acidosis
   C. Acidifying the urine enhances aspirin excretion by the kidney
   D. Activated charcoal may be useful up to 12 hours after ingestion
   E. N-acetylcysteine improves prognosis in large overdoses

Short answers questions

1. Write short notes on the following:
   A. Dose–response curves
   B. Volume of distribution
   C. Phase I metabolism of drugs
   D. Pharmacogenetics
   E. Prescription of controlled drugs
   F. Cytochrome P450 oxidative enzymes

Essay questions

1. Write an essay on pharmacodynamics illustrating the principles of drug actions with examples.

2. Describe the immediate management of a patient presenting with a suspected drug overdose.

3. Describe the main features of the different types of adverse reaction to drugs with examples.

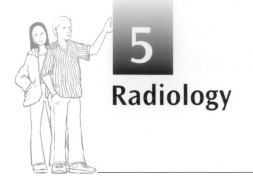

Radiology

Medical imaging remains a vital part of disease diagnosis. Diagnostic imaging is complemented by therapeutic procedures carried out by the radiologist. Interpretation of chest X-rays, abdominal X-rays and CT scans of the head, combined with the role of imaging in diagnosis and the risks of radiological procedures are important subjects in examinations.

Many radiological procedures involve exposure to X-radiation. They should therefore only be used when a strong indication is present. Care must be taken in women of childbearing age in order to avoid risk to the fetus.

Types of imaging

X-rays
▌ Utilize electromagnetic radiation
▌ Commonest form of medical imaging
▌ Image illustrates the variations in radiodensity of tissues to X-rays

Contrast studies
▌ Introduction of radiopaque contrast
▌ Outlines hollow organs, e.g. Barium enema
▌ Water-soluble contrast substances allow
— Examination of vasculature containing the agent, e.g. angiography
— excretion of the contrast agent, e.g. intravenous urogram

Computerized axial tomography (CT)
- Utilizes X-rays
- Integrates large quantities of data
- Allows computerized reconstruction of cross-sectional images

Ultrasound
- Utilizes high-frequency sound
- Measures reflection of sound waves
- Non-invasive and no radiation exposure
  — Obstetric ultrasound
  — Hepatic and pancreatic imaging

Magnetic resonance imaging (MRI)
- Magnetic fields used to produce 'proton spin'
- Data reconstruction allows detailed images
- Signal depends on water content of tissue

Nuclear medicine
- Use of isotopes in imaging
  — $\dot{V}/\dot{Q}$ scan for pulmonary embolus
  — Renal function studies
  — White cell scans for occult infection
  — Bone scans for malignancy

The chest X-ray (Fig. 5.1)

ORDER OF ANALYSIS

Basic details
- State name and age of the patient
- Date of the X-ray
- Antero-posterior (AP) or postero-anterior (PA) (describes the direct of travel of the X-rays)
- Check left and right markers

Rotation of film
- Look at medial ends of the clavicle
- Symmetry either side of spinous processes
- Sternum and vertebral column should be in line

Check
Is there a pneumothorax?
(Fig. 5.2)
- Lack of lung markings (notably in the apices)
- Visible lung margin separate from ribs
- Mediastinal shift

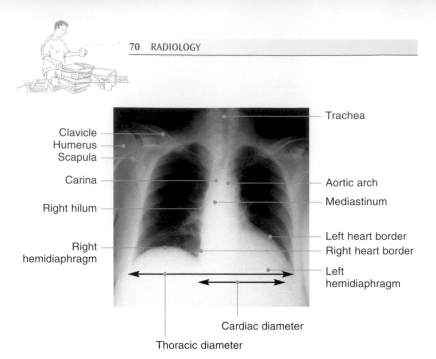

Fig. 5.1   The normal chest X-ray.

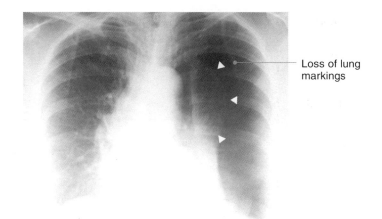

Fig. 5.2   Pneumothorax. The arrows show the edge of the collapsed lung. (*K&C*, p. 917)

Is there air under the diaphragm? (Fig. 5.3)	**I** Black line immediately under diaphragm **I** Indicates perforation
Expansion	**I** Count posterior ribs visible in the lung field **I** Normal is 6–7

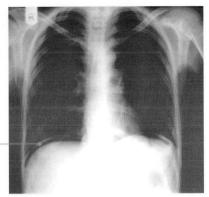

Right hemidiaphragm (thin white line) with air (black shadow) beneath it

Fig. 5.3   Air under the diaphragm indicates an intra-abdominal perforation.

Trachea	▌ Is the trachea deviated? Mediastinal shift ▌ Is the carina splayed? Right atrial enlargement
Hilar shadows	▌ Look for mass lesions
Diaphragm	▌ Flattening – over-expansion ▌ Calcification – asbestosis

Lung fields	▌ Look at lung markings
	▌ Dark areas
	  — Loss of vascular markings
	  — Hyperinflation (chronic obstructive pulmonary disease, COPD – Fig. 5.4)
	▌ White shadows
	  — Collapse (loss of air volume)
	  — Consolidation (infection)
	  — Mass lesion
	  — Fluid in pleural space – pleural effusion
	  — Alveolar fluid – pulmonary oedema
	  — Calcification
	▌ Check the lung apices – old tuberculosis

Cardiac shadow	▌ Look at heart size
	  — PA film only
	  — Normal < 50% thoracic diameter
	▌ Shape of cardiac outline

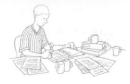

Fig. 5.4
Chronic obstructive
pulmonary disease.
(*K&C*, p. 862)

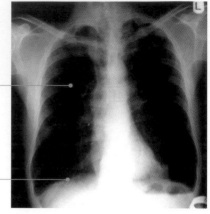

Dark
hyperinflated
lung fields

Flattened
hemidiaphragm

I Presence of mechanical valves
I Double right heart shadow – enlarged right atrium

Bones   I Look for rib fractures
I Bone lesions, e.g. metastases

INFECTIONS

Lobar pneumonia   I White patches of consolidation in lung field
(Fig. 5.5)   I Collapse of lobe → loss of lung volume
I → Local structures may be moved, e.g.
  — Elevated hemidiaphragm
  — Reduced rib spacing

Fig. 5.5
Lobar collapse.
(*K&C*, p. 886)

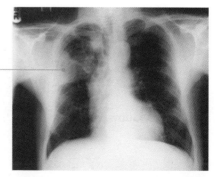

Collapsed right
upper lobe

Fig. 5.6
Right
bronchopneumonia.
(*K&C*, p. 890)

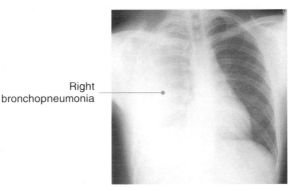

Right
bronchopneumonia

Bronchopneumonia (Fig. 5.6)
▌ Diffuse shadowing across more than one lobe

Lung abscess
(Fig. 5.7)
▌ Circular lesion with air fluid level

Tuberculosis
(Fig. 5.8)
▌ Apical shadowing or discrete lesion
▌ May show calcification
▌ Chest wall deformity due to thoracoplasty (removal of ribs)

Miliary shadows
(Fig. 5.9)
▌ Miliary (blood-spread) tuberculosis
▌ Old chickenpox pneumonia
▌ Metastatic cancer

Fig. 5.7
Left lung abscess.
(*K&C*, p. 795)

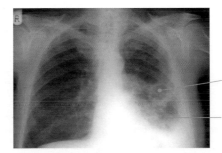

Lung abscess
with air fluid
level

Left base
consolidation

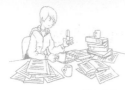

Fig. 5.8
Tuberculosis. Old sites of infection appear as apical shadows. Thoracoplasty was a surgical deflation of the infected lobe used prior to antituberculous therapy. (*K&C*, p. 892)

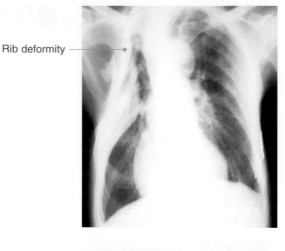

Rib deformity

Fig. 5.9
Miliary shadowing. This is classically seen after chickenpox pneumonia or miliary tuberculosis; however, it can also occur due to lung metastases.

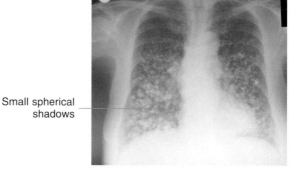

Small spherical shadows

NEOPLASMS

Bronchogenic carcinoma (Fig. 5.10)
▌ Dense white shadows in lung field
▌ Mediastinal lymphadenopathy
▌ Hilar enlargement

Lymphoma (Fig. 5.11)
▌ Mediastinal masses

Metastases (Fig. 5.12)
▌ Cannonball lesions – discrete masses

Bony infiltration (Fig. 5.13)
▌ Mottling or radiolucent areas in bones

Fig. 5.10
Bronchogenic
carcinoma.
(*K&C*, p. 911)

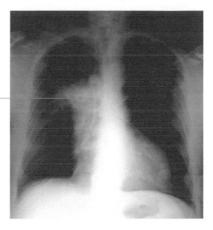

Mass arising
from right hilum

Fig. 5.11
Mediastinal mass.
Masses may be due to
lymphadenopathy
(malignancy,
lymphomas or
tuberculosis), tumours
(thymomas, germ cell
tumours) or large
retrosternal goitres.

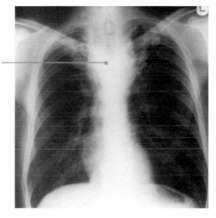

Mediastinal
mass

Fig. 5.12
A single pulmonary
metastasis.

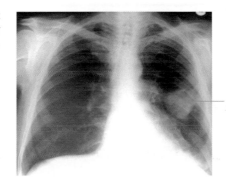

Cannonball
lesion in left
midzone

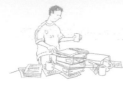

Fig. 5.13
Bony infiltration by
tumour.

Mottled
shadowing of
humerus

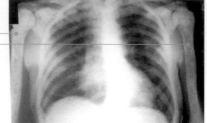

CARDIAC LESIONS

Mechanical valves

▌ Visible metal valve ring or cage

Cardiac surgery
(Fig. 5.14)

▌ Midline sternotomy wires

Enlarged heart
(Fig. 5.15)

▌ Cardiac:thoracic ratio > 50% (PA film)
▌ Loss of atrial appendage shadow
▌ Atrial enlargement
    — Splayed carina
    — Double right heart border

Abnormal cardiac outline

▌ Boot-shaped heart – tetralogy of Fallot
▌ Globular heart – pericardial effusion

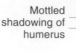

Pacemaker

Sternotomy wires

Large pleural
effusion

Fig. 5.14   Sternotomy wires from a previous coronary artery bypass graft are clearly visible.
A large left pleural effusion can also be seen.

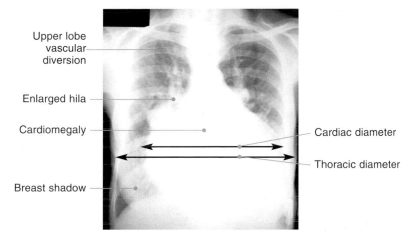

Upper lobe vascular diversion

Enlarged hila

Cardiomegaly

Breast shadow

Cardiac diameter

Thoracic diameter

Fig. 5.15 Pulmonary oedema. The heart is enlarged, and the vascular engorgement is visible as increased upper zone vascular markings. The hila are also engorged. (*K&C*, p. 718)

Pulmonary oedema
(Figs. 5.15 and 5.16)

- Enlarged heart
- Pleural effusions
- Enlarged hilum
- Fluid in the horizontal fissure
- Kerley B lines (interstitial oedema)
- Upper lobe pulmonary diversion
- Peribronchiolar cuffing

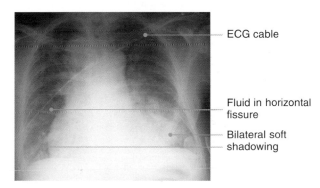

ECG cable

Fluid in horizontal fissure

Bilateral soft shadowing

Fig. 5.16 Pulmonary oedema. There are bilateral fluffy basal shadows and fluid in the horizontal fissure.

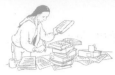

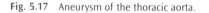

Trachea
displaced by
aorta

Fluid in
horizontal
fissure
(pulmonary
oedema)

Aneurysmal
thoracic aorta

Fig. 5.17   Aneurysm of the thoracic aorta.

**Thoracic aortic
aneurysm**
(Fig. 5.17)

❚ Dilated aortic arch

PLEURAL EFFUSIONS

❚ Loss of costophrenic angle
❚ Dense white shadow with no lung markings

Unilateral
(Fig. 5.18)

❚ Pneumonia
❚ Malignancy
❚ Pulmonary embolus
❚ Cardiac failure

Fig. 5.18
Right pleural effusion.
(*K&C*, p. 916)

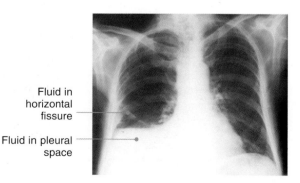

Fluid in
horizontal
fissure

Fluid in pleural
space

Bilateral	▌ Cardiac failure
	▌ Vasculitis, e.g. rheumatoid arthritis
	▌ Hypoalbuminaemia

PNEUMOTHORAX

▌ Collapse of lung → free air in the pleural space

| **Simple** (Fig. 5.2) | ▌ Lung collapse |
| | ▌ No mediastinal shift |

| **Tension** | ▌ Mediastinal shift away from the side of the pneumothorax |

MISCELLANEOUS

| **Hiatus hernia** (Fig. 5.19) | ▌ Air fluid level in a viscus visible behind or to the left of the heart shadow |

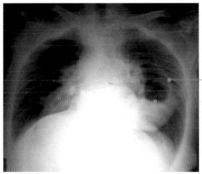

Fig. 5.19 Large hiatus hernia. A hiatus hernia may be seen as a hollow viscus with an air fluid level behind or to the left of the heart. (K&C, p 263)

Stomach wall

Air fluid level

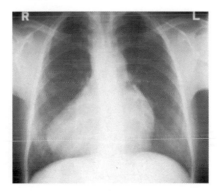

Fig. 5.20 Dextrocardia. A right-sided cardiac shadow, sometimes as part of situs inversus. Always check the side markers on an X-ray.

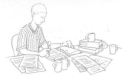
Dextrocardia
(Fig. 5.20)

❚ A right-sided heart shadow may represent true dextrocardia or incorrectly placed side markers

The plain abdominal X-ray (Fig. 5.21)

ORDER OF ANALYSIS

Introduction
❚ Patient's name, age, date of X-ray
❚ Erect or supine

Bones
❚ Thoracic and lumbar spine

Gas shadows
❚ Gastric shadow – under left hemidiaphragm
❚ Small bowel loops – fold lines extend across the full width of the bowel
❚ Colonic shadow – haustral pattern does not extend across the full width of bowel

Fig. 5.21
Normal abdominal X-ray.

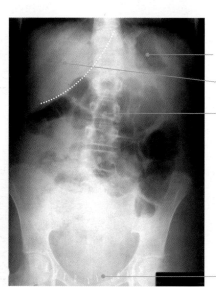

Gastric fundus

Liver

Small intestinal gas-filled loops

Skin staples from previous surgery

Organ shadows
- Liver (right upper quadrant)
- Gallbladder (if calcified gallstones present)
- Kidneys (and presence of calcification)
- Pancreatic calcification (chronic pancreatitis)

GASTROINTESTINAL ABNORMALITIES

Stomach
(Fig. 5.22)
- Dilated stomach
  - Ileus
  - Pyloric stenosis

Small intestine
(Fig. 5.23)
- Obstruction
  - Multiple air fluid levels
  - Dilatation
- Inflammation – separated bowel loops (due to thickened bowel wall)

Colon
(Figs 5.24–5.27)
- Faeces – speckled appearance
- Toxic megacolon – dilated colon
- Volvulus   sigmoid dilatation (coffee bean sign)
- Colitis
  - Featureless colon
  - Ulceration
  - Mucosal islands

Fig. 5.22
Gastric dilatation. The stomach is grossly distended. There is accompanying small bowel distension.

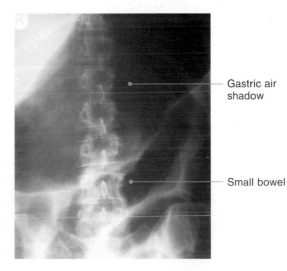

Gastric air shadow

Small bowel

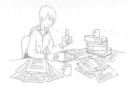

Fig. 5.23
Small bowel obstruction with ileus. Multiple air fluid levels are seen in the small bowel (erect film).

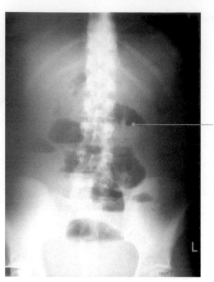

— Air fluid level

Liver
❙ Enlargement
❙ Gallstones
❙ Ascites – diffuse ground glass appearance

Pancreas
❙ Speckled calcification (chronic pancreatitis)

Fig. 5.24
Bowel distension due to obstruction. The loops are markedly dilated (arrow).

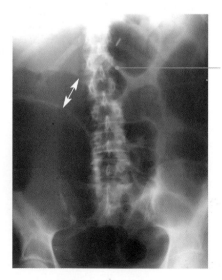

— Small bowel, with folds extending across width of bowel

Fig. 5.25
Toxic megacolon. The transverse colon is dilated (arrow). Classically, the transverse colon is the site of the dilatation. This is a medical emergency as there is a high risk of perforation and peritonitis.
(*K&C*, p. 307)

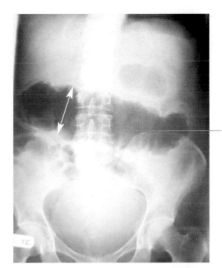

Transverse colon

Fig. 5.26
Ulcerative colitis. The colon is smooth and featureless.
(*K&C*, p. 305)

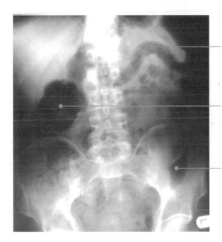

Loss of haustral pattern in transverse colon

Dilated proximal colon

Featureless sigmoid colon

URINARY TRACT

Kidneys
(Fig. 5.28)
▌ Calcification
▌ Staghorn calculi
▌ Stone in ureter

Bladder
▌ Stones

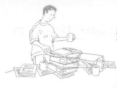

Fig. 5.27
Constipation. Faeces
appear as a speckled
pattern in the colon.
(*K&C*, p. 309)

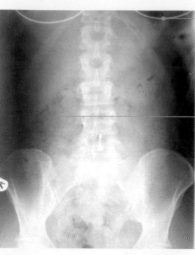

Bra wire

Faecal loading

Fig. 5.28
Staghorn renal
calculus. (*K&C*, p. 626)

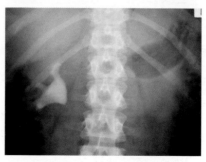

Contrast studies

Contrast (oral or rectal barium or intravenous water-
soluble contrast) is used to define specific organs
radiologically.

BARIUM STUDIES

Barium swallow

I Visualizes the pharynx and oesophagus
I Achalasia
— Rat's tail appearance (Fig. 5.29)
— Dilated oesophagus
I Strictures
— Benign – short and smooth
— Malignant – long and ragged (Fig. 5.30)

Fig. 5.29
Achalasia. This barium swallow shows the classical rat's tail appearance of the distal oesophagus in achalasia. (*K&C*, p. 266)

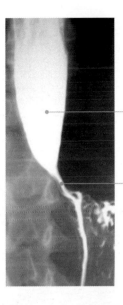

Dilated oesophagus

Narrowed lower oesophageal sphincter

Fig. 5.30
Barium swallow showing a malignant oesophageal stricture. (*K&C*, p. 268)

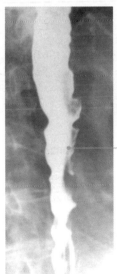

Long irregular malignant stricture

Barium meal
- Visualizes the stomach and duodenum
- Ulcer – discrete collections of barium
- Cancers – filling defects

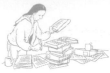

Barium follow-through
(Fig. 5.31)

❙ Visualizes small bowel
❙ Strictures ⎫
❙ Inflammation ⎬ Crohn's disease
⎭
❙ Tumours
❙ Diverticulae – Meckel's diverticulum

Barium enema
(Figs 5.32–5.34)

❙ Visualizes colon
❙ Malignancy – apple-core lesions
❙ Diverticular disease
❙ Inflammatory colitis
❙ Polyps

Fig. 5.31
Barium meal and follow-through showing a terminal ileal stricture (the string sign of Kantor) in Crohn's disease.
(*K&C*, p. 302)

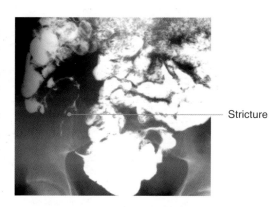

Stricture

Fig. 5.32
Barium enema of a colonic carcinoma demonstrating an 'apple-core' stricture.
(*K&C*, p. 316)

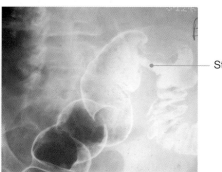

Stricture

Fig. 5.33
Barium enema in
ulcerative colitis. The
colon is featureless
with a loss of the
normal haustral
pattern. (*K&C*, p. 305)

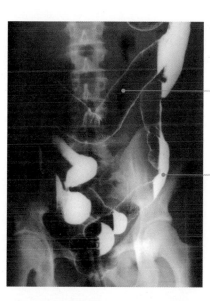

Transverse
colon

Barium (patient
lying on left
side)

Fig. 5.34
Diverticular disease
on a barium enema.
(*K&C*, p. 312)

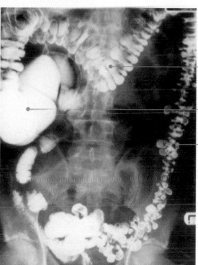

Normal
transverse
colon

Caecum

Diverticulae
with stricturing
in ascending
colon

INTRAVENOUS CONTRAST STUDIES

Angiograms   ❙ Outline vascular tree
❙ Coronary arteries for ischaemic heart disease
❙ Renal arteries for hypertension
❙ Cerebral arteries for subarachnoid haemorrhage

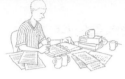
Digital subtraction angiography
I The digitized image prior to contrast is electronically subtracted from that with contrast, leaving just the contrast-outlined vascular bed
I Removes any overlying anatomical features

Urograms
I Intravenous contrast excreted by kidneys
I Outlines the collecting ducts, renal pelvis, ureters and bladder
I Detects:
— Non-functioning kidney
— Hydronephrosis
— Tumours
— Calculi

Computed axial tomography (CT)

Computerized axial tomography (CT or CAT scans) utilize computer-generated images captured using an array of X-ray beams. They have a high radiation dose. Intravenous contrast can be given to enhance vascular lesions. Oral contrast can be given to enhance the bowel.

CT SCANS OF THE HEAD

Cerebrovascular accidents
(Fig. 5.35)
(*K&C*, p. 1154)
I Ischaemic strokes may not be apparent for 48 hours; they appear as dark areas
I Haemorrhagic strokes appear as white areas

Intracranial bleeds
(Figs 5.36–5.37)
I Acutely blood appears white
I Extradural haemorrhages are biconvex
I Subdural haemorrhages are crescent-shaped
I Intracerebral bleeds are within the substance of the brain
I Subarachnoid bleeds appear as white areas in the ventricular system of the brain

Mass lesions
(Fig. 5.38)
I Malignancies (primary or secondary)
I Local oedema appears black
I Look for midline shift

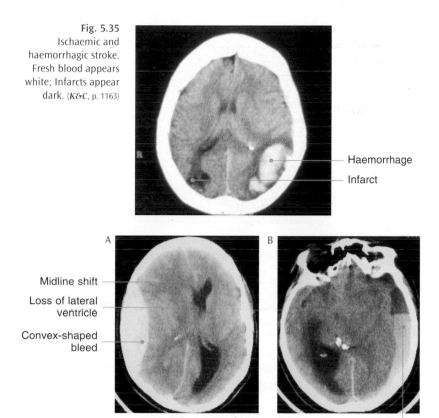

Fig. 5.35 Ischaemic and haemorrhagic stroke. Fresh blood appears white; Infarcts appear dark. (*K&C*, p. 1163)

Haemorrhage

Infarct

A

B

Midline shift

Loss of lateral ventricle

Convex-shaped bleed

Biconcave bleed

Fig. 5.36   Intracranial bleeds. A. Extradural haematoma. B. Subdural haematoma. (*K&C*, p. 1172)

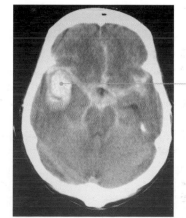

Fig. 5.37 Subarachnoid haemorrhage. Fresh blood appears white and is seen in the cortex and fissures. (*K&C*, p. 1171)

Blood

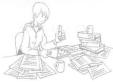

Fig. 5.38
Intracerebral mass
lesion (contrast-
enhanced CT of the
head). There is an
enhancing mass with
surrounding oedema
and obliteration of
the right lateral
ventricle with midline
shift. (*K&C*, p. 1198)

Left lateral ventricle

Oedema

Enhancing mass

Mass in liver

Right lobe of
liver

Stomach
Rib

Aorta
Renal cortex

Renal pelvis
Vertebral column

Fig. 5.39   CT of the abdomen. There is a mass lesion in the liver.

CT SCANS OF THE BODY (Figs 5.39 and 5.40)

CT scans of the body are useful for a very wide range
of diseases. Staging of malignancy and location of
occult malignancy are common uses.

Magnetic resonance imaging (MRI)

MRI provides high-resolution imaging of internal
structures based on the water content of the tissue.
It is useful for accurate localization of pathology and

Fig. 5.40
Calcified gallstones on
abdominal CT.
(*K&C*, p. 387)

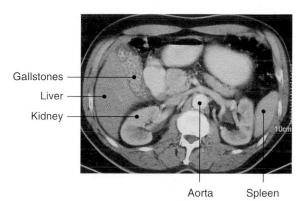

Gallstones

Liver

Kidney

Aorta   Spleen

its relationship to surrounding structures, notably in
the central nervous system.

Ultrasound

Ultrasound utilizes sound waves and their reflections
in order to image structures. It is safe, quick and non-
invasive. Boundaries between solids and fluids give
strong signals, making ultrasound useful for identifying
collections such as abscesses and pleural effusions.

**Liver, pancreas
and biliary tree**
(Fig. 5.41)

I Mass lesions in the liver
I Stones in the biliary tree
I Biliary obstruction
I Pancreatic cysts
I Carcinoma of the pancreas

Fig. 5.41
Hepatic ultrasound
showing liver cysts.
(*K&C*, p. 381)

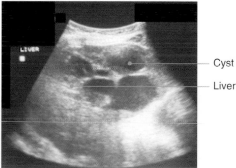

Cyst

Liver tissue

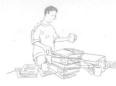

Renal ultrasound
▮ Renal masses
▮ Hydronephrosis
▮ Renal stones
▮ Congenital renal abnormalities

Vascular tree
▮ Doppler ultrasound of leg veins for deep vein thrombosis
▮ Carotid dopplers for stenosis in cerebrovascular disease

Nuclear medicine

Isotopes can be detected with photosensitive films or a gamma camera. The isotope is incorporated into a molecule designed to be picked up by a specific organ or excreted by the liver or kidney. Alternatively, blood cells can be labelled.

Red cell scan
▮ The patient's erythrocytes are labelled and reinjected
▮ May detect a site of occult blood loss

White cell scan (Fig. 5.42)
▮ Labelled leucocytes are injected
▮ Localize at site of infection or inflammation, e.g. abscesses

Bone scan (Fig. 5.43)
▮ Shows sites of high bone turnover, e.g. bone metastases

Fig. 5.42 White cell scans. The colon is outlined due to an acute pancolitis (ulcerative colitis).

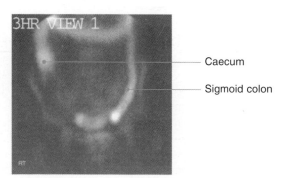

Caecum

Sigmoid colon

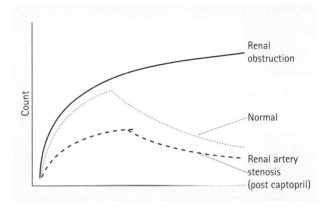

Fig. 5.43 Renal scintigraphy. The strength of signal over the kidney is measured. A normal kidney reaches a peak signal at 10–12 minutes. With an obstructed kidney the count plateaus rather than reducing, as the technetium does not pass into the bladder. Renal artery stenosis results in a delay in reaching a signal peak, with a lower peak. This is most marked after captopril is given.

Renal function scans

[^{99}Tc]DTPA scans
- Technetium diethylenetriaminepentaacetic acid
- Measures glomerular filtration
- Each kidney measured separately

[^{99}Tc]DMSA scans
- Tc-labelled dimercaptosuccinic acid
- Measure renal tubular function

Captopril scans
(Fig. 5.43)
- DTPA scan with captopril given
- May reveal renal artery stenosis
- Indicated by a delay in peak signal

Interventional radiology

Interventional radiology allows therapeutic and diagnostic procedures to be carried out without the need for general anaesthetic and in a less invasive way than surgery, although haemorrhage and perforation of a viscus or a blood vessel are important risks. Vascular procedures carry the risk of arterial spasm or occlusion and therefore tissue ischaemia.

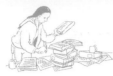

Directed biopsy	▌ Masses can be biopsied under CT or ultrasound control rather than requiring a general anaesthetic
Vascular procedures	▌ Angioplasty of arterial stenosis ▌ Insertion of filters to prevent embolism ▌ Insertion of coils into berry aneurysms to prevent subarachnoid haemorrhage
Biliary stenting	▌ Insertion of a stent to overcome obstruction of the biliary tree, e.g. in cholangiocarcinoma ▌ Percutaneous transhepatic cholangiography (PTCA)
Drain insertion	▌ Nephrostomies to relieve hydronephrosis ▌ Insertion of drains into abscesses

Self-assessment questions

Multiple choice questions

1. The following are accepted risks of CT-guided biopsy:
   A. Haemorrhage
   B. Secondary tumours along the path of the biopsy needle
   C. Radiation mucositis
   D. Hypothyroidism
   E. Abscess formation

2. The following are true of CT scans of the head:
   A. A CT scan carried out within 24 hours of an ischaemic stroke is often normal
   B. Fresh blood appears dark on an unenhanced CT scan
   C. Acoustic neuromas are seen as masses arising from the pituitary fossa
   D. Oedema around mass lesions appears black
   E. Intravenous contrast is useful in the diagnosis of intracerebral mass lesions

Objective structured clinical examination questions

1. A 67-year-old man is admitted with anorexia and a productive cough. He has been feeling unwell for about 2 weeks with a cough productive of blood-stained sputum. His chest X-ray is shown. His temperature on admission is 36.7°C, oxygen saturation 93% on air.

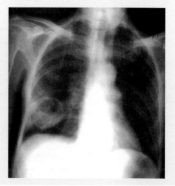

A. Describe the abnormality seen.
B. Suggest three diagnoses in order of likelihood.
C. Name two further appropriate investigations.

2. A 76-year-old man is admitted with back pain and pain in his left thigh. He has had previous treatment for a renal cell carcinoma. Which of the following tests would be appropriate in his further investigation?
A. Plain X-rays of the thoracic and lumbar spine
B. Nucleotide bone scan
C. CT scan of the abdomen
D. Venogram of the left leg
E. MRI scan of the spine

3. A 58-year-old woman is admitted for a CT-guided biopsy of a mass in the liver. List the important complications about which she should be advised and explain the procedure to her in order to gain informed consent.

4. A 76-year-old man presents with right loin pain and haematuria. His abdominal X-ray is shown.

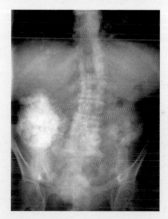

A. Describe the abnormality seen.
B. Suggest two possible diagnoses.
C. Suggest two useful radiological investigations.

Short answer questions

1. Write short notes on the following:
A. Causes of pleural effusions
B. Signs of pulmonary oedema on a chest X-ray
C. Causes of superior mediastinal masses

2. Outline the role of the following modalities in radiology:
A. Ultrasound
B. CT scans of the head
C. Renal scintigraphy

Essay questions

1. Discuss the role of isotopes in imaging in medicine. In your answer outline the indications, diagnostic utility and risks of the techniques.

2. Discuss the role of modern interventional radiology in the diagnosis and treatment of disease. Outline the risks of such techniques.

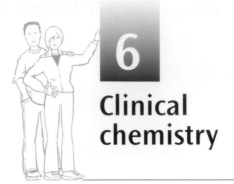

6

Clinical chemistry

Throughout this chapter the following simple abbreviations will be used:

▎ Sodium – Na⁺
▎ Potassium – K⁺

Fluid and electrolyte balance (K&C, p. 667)

If you need more detailed explanation refer to Kumar & Clark, Clinical Medicine, Chapter 12.

WATER

Total body water
▎ 50–60% of lean body weight ♂
▎ 45–50% of lean body weight ♀
▎ In a 70 kg male total body water is 42 litres
  — 28 litres intracellular
  — 9.4 litres interstitial
  — 4.6 litres plasma

Distribution of water
▎ Osmotic pressure is the primary determinant of water distribution between compartments
▎ In each compartment the following are responsible for osmotic pressure
  — Intracellular compartment – K⁺
  — Extracellular fluid compartment – Na⁺
  — Vascular compartment – proteins

Distribution of 1 litre of standard intravenous replacement fluids
▎ 5% dextrose distributes equally across all three compartments
▎ 0.9% saline remains in the extracellular compartment
▎ Colloid stays in the vascular compartment

Normal fluid and electrolyte requirements

I Normal daily fluid requirement is 2–3 litres with 100 mmol Na^+ and 70 mmol K^+ which allows for urinary, faecal and insensible loss

Sodium content of standard intravenous replacement fluids

I 1 litre of 0.9% (physiological) saline contains 150 mmol Na^+
I 1 litre of 5% dextrose contains no Na^+
I 1 litre of dextrose saline contains 30 mmol Na^+

An example of a standard 24-hour fluid regime

I 1 litre 0.9% saline
I + 2 litres 5% dextrose
I Each with 20 mmol KCl added

When to decrease the above fluid regime

I Elderly patients – require less volume, particularly if in heart failure
I Acute renal failure – replace fluids as the previous day's urine output + 500 mL (remember these patients are often hyperkalaemic and will not require KCl supplements)
I Heart failure – reduce the volume
I Drugs – can alter water and electrolyte excretion, e.g. ACE inhibitors induce K^+ retention

When to increase the above fluid regime

I Dehydration
I Shock
I Increased GI losses – replace nasogastric losses with KCl supplemented 0.9% saline
I Increased insensible losses – fever/burns
I Pancreatitis
I Drugs – can alter water and electrolyte losses, e.g. diuretics increase Na^+ and water loss

Regulation of extracellular fluid volume (Fig. 6.1) (K&C, p. 668)

I Extracellular fluid volume is regulated by Na^+ excretion from the kidneys which is dependent on the circulating blood volume
I Circulating volume is determined by neurohumoral mechanisms via
— Volume receptors

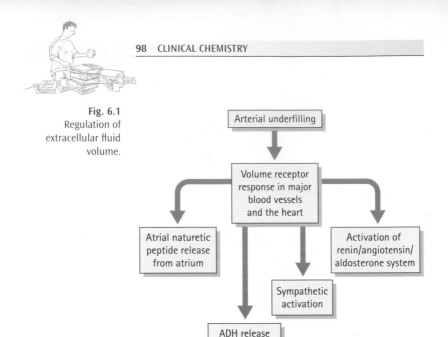

Fig. 6.1
Regulation of extracellular fluid volume.

— Catecholamines
— Atrial natriuretic peptide
— Renin/angiotensin/aldosterone

Regulation of water homeostasis (*K&C*, p. 671)

❙ Water homeostasis is effected by thirst and the concentrating and diluting functions of the kidney via the effects of antidiuretic hormone (ADH)

Increased extracellular volume (*K&C*, p. 673)

Aetiology ❙ Heart failure
❙ Hypoalbuminaemia
❙ Cirrhosis
❙ Renal sodium retention
— Acute nephritis
— Chronic renal failure
— Mineralocorticoids
— NSAIDs

Clinical features ❙ Peripheral oedema
❙ Pulmonary oedema
❙ Pleural effusion

I Ascites
I Raised jugular venous pressure
I Raised blood pressure
I Third heart sound

Management I Diuretics
I Treat underlying cause where possible

Decreased extracellular volume (*K&C*, p. 676)

Aetiology I Haemorrhage
I Burns
I GI losses
— Vomiting
— Diarrhoea
— Ileostomy
— Ileus
I Renal losses
Polyuria
— Diuretics
I Reduced renal tubular Na^+ conservation
— Reflux nephropathy
— Papillary necrosis – NSAIDs, diabetes mellitus, sickle cell disease

Clinical features I Loss of skin turgor
I Postural hypotension – a fall in BP from lying to standing (normally the blood pressure rises on standing). May be due to reduced circulating volume, altered autonomic function or prolonged bed rest (Table 6.1)

Table 6.1 Causes of postural hypotension

Hypovolaemia	
Autonomic failure	**Drugs altering peripheral**
Diabetes mellitus	**vasoconstriction**
Shy–Drager syndrome	Nitrates
Systemic amyloidosis	Calcium channel blockers
	α-blockers
Drugs altering autonomic	
function	**Prolonged bed rest**
Ganglion blockers	
Tricyclic antidepressants	

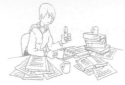
I Low jugular venous pressure
I Peripheral vasoconstriction (cold skin and empty veins in the peripheries)
I Tachycardia
I Hypotension

Septicaemia
I Note that in septicaemia the physical signs listed above occur despite normal body water/Na^+ because of vasodilatation and increased capillary permeability

Management I Replacement of fluid/electrolytes lost
I Treat underlying cause

SODIUM (*K&C*, p. 679)

I Disorders of Na^+ concentration are caused by disturbance of water balance
I In all disorders of Na^+ concentration treatment should aim for slow changes in Na^+ concentrations to avoid precipitating cerebral oedema
I Plasma and urine osmolality are often useful measures to investigate the cause of altered sodium concentrations
I Plasma osmolality can be estimated as:

$$2\,[Na^+] + [urea] + [glucose]$$

Hyponatraemia I May be associated with normal extracellular volume and body Na^+ content, salt deficiency or water excess

Hyponatraemia with normal extracellular volume
Aetiology I Abnormal ADH release
— Syndrome of inappropriate antidiuretic hormone (ADH) (see Ch. 13)
— Addison's disease
— Hypothyroidism
— Vagal neuropathy
— Stress

— Osmotically active substances causing ADH release, e.g. glucose, mannitol, alcohol, sickle cell syndrome
▌ Psychiatric illness
— Psychogenic polydipsia
— Tricyclic antidepressants
▌ Drugs
— DDAVP
— Oxytocin
— Tolbutamide/chlorpropamide

Clinical features ▌ Normovolaemia
▌ Signs of underlying cause

Management ▌ Treat underlying cause

Salt-deficient hyponatraemia
Aetiology ▌ GI losses
— Vomiting
— Diarrhoea
— Haemorrhage
▌ Renal losses
— Osmotic diuresis (e.g. hyperglycaemia)
— Diuretics
— Adrenocortical insufficiency
— Tubulo-interstitial renal disease
— Unilateral renal artery stenosis
— Recovery phase of acute tubular necrosis

Clinical features ▌ Hypovolaemia (see above)

Management ▌ Replace lost fluid/electrolytes
▌ Treat underlying cause

Hyponatraemia due to water excess
Aetiology ▌ Heart failure
▌ Liver failure
▌ Oliguric renal failure
▌ Hypoalbuminaemia
▌ Excess fluids (iatrogenic)

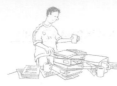

Clinical features	❙ Volume overload (see above) ❙ If severe can cause drowsiness, convulsions and coma ❙ Signs of underlying disease
Management	❙ Fluid restriction ❙ Treat underlying cause

Pseudohyponatraemia

❙ Rarely hyperlipidaemia or hyperproteinaemia produces a spuriously low measured Na^+ concentration
❙ Plasma osmolality is normal

Hypernatraemia

❙ Hypernatraemia nearly always indicates water deficiency
❙ In normal individuals with an intact thirst axis and free access to water hypernatraemia is rare
❙ Thirst is frequently deficient in elderly patients which makes them more prone to hypernatraemia

Aetiology

❙ Inadequate water intake *PLUS*
❙ ADH deficiency
— Diabetes insipidus
❙ Insensitivity to ADH (nephrogenic diabetes insipidus)
— Drugs (e.g. lithium, tetracyclines, amphotericin B)
— Acute tubular necrosis
❙ Osmotic diuresis
— Hyperosmolar diabetic coma
— Total parenteral nutrition

Clinical features

❙ Volume depletion (see above)
❙ Confusion/convulsions
❙ Fever
❙ Features of underlying cause

Investigations

❙ Plasma osmolality will be high
❙ A low urine osmolality indicates diabetes insipidus

Management I Replace fluid
I Treat underlying cause

POTASSIUM (*K&C*, p. 682)

Serum K^+ concentrations are determined by
I Uptake of K^+ into cells (Fig. 6.2)
I Renal excretion (controlled by aldosterone)
I Extrarenal losses, e.g. gastrointestinal

Hypokalaemia

Aetiology I See Table 6.2

Clinical features I If severe, muscle paralysis
I Cardiac arrhythmias in abnormal hearts
I Potentiation of digoxin toxicity

Management I Give supplements
I Potassium-sparing drugs
I Treat underlying cause

Hyperkalaemia

Aetiology I See Table 6.3

Fig. 6.2
Regulation of uptake
of potassium into
cells.

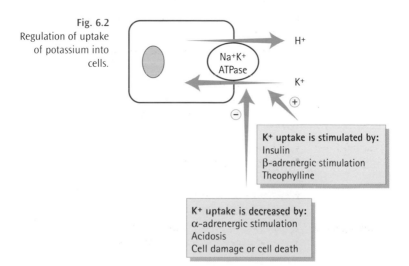

K+ uptake is stimulated by:
Insulin
β-adrenergic stimulation
Theophylline

K+ uptake is decreased by:
α-adrenergic stimulation
Acidosis
Cell damage or cell death

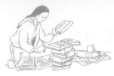

Table 6.2 Causes of hypokalaemia

Increased renal excretion
Diuretics – thiazide and loop

Increased aldosterone secretion
Liver failure
Heart failure
Nephrotic syndrome
Cushing's syndrome
Conn's syndrome
Adrenocorticotrophic hormone (ACTH) producing tumours

Exogenous mineralocorticoid
Corticosteroids
Carbenoxolone
Liquorice

Renal disease
Renal tubular acidosis types 1 and 2
Renal tubular damage
  Acute leukaemia
  Cytotoxics

Nephrotoxic drugs, e.g. gentamicin
Release of urinary tract obstruction

Severe dietary deficiency

Redistribution into cells
β-adrenergic stimulation
  acute myocardial infarct
  β-agonists, e.g. salbutamol
Insulin, e.g. treatment of diabetic ketoacidosis
Correction of vitamin B_{12} deficiency
Alkalosis

GI losses
Vomiting
Diarrhoea
Purgative abuse
Villous adenoma
Ileostomy/ uterosigmoidostomy
Fistulae
Ileus/intestinal obstruction

Table 6.3 Causes of hyperkalaemia

Decreased excretion
Renal failure
Drugs
  Spironolactone
  Amiloride
Aldosterone deficiency
Renal tubular acidosis type 4
Addison's disease
ACE inhibitors
NSAIDs
Ciclosporin
Heparin
Acidosis

Increased release from cells
Acidosis

Diabetic ketoacidosis
Rhabdomyolysis
Tissue damage
Tumour lysis
Succinylcholine
Digoxin poisoning
Vigorous exercise

Increased extraneous load
Potassium chloride administration
Blood transfusion

Spurious
Increased *in vitro* release (haemolysed sample)

Clinical features   ▌ Cardiac arrhythmias
▌ Hypotension/bradycardia if severe
▌ Kussmaul breathing (associated acidosis)
▌ Widened QRS/tented T waves on ECG

Management   ▌ See page 374 for emergency treatment
▌ Calcium resonium – exchange resin given orally or rectally
▌ Dialysis
▌ Treat cause

CALCIUM

Disorders of calcium metabolism are discussed in Chapter 11 (page 303).

MAGNESIUM (*K&C*, p. 686)

▌ Serum magnesium concentrations are determined by uptake in the small bowel and renal excretion
▌ Disordered magnesium concentrations occur in association with other electrolyte imbalance

Hypomagnesaemia

Aetiology   ▌ See Table 6.4

Clinical features   ▌ Irritability
▌ Tremor
▌ Ataxia
▌ Carpopedal spasm
▌ Hyperreflexia
▌ Confusion/hallucinations
▌ Convulsions
▌ ECG shows prolonged QT interval, flat T waves

Management   ▌ Give supplements
▌ Treat underlying cause

Hypermagnesaemia

Aetiology   ▌ See Table 6.4

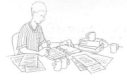

Table 6.4   Causes of hypo/hypermagnesaemia

HYPOMAGNESAEMIA	
Decreased magnesium absorption	Cisplatin
	Ciclosporin
Malabsorption	**GI losses**
Malnutrition	Prolonged nasogastric
Alcohol excess	suction
Increased renal excretion	Excessive purgatives
Drugs	GI/biliary fistulae
Diuretics – loop and	Severe diarrhoea
thiazide	**Acute pancreatitis**
Digoxin	
Diabetic ketoacidosis	**HYPERMAGNESAEMIA**
Bartter's syndrome	**Impaired renal excretion**
Hyperaldosteronism	Chronic renal failure
SIADH	Acute renal failure
Alcohol excess	
Hypercalciuria	**Increased magnesium intake**
1,25-(OH)-vitamin D	Purgatives
deficiency	Antacids
Drug toxicity	
Amphotericin	**Haemodialysis with high**
Aminoglycosides	**magnesium concentration dialysate**

Clinical features
I Lethargy
I Muscle weakness
I Hyporeflexia
I Narcosis
I Respiratory paralysis
I Cardiac conduction defects

Management
I Calcium gluconate, dextrose and insulin
I Dialysis
I Remove cause

PHOSPHATE (K&C, p. 688)

I The regulation of phosphate concentrations is closely linked to that of calcium

Hypophosphataemia

Aetiology I See Table 6.5

Table 6.5   Causes of hypo/hyperphosphataemia

HYPOPHOSPHATAEMIA	Decreased intake/absorption
Redistribution	Dietary
Respiratory alkalosis	Malabsorption
Treatment of diabetic ketoacidosis	Vomiting
Carbohydrate administration after starvation (refeeding syndrome)	Gut phosphate binders, e.g. aluminium hydroxide
Post-parathyroidectomy	Vitamin D deficiency
	Alcohol withdrawal
Renal losses	**HYPERPHOSPHATAEMIA**
Hyperparathyroidism	Chronic renal failure
Renal tubular defects	Phosphate-containing enemas
Diuretics	Tumour lysis
	Rhabdomyolysis
	Myeloma

Management
 ▌ If mild, rarely requires treatment
 ▌ If severe, give i.v. replacement slowly

Hyperphosphataemia

Aetiology ▌ See Table 6.5

Management
 ▌ If acute, rarely requires treatment
 ▌ If chronic, give gut phosphate binders or dialyse

Acid–base disorders (K&C, p. 689)

 ▌ Acid–base disturbance may be caused by:
   — Abnormal carbon dioxide removal in the lungs (respiratory alkalosis/acidosis)
   — Abnormalities of the regulation of bicarbonate and other buffers in the blood (metabolic alkalosis/acidosis)
 ▌ Arterial blood gas analysis provides information on
   — pH
   — Bicarbonate concentrations
   — Partial pressures of oxygen and carbon dioxide

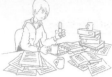

Respiratory acidosis
- Caused by retention of carbon dioxide
- Renal retention of bicarbonate may partly compensate (see Ch. 8)

Respiratory alkalosis
- Caused by increased removal of carbon dioxide as a result of hyperventilation (see Ch. 8)

Metabolic acidosis
- Caused by accumulation of acid
- Demonstrated by a fall in plasma bicarbonate
- Arises from:
  — Acid administration
  — Acid generation
  — Impaired acid excretion by kidneys
  — Bicarbonate losses from GI tract
- Anion gap (unmeasured anions) helps differentiate the causes

$$\text{Anion gap} = (\,[Na^+] + [K^+]\,) - (\,[HCO_3^-] + [Cl^-]\,)$$

- Normal anion gap = 10–18 mmol/L^{-1}
- Note that albumin is a major part of this anion gap; a fall in albumin will reduce the anion gap

Metabolic acidosis with a normal anion gap
- Suggests that either hydrochloric acid is being generated or bicarbonate is being lost
- In all cases plasma bicarbonate is low and plasma chloride high

Aetiology
- Increased GI bicarbonate losses
  — Diarrhoea
  — Ileostomy
  — Ureterosigmoidostomy
- Increased renal bicarbonate losses
  — Acetozolamide
  — Proximal (type 2) renal tubular acidosis
  — Hyperparathyroidism
  — Renal tubular damage – heavy metal poisoning, paraproteins, drugs
- Decreased renal hydrogen ion losses
  — Distal (type 1) renal tubular acidosis
  — Type 4 renal tubular acidosis

I Increased hydrochloric acid production
— Ammonium chloride ingestion
— Increased catabolism of lysine/arginine

Metabolic acidosis with a high anion gap

I Suggests presence of unmeasured endogenous or exogenous anions

Aetiology   I Renal failure
I Lactic acidosis
I Ketoacidosis
I Exogenous acid such as salicylate (aspirin)

Metabolic   I Rarer than metabolic acidosis because renal
alkalosis   excretion of bicarbonate is normally very efficient
I Can occur in
— Extracellular fluid depletion
— Potassium deficiency
— Excess mineralocorticoids
— Thiazide/loop diuretics
— Vomiting
— Exogenous alkalis, e.g. antacids plus one of the above

Cardiac markers (K&C, p. 777)

If you need more detailed explanation refer to Kumar & Clark, Clinical Medicine, Chapter 13.

These are enzymes whose elevated levels can be measured in the serum to help diagnose cardiac ischaemia; they are also abnormal in other situations as listed below.

CREATINE KINASE (CK)

Sources   I Heart and skeletal muscle

Raised in   I Myocardial infarction
I Muscle dystrophies
I Polymyositis

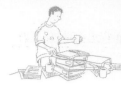

▌ Pulmonary embolus
▌ Postoperative period
▌ Myocarditis
▌ Muscle trauma, e.g. fits, injections, exercise

ASPARTATE AMINOTRANSFERASE (AST)

Sources ▌ Heart, liver, muscle and kidney

Raised in ▌ Myocardial infarction
▌ Liver disease (hepatitis of any cause)
▌ Haemolytic anaemia
▌ Muscle trauma, e.g. fits, injections, exercise

Lowered in ▌ Renal failure

LACTATE DEHYDROGENASE (LDH)

Sources ▌ All cells release LDH when damaged

Raised in ▌ Myocardial infarction
▌ Tissue necrosis of any cause
▌ Liver disease
▌ Kidney disease
▌ Haematological diseases, e.g. lymphoma
▌ Muscle trauma, e.g. fits, injections, exercise

CARDIAC TROPONINS (TROPININ T AND I)

▌ Regulatory proteins which have a high specificity
for cardiac injury
▌ Released early (2–4 hours) after injury and persist
for up to 7 days
▌ Can be useful indicators of critical cardiac disease
when elevated in patients presenting with chest
pain

Liver biochemistry (K&C, p. 340)

Liver function tests in the blood can be divided into
3 groups. Note that in severe disease the first two

groups can both be elevated and that drugs can induce liver enzymes (see Ch. 4).

I Tests suggesting bile duct obstruction
— Bilirubin
— Alkaline phosphatase
— γ–glutamyltranspeptidase
I Tests suggesting disease of hepatocytes
— Aminotransferases ALT and AST
I Tests of liver synthetic function. Albumin and clotting factors are made in the hepatocyte and so reflect synthetic function
— Albumin
— Prothrombin time

Further information is given in Chapter 10.

BILIRUBIN

Sources   I Mainly haemoglobin destruction

Raised in   I Bile duct obstruction of any cause
I Hepatitis of any cause
I Haemolytic anaemia
I Gilbert's syndrome

ALKALINE PHOSPHATASE

Sources   I Bile ducts, bone and placenta
I If source is the liver
— γ-glutamyl transpeptidase is elevated
I If source is bone
— γ-glutamyl transpeptidase is not elevated
— Calcium/phosphate may be abnormal

Raised in   I Bile duct obstruction of any cause
I Liver malignancy/space-occupying lesion
I Bony metastases

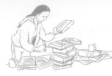
▌ Osteomalacia
▌ Paget's disease of bone
▌ Haematological malignancy, e.g. lymphoma
▌ Heart failure (liver congestion)
▌ Also normally higher in children and pregnancy
▌ Hepatitis of any cause

Lowered in   ▌ Hypothyroidism

GAMMA GLUTAMYL TRANSPEPTIDASE (γ-GT)

Sources   ▌ Bile ducts and kidney

Raised in   ▌ Alcohol excess
▌ Bile duct obstruction of any cause including malignancy/SOL
▌ Hepatitis of any cause if severe
▌ Renal carcinoma

ALANINE AMINOTRANSFERASE (ALT)

Sources   ▌ Liver and heart

Raised in   ▌ Hepatitis of any cause
▌ Bile duct obstruction of any cause

Tests of renal function *(K&C, p. 593)*

This is covered in detail in Chapter 14. If you need more detailed explanation refer to Kumar & Clark, Clinical Medicine, Chapter 11.

UREA

▌ Plasma urea varies with protein intake and renal excretion

Raised in
- Renal disease of any cause
- Dehydration
- GI bleeding
- Shock
- Cardiac failure
- Adrenal insufficiency
- Old age

Lowered in
- Liver failure
- Nephrotic syndrome
- Cachexia/kwashiorkor
- Pregnancy
- Overhydration

CREATININE

- Retention of creatinine indicates glomerular insufficiency

Raised in
- Renal disease of any cause
- Large meat intake
- Old age

Lowered in
- Muscle-wasting
- Pregnancy

URATE

- End-product of protein metabolism
- Excreted by kidneys

Raised in
- Gout
- Eclampsia
- Leukaemia/myeloma/lymphoma
- Renal insufficiency
- Thiazide diuretic therapy

Lowered in
- Allopurinol therapy
- Acute hepatitis of any cause
- Salicylate therapy

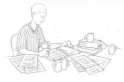

Acute phase reactants

❚ Non-specific tests for inflammation/infection
❚ Include
— Erythrocyte sedimentation rate (ESR)
— C-reactive protein (CRP)

Self-assessment questions

Multiple choice questions

1. The following abnormalities occur in diabetic ketoacidosis:
A. Postural hypotension
B. Peripheral oedema
C. Hyponatraemia
D. Hypokalaemia
E. Hyperkalaemia

2. The following diuretics induce hypokalaemia:
A. Furosemide (frusemide)
B. Bendroflumethiazide (bendrofluazide)
C. Spironolactone
D. Amiloride
E. Bumetanide

3. The following statements are correct for standard i.v. fluid solutions:
A. Normal saline distributes to all three fluid compartments
B. 5% dextrose remains in the vascular compartment
C. Colloid is used in hypovolaemia
D. Normal saline is indicated in most cases of hyponatraemia
E. Normal saline is useful i.v. fluid replacement therapy in patients with chronic liver disease

4. Causes of a metabolic acidosis with a high anion gap include:
A. Sepsis
B. Diabetic ketoacidosis
C. Aspirin overdose
D. Acute renal failure
E. Type 4 renal tubular acidosis

5. Causes of a metabolic acidosis with a normal anion gap include:
A. Diabetic ketoacidosis
B. Type 4 renal tubular acidosis
C. Diarrhoea
D. Lead poisoning
E. Hyperparathyroidism

6. Causes of metabolic alkalosis include:
A. Vomiting
B. Hypokalaemia
C. Acute renal failure
D. Furosemide (frusemide)
E. Hyperkalaemia

7. An elevated creatine kinase occurs in the following circumstances:
A. Day 5 of uncomplicated acute myocardial infarct
B. Day 2 after hip replacement
C. Following a tonic-clonic seizure
D. Polymyositis
E. Rhabdomyolysis

8. Serum bilirubin would be elevated in patients with:

A. Gilbert's syndrome

B. A gallstone obstructing the common bile duct

C. Gallstones in the gallbladder

D. Autoimmune haemolytic anaemia

E. Acute fulminant hepatitis A

9. An elevated blood urea would be expected in:

A. Pregnancy

B. GI bleeding

C. Nephrotic syndrome

D. Acute renal failure

E. Dehydration

Extended matching questions

Question 1 *Theme: abnormal blood test results*

A. Shock

B. Cardiac failure

C. Cardiac failure treated with loop diuretics

D. Pneumonia

E. Renal failure

F. Nephrotic syndrome

G. Renal tubular acidosis

H. Diarrhoea

I. High ileostomy volumes

For each of the following questions, select the most likely answer from the list above:

I. An 84-year-old female presents with confusion and ankle oedema. Blood results show the following: Na^+ 132, K^+ 2.8, Urea 9.8, Creat 128. What is the most likely diagnosis?

II. A 37-year-old patient with Crohn's disease presents with malaise. Blood tests reveal the following: Na^+ 132, K^+ 2.8, Urea 10, Creat 60, Mg^{2+} 0.54 (low), Cl^- 105, pH 7.3, Bicarbonate 15. What is the most likely diagnosis?

III. A 56-year-old male presents with fever and malaise. Blood tests reveal the following: Na^+ 124, K^+ 4.5, Urea 7.6, Creat 98, pH 7.54, Po_2 8.2, Pco_2 3.2. What is the most likely diagnosis?

Question 2 *Theme: acid–base disturbance*

A. Acute renal failure

B. Acute liver failure

C. Aspirin overdose

D. Recurrent vomiting

E. Renal tubular acidosis

F. Diabetic ketoacidosis

G. Respiratory alkalosis

H. Type II respiratory failure

For each of the following questions, select the most likely answer from the list above:

I. A 64-year-old female presents with confusion and breathlessness. Blood gas analysis shows the following: pH 7.3, Pco_2 9.6, Po_2 4.5, Bicarbonate 28. What is the most likely diagnosis?

II. A 37-year-old patient with diabetes presents with a history of vomiting and confusion. Blood gas analysis shows the following: pH 7.15, Pco_2 2.5, Po_2 12.5, Bicarbonate 10. What is the most likely diagnosis?

III. An 18-year-old male is found collapsed at home. There is no history available. Blood tests reveal the following: pH 7.25, Pco_2 3.6, Po_2 13.5, Bicarbonate 8, Na^+ 135, K^+ 4, Cl^- 101. What is the most likely diagnosis?

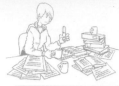

Short answer questions

1. Write short notes on the following:
   A. Hypomagnesaemia
   B. Treatment of hyperkalaemia
   C. Causes of extracellular volume depletion

2. Write short notes on the following:
   A. The anion gap
   B. Metabolic acidosis
   C. Arterial blood gases

3. Write short notes on the following:
   A. Cardiac troponins
   B. Liver function tests
   C. Acute phase proteins

Essay questions

1. Outline the common causes of hyponatraemia.

2. Describe how you would investigate a patient found to have a low pH and low bicarbonate on blood gas analysis.

3. Outline how you would initiate investigation of a patient presenting with jaundice. Limit your answer to blood tests only.

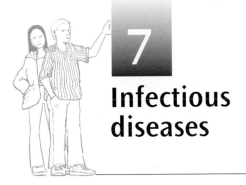

7

Infectious diseases

Infectious disease remains the most common cause of morbidity and mortality worldwide. In order for an infectious agent to propagate within the population, there must be a reservoir of infection and a mode of transmission. Thus avoidance of infection starts with reduction of the reservoir and limiting or avoiding the transmission of an organism.

System-specific infections are discussed in the appropriate chapters.

Diagnosis of infectious disease (K&C, p. 29)

History
❚ Exposure to the causative agent
— Travel to a high-risk area
  Contact with an infected individual
— Occupation history
— Animal exposure
— Sexual history
— Intravenous drug abuse
— Blood transfusion
❚ Vaccination history

Examination
❚ Presence of a fever (Table 7.1)
❚ Rashes
❚ Lymphadenopathy
❚ Hepatosplenomegaly

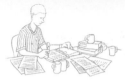

Table 7.1   Causes of fever of unknown origin (FUO) (K&C, p. 33)

Infections (40%)	Immune (20%)
Abscess	Drugs
Tuberculosis	Connective tissue disease
Urinary infection	Sarcoidosis
Biliary infection	**Other**
Endocarditis	Thyrotoxicosis
Epstein–Barr virus	Ulcerative colitis
Malignancy (30%)	Crohn's disease
Lymphomas	Factitious
Leukaemia	
Solid tumours	*5–10% remain undiagnosed*

Investigations

Full blood count and blood film

- Neutrophilia suggests bacterial infection
- Lymphocytosis suggests viral infection
- Neutropenia may suggest viral infection
- Eosinophilia suggests parasitic infection
- Parasites on blood film, e.g. malaria

Blood culture

- Aerobic and anaerobic bottles
- Follow sterile procedure
- May require repeated samples

Liver function

- Elevated transferases in viral hepatitis

TAKING BLOOD CULTURES

An aseptic technique is vital to avoid skin contaminants
Repeat cultures from different sites at different times
Wear gloves for the procedure
Select an appropriate vein
Thoroughly clean the overlying skin
Do not touch the skin
Take 15–20 ml of blood
Open the tops of the culture bottles
Clean the top of the bottle with a sterile wipe
Place a fresh needle on the syringe and insert through the seal of each bottle, placing 8–10 ml of blood in each bottle
Clearly label the samples
Send to laboratory or place in incubator

> ### MICROBIOLOGY REQUEST FORMS
> In order to make an accurate diagnosis, the following information is vital:
>
> - Patient details
> - Clinical details: duration and type of illness, other related features
> - Antibiotic therapy: duration and type of treatment
> - History of foreign travel
> - Type of specimen
> - Requested investigation
> - Clinical risks – viral hepatitis/HIV

Microscopy, culture and sensitivity

▌ Can be performed on stool, urine, CSF, sputum, ascitic fluid, pleural fluid, joint aspirates
▌ Provides organism identification and antibiotic sensitivity

Immunological diagnosis

▌ Presence of antibodies against specific antigens
▌ Presence of specific antigens due to their reaction with a known antibody

Genetic diagnosis

▌ Detection of genome of organism, e.g. hepatitis C virus RNA

Histological examination

▌ Pathology of specific infections on tissue biopsy

Imaging

▌ Localization of an infection, e.g. by ultrasound or CT scanning
▌ Labelled white cell scanning localizes the source of an infection

Treatment of infectious disease (K&C, p. 34)

ANTIBACTERIAL DRUGS (Fig. 7.1) (K&C, pp. 36–42)

β-lactams
Penicillins

▌ Block cell wall growth
▌ Group 1: parenteral formulations
— e.g. Benzylpenicillin

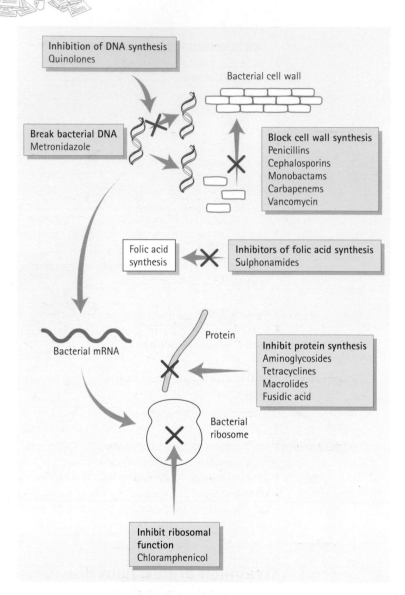

Fig. 7.1   Mechanism of action of antibacterial drugs.

▌ Group 2: oral penicillin
    — e.g. Phenoxymethylpenicillin (penicillin V)
▌ Group 3: β-lactamase-stable penicillins
    — e.g. Flucloxacillin

■ Group 4: extended spectrum
— e.g. Amoxicillin, ampicillin
■ Group 5: β-lactamase-resistant penicillin
— e.g. Temocillin

Cephalosporins
■ Inhibit cell wall synthesis
■ Penicillinase-resistant
■ Broader antibacterial range

First generation
■ Gram-positive cocci and Gram-negative
— Cefalexin, Cefradrine

Second generation
■ Gram-negative infections
— Cefuroxime, cefaclor

Third generation
■ Gram-negative infections
— Ceftazidime, ceftriaxone

Monobactams
■ Aztreonam

Carbapenems
■ Imipenem, meropenem

Aminoglycosides
■ Inhibit bacterial protein synthesis
■ Gram negatives, e.g. *Pseudomonas*
— Gentamicin, neomycin
■ N.B. Renal and ototoxicity, therefore serum levels need monitoring

Tetracyclines
■ Inhibit bacterial protein synthesis
■ Atypical pneumonias, acne
— Tetracycline, doxycycline
■ N.B. Contraindicated in children and during pregnancy as they cause permanently stained teeth

Macrolides
■ Inhibit bacterial protein synthesis
■ Useful in atypical pneumonia
— Erythromycin, clarithromycin

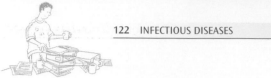

❙ Gram-negative infection
    — Clarithromycin, azithromycin

Chloramphenicol ❙ Inhibits bacterial ribosome function
    ❙ *Salmonella* enteric fevers
    ❙ Conjunctivitis (local therapy)

Fusidic acid ❙ Inhibits bacterial protein synthesis
    ❙ *Staphylococcus aureus* osteomyelitis

Sulphonamides ❙ Inhibit bacterial folic acid synthesis
    ❙ Used with trimethoprim in urinary tract and
    Pneumocystis carinii infection

Quinolones ❙ Inhibit DNA synthesis
    ❙ Gram-negative infections
    — Ciprofloxacin

Nitroimidazoles ❙ Break bacterial DNA
    ❙ Anaerobic infections
    — Metronidazole

Glycopeptides ❙ Inhibit cell wall synthesis
    ❙ Gram-positive bacteria
    — Vancomycin

ANTIFUNGAL DRUGS (*K&C*, p. 42)

Polyenes ❙ Disrupt fungal membranes
    — Amphotericin B – systemic disease
    — Nystatin – oral and enteric *Candida*

Azoles ❙ Broad-spectrum antifungals
    — Clotrimazole – ringworm
    — Ketoconazole – candidiasis

Triazoles — Fluconazole – penetrates CSF
    — Itraconazole

Others — Terbinafine
    — Griseofulvin

ANTIVIRAL DRUGS (K&C, p. 43)

Aciclovir	❚ Terminates viral DNA synthesis ❚ Herpes simplex and varicella zoster virus
Ganciclovir	❚ Cytomegalovirus infection
Amantadine	❚ Influenza virus
Interferons	❚ Hepatitis B and C
Ribavirin	❚ Combination therapy (with interferon) for chronic hepatitis C
Antiretrovirals	❚ See page 134

Vaccination (Table 7.2) (K&C, p. 44)

Passive	❚ Antibody raised against the infecting organism ❚ e.g. Tetanus immunoglobulin, diphtheria, rabies
Active	❚ Immunogenic antigen induces antibody production

Table 7.2 Vaccination schedule

2 months	**3 years**
Diphtheria ⎫	Diphtheria, tetanus
Pertussis ⎬ 3 doses	MMR and oral polio
Tetanus ⎭	
Haemophilus influenzae b	**10–14 years**
Oral polio	BCG if tuberculin-negative
Meningococcus gp C	
	18 years
Tuberculosis (BCG) for infants at high risk	Diphtheria, tetanus and oral polio
1 year	
Measles ⎫	
Mumps ⎬ MMR	
Rubella ⎭	

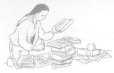

Live attenuated vaccines	▌ Oral polio ▌ Measles, mumps, rubella ▌ BCG
Inactivated (killed) vaccines	▌ Hepatitis A ▌ Pertussis (whooping cough) ▌ *Haemophilus influenzae b* ▌ Meningococcus A and C ▌ Pneumococcus ▌ Influenza
Toxoids	▌ Tetanus ▌ Diphtheria
Recombinant vaccines	▌ Hepatitis B

Bacterial infection (K&C, p. 64)

GRAM-POSITIVE COCCI

Staphylococcus
▌ *Staph. aureus, epidermidis, saprophyticus*
▌ Skin:cellulitis, impetigo
▌ Lungs: pneumonia, abscesses
▌ Heart: endocarditis
▌ CNS: meningitis, abscesses
▌ Bones: osteomyelitis
▌ Gut: enterocolitis
▌ *Staph. aureus* produces a toxin, which may cause:
— Food poisoning
— Toxic shock syndrome
— Scalded skin syndrome

Management
▌ Much community-acquired infection is penicillin-sensitive
▌ However, hospital spread of methicillin-resistant *Staph. aureus* (MRSA) is increasing

Streptococcus
▌ Majority of infections are due to β-haemolytic *Strep. pyogenes*
▌ Skin: impetigo, erysipelas
▌ Mouth: pharyngitis, tonsillitis
▌ Lungs: pneumonia – *Strep. pneumoniae*
▌ Other: endocarditis – *Strep. viridans,* scarlet fever, rheumatic fever

Management ▌ Majority are sensitive to penicillins

GRAM-NEGATIVE COCCI

Neisseria ▌ *Neisseria meningitidis* → Meningitis and
septicaemia
▌ *Neisseria gonorrhoeae* → gonorrhoea

Management ▌ Penicillin or cefotaxime

GRAM-POSITIVE BACILLI

Corynebacterium ▌ *C. diphtheriae*
▌ Toxin-producing forms → diphtheria
▌ Nasal discharge
▌ Pharyngeal inflammation
▌ Laryngeal inflammation → husky voice
▌ → Respiratory obstruction
▌ Myocarditis
▌ Neurological manifestations – cranial nerve palsies,
polyneuropathy

Management ▌ Antitoxin + penicillin

Listeria ▌ *L. monocytogenes*
▌ → Abortions, meningitis or septicaemia

Management ▌ Ampicillin and gentamicin

Clostridium ▌ *C. botulinum, C. difficile* – see Ch. 10
▌ *C. tetani* → tetanus
— Infects puncture wounds and bites
— Neurotoxin production
— → Neuromuscular blockade, lockjaw, muscle
spasm, autonomic neuropathy

Management ▌ Antitoxin, penicillin, ITU care

Bacillus group
B. anthracis ▌ Anthrax
▌ → Erythematous skin lesion that ulcerates
▌ → Black central eschar
▌ Pulmonary and GI tract involvement

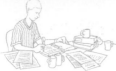

Management	❚ Penicillin
B. cereus	❚ → Toxin mediated food poisoning

GRAM-NEGATIVE BACILLI

Brucella	❚ *B. abortus, melitensis, suis* ❚ Endotoxin → headache, fever, weakness ❚ Lymphadenopathy, hepatosplenomegaly ❚ Arthritis, encephalitis and endocarditis ❚ Contracted from non-pasteurized milk
Management	❚ Doxycycline
Bordetella	❚ *B. pertussis* – whooping cough ❚ Childhood disease ❚ Catarrhal phase – rhinorrhoea and conjunctivitis ❚ Paroxysmal phase – coughing attacks
Management	❚ Erythromycin in catarrhal phase
Haemophilus	❚ *H. influenzae, ducreyi, parainfluenzae* ❚ Increased risk of infection post-splenectomy ❚ Pneumonia, bronchitis ❚ Meningitis (*H. influenzae b*) ❚ Epiglottitis
Management	❚ Cefotaxime, cefuroxime
Prevention	❚ Hib vaccine
Cholera	❚ *Vibrio cholerae* (see Ch. 10)
Enterobacteria	❚ *Escherichia coli* ❚ *Salmonella* ❚ *Campylobacter* ⎫ see Chapter 10 ❚ *Shigella* ❚ *Helicobacter* ❚ *Yersinia*

Mycobacterial disease

Mycobacterium tuberculosis	❚ Acid-fast aerobic bacillus ❚ Droplet spread

▌ → Caseating granuloma
— Lung
— Adrenals
— Terminal ileum
— Lymph nodes
▌ → Cough, fever, weight loss, night sweats
▌ Immunosuppression → haematogenous spread
(miliary TB)

Complications ▌ TB meningitis
▌ TB peritonitis
▌ Arthritis and osteomyelitis
▌ Constrictive pericarditis

Investigations ▌ Imaging – X-ray/CT scan of the chest
▌ Microbiology – Ziehl–Nielsen staining of sputum
▌ Bronchoscopy and washings
▌ Biopsy of solid lesions
▌ CSF examination in meningitis

Management ▌ Combination therapy (Table 7.3)

Contact tracing ▌ X-ray and tuberculin testing in close contacts

---

Table 7.3   Drug regimens in tuberculosis

Pulmonary TB
Rifampicin and isoniazid for 6 months, pyrazinamide for first
2 months (add ethambutol if previously treated for TB)

TB osteomyelitis and ileal TB
Rifampicin and isoniazid for 9 months, pyrazinamide for
2 months

TB meningitis
Rifampicin, isoniazid for 12 months, pyrazinamide for
2 months

Drug resistance and HIV
Start standard therapy as above but alter based on
sensitivities. Treat for a total of 2 years, or 1 year after the last
positive culture result

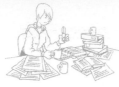

Immunization
- Bacille Calmette–Guérin (BCG)
- Bovine strain of TB with very low virulence after tuberculin testing

Mycobacterium leprae
- Leprosy (Hansen's disease)
- Immune response determines disease type (there are two ends of a clinical spectrum)

Tuberculoid
- High cell-mediated immunity
- Hypopigmented skin patches
- Loss of sensation over patch
- Tender thickened nerves

Lepromatous
- Macules, papules or nodules in the skin
- Laryngitis and hoarse voice
- Collapse of nasal cartilage
- Leonine face

Investigations
- Impossible to culture organism
- Diagnosis is basically clinical

Management
- Dapsone, rifampicin and clofazimine for 2 years

Spirochaetes

Syphilis
- *Treponema pallidum*

Primary syphilis (10–90 days post-infection)
- Painless ulcer (chancre) at infection site

Secondary syphilis (4–10 weeks)
- Lymphadenopathy
- Rash – papules or pustules
- Warty skin lesions (condylomata lata)
- Oral 'snail track' ulcers

Tertiary syphilis
- Granulomatous lesions
- Skin, bones, liver

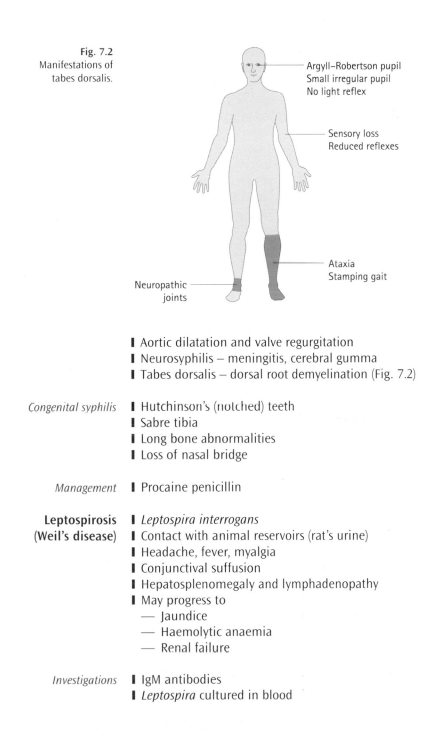

Fig. 7.2 Manifestations of tabes dorsalis.

Argyll–Robertson pupil
Small irregular pupil
No light reflex

Sensory loss
Reduced reflexes

Ataxia
Stamping gait

Neuropathic joints

❚ Aortic dilatation and valve regurgitation
❚ Neurosyphilis – meningitis, cerebral gumma
❚ Tabes dorsalis – dorsal root demyelination (Fig. 7.2)

Congenital syphilis   ❚ Hutchinson's (notched) teeth
❚ Sabre tibia
❚ Long bone abnormalities
❚ Loss of nasal bridge

Management   ❚ Procaine penicillin

Leptospirosis (Weil's disease)   ❚ *Leptospira interrogans*
❚ Contact with animal reservoirs (rat's urine)
❚ Headache, fever, myalgia
❚ Conjunctival suffusion
❚ Hepatosplenomegaly and lymphadenopathy
❚ May progress to
  — Jaundice
  — Haemolytic anaemia
  — Renal failure

Investigations   ❚ IgM antibodies
❚ *Leptospira* cultured in blood

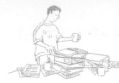

Management | Penicillins
| Erythromycin

Lyme disease | *Borrelia burgdorferi*
| Carried by ixodid ticks (from deer and sheep)
| Erythema chronicum migrans
| Headache, fever and malaise
| Meningoencephalitis
| Cranial nerve palsies
| Cardiac arrhythmias, myocarditis
| Arthritis

Investigations | IgM antibodies against organism

Management | Amoxicillin/penicillin

Viral infections

| Viral hepatitis is discussed in Chapter 10

DNA VIRUSES

Adenoviruses | Croup
| Gastroenteritis
| Mesenteric adenitis in children

α-herpesvirus
Herpes simplex-1 | Stomatitis (primary infection)
(HSV-1) | Cold sores
| Erythema multiforme

Herpes simplex-2 | Genital herpes
(HSV-2)

Varicella zoster | Chickenpox (primary infection)
virus (VZV) | Shingles (see Ch. 12)

β-herpesvirus
Cytomegalovirus | Retinitis ⎫
(CMV) | Pneumonitis ⎬ in
| Gastrointestinal ulcers ⎭ immunocompromised

Human herpes viruses 6 and 7 **I** Roseola infantum (children)

γ-herpesvirus
Epstein–Barr virus (EBV)
I Infectious mononucleosis
I Burkitt's lymphoma
I Nasopharyngeal carcinoma
I Gastric carcinoma

Human herpes virus 8 **I** Kaposi's sarcoma

Parvovirus B19
I Erythema infectiosum in children (fifth disease/slapped cheek syndrome)
I Aplastic crisis in sickle cell disease
I Anaemia, leucopenia and thrombocytopenia

Poxvirus
I Smallpox
I Molluscum contagiosum

RNA VIRUSES

PicoRNAviruses
Poliovirus
I Poliomyelitis
I 95% asymptomatic
I 0.1% suffer paralytic poliomyelitis
I Asymmetric paralysis
I No sensory involvement

Coxsackievirus
I Hand, foot and mouth disease (vesicular rash)
I Meningitis and encephalitis
I Myocarditis and pericarditis

Togaviruses
Rubella (German measles)
I Conjunctivitis
I Lymphadenopathy
I Macular pink/red rash
I Fetal infection → cardiac defect, cataracts, mental retardation and deafness

Yellow fever
I Mosquito spread
I Africa and Asia
I High fever

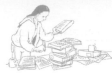
❚ Bradycardia
❚ Jaundice
❚ Clotting abnormalities → bleeding

Orthomyxovirus

Influenza
❚ Type A → epidemics and pandemics
❚ Type B → localized outbreaks
❚ Type C → rarely produces disease

Paramyxovirus

Measles (rubella)
❚ Incubation 8–14 days
❚ Malaise, fever, cough
❚ Koplik's spots in the mouth
❚ Erythematous rash
❚ Complications
— Pneumonia
— Myocarditis
— Encephalomyelitis
— Subacute sclerosing panencephalitis

Mumps
❚ Incubation 18 days
❚ Fever, headache, anorexia
❚ Parotid gland swelling ± submandibular involvement
❚ Epididymo-orchitis after puberty

Rhabdovirus

Rabies
❚ Contracted in animal bites
❚ Anxiety, agitation, hydrophobia and aerophobia
❚ Hyperreflexia and muscle spasm
❚ Death at 10–14 days
❚ No effective treatment

Human immunodeficiency virus (HIV) and acquired immune deficiency syndrome (AIDS) (*K&C*, p. 131)

Epidemiology
❚ Young adults and children in developing world – heterosexual and vertical spread, breast-feeding
❚ Sexual intercourse (vaginal and anal)
❚ Blood spread (shared needles, transfusions)

HIV	❚ Two subtypes (1 & 2) ❚ Retrovirus (reverse transcriptase allows DNA synthesis from RNA) ❚ Binds to CD4 lymphocyte surface marker ❚ Enters lymphocyte → viral synthesis
Clinical features	❚ Seroconversion illness 2 weeks after infection ❚ Fever, lymphadenopathy, headache
Investigations	❚ IgG against gp120 ❚ IgG against p24 ⎫ ❚ Viral p24 antigen ⎬ after appropriate ❚ Viral culture ⎭ counselling ❚ Viral load (RNA copies per ml)
Clinical latency	❚ Median time of 10 years until clinical presentation of AIDS
AIDS (K&C, p. 135)	❚ Infections due to low CD4 lymphocyte count ❚ Diagnosis based on low CD4 count and the presence of an AIDS-defining illness
Neurological disease	❚ HIV-related dementia ❚ Distal sensory polyneuropathy ❚ Autonomic neuropathy ❚ Progressive multifocal leucoencephalopathy ❚ Cryptococcal meningitis ❚ Cerebral lymphoma ❚ Cerebral toxoplasma
Eye disease	❚ CMV retinitis
Mucocutaneous disease	❚ Kaposi's sarcoma ❚ Molluscum contagiosum ❚ Shingles ❚ Oral hairy leucoplakia (tongue) ❚ Oral/oesophageal candidiasis ❚ Squamous cell carcinomas
Haematological disease	❚ Low CD4 (< 200) ❚ Anaemia ❚ Neutropenia ❚ Isolated thrombocytopenia

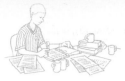

Gastrointestinal disease	**I** Weight loss
	I *Cryptosporidium*
	I *Microsporidium*
	I HIV enteropathy
	I CMV colitis
	I Bacterial infection
	I *Mycobacterium*
	I Sclerosing cholangitis
	I Oesophageal candidiasis

Gastrointestinal
disease

I Weight loss
I *Cryptosporidium* ⎫
I *Microsporidium* ⎪
I HIV enteropathy ⎬ HIV-related
I CMV colitis ⎪ diarrhoea
I Bacterial infection ⎪
I *Mycobacterium* ⎭
I Sclerosing cholangitis
I Oesophageal candidiasis

Renal disease

I HIV nephropathy
I Focal glomerulonephritis

Respiratory disease

I Pneumonia
I *Pneumocystis carinii* pneumonia (PCP)

Disease monitoring

I CD4 lymphocyte count
I HIV viral load (HIV RNA)

Management
(Table 7.4)

Antiretroviral drugs
I Nucleoside analogues, e.g. zidovudine
I Protease inhibitors, e.g. ritonavir
I Non-nucleoside reverse transcriptase inhibitors,
e.g. nevirapine
I HAART: highly active antiretroviral therapy –
combination therapy that significantly reduces viral
load and improves survival

Early management of opportunistic infections
I Screening for infection, e.g. ophthalmoscopy for
CMV retinitis

Table 7.4   Post-exposure prophylaxis

Post-needlestick injury
Blood from patient and injured person

Then 4–6 weeks of
Zidovudine
Lamivudine
± Indinavir

Monitoring
▌ Immune status (CD4 count)
▌ Viral replication (HIV DNA measurement)

Prevention of infection
▌ Safe sex practices
▌ Needle exchanges
▌ Screening of blood transfusions

Fungal disease (K&C, p. 94)

Candidiasis
▌ *Candida albicans*
▌ Vaginal and oral thrush
▌ Oesophagitis
▌ Increased in the immunocompromised, by antibiotics and steroids and in the elderly

Diagnosis
▌ Microscopy
▌ Clinical appearance

Management
▌ Nystatin for oral lesions
▌ Ketoconazole

Histoplasmosis
▌ *Histoplasma capsulatum*
▌ Pulmonary focus
▌ Erythema nodosum and multiforme
▌ TB-like disease

Aspergillosis
Bronchopulmonary allergic aspergillosis
▌ Mimics asthma
▌ Bronchiectasis and eosinophilia

Aspergilloma
▌ Fungus ball in cavity in lung
▌ Often in old TB focus

Invasive aspergillosis
▌ Immunocompromised patients
▌ Pneumonia
▌ Meningitis and intracerebral abscess

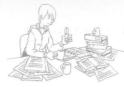

Protozoal disease (K&C, p. 98)

Leishmaniasis

Visceral leishmaniasis (kala-azar)
- Fever, cough, diarrhoea
- Pigmented rough skin
- Splenomegaly (often massive)
- Hypersplenism → pancytopenia
- Hepatomegaly

Cutaneous leishmaniasis
- Transmitted by sandfly
- Multiple painless nodules → ulceration

Trypanosomiasis

Sleeping sickness (African disease)
- Tsetse fly transmission
- Meningoencephalitis
- Apathy and somnolence

Chagas disease (American disease)
- Lymphadenopathy
- Hepatosplenomegaly
- Conjunctivitis
- GI motility disturbance
- Neurological complications

Toxoplasmosis
- *Toxoplasma gondii*
- Transmission by cats
- Lymphadenopathy
- Neck stiffness and headache
- Acute febrile illness

Malaria

Epidemiology
- 250 million people worldwide
- Hot humid countries

Aetiology
- *Plasmodium – vivax, ovale, falciparum, malariae*
- Transmitted by ♀ *Anopheles* mosquito

Clinical features
- High fever
- Splenomegaly
- *Vivax, ovale* and *malariae* → milder chronic disease
- *Falciparum* → more serious acute disease:
- Blackwater fever: haemolysis → black urine
- Cerebral malaria: convulsions, coma

Table 7.5 Prevention of malaria

Avoid insect bites
Repellents
Mosquito nets

Chemoprophylaxis
Seek advice prior to travel due to changes in resistance patterns

Proguanil daily + chloroquine weekly
or
Mefloquine weekly
or
Maloprim daily + chloroquine weekly

▌ Severe malaria: 1% erythrocytes infected (*falciparum* malaria)
▌ → Cerebral, renal and GI involvement
  — Risk of splenic rupture
  — Renal failure
  — Haemolysis and thrombocytopenia
  — Hypoglycaemia and acidosis

Investigations ▌ Thick and thin blood film shows parasites and allows identification
▌ Blood count, liver function tests, urea and electrolytes for complications

Management ▌ Falciparum: quinine sulphate orally (consider i.v. quinine if severe malaria) plus single dose of pyrimethamine and sulfadoxine (Fansidar®)
▌ Other species: chloroquine

Prevention ▌ See Table 7.5

Nematode, trematode and cestode infections (K&C, p. 109)

NEMATODES

Filariasis ▌ Lymphangitis and elephantiasis

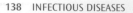

| Toxocara | I Transmitted by dogs and cats |
| | I Abdominal pain and hepatomegaly |

| Intestinal infections | I See Chapter 10 |

TREMATODES

Schistosomiasis (bilharzia)

Schistosoma japonicum/mansoni	I Intestinal ulceration and fibrosis
	I Granulomatous hepatitis
	I Hepatosplenomegaly
	I Portal hypertension

| *S. haematobium* | I Dysuria and haematuria |
| | I Bladder carcinoma |

CESTODES

I Tapeworms

Sexually transmitted disease (K&C, p. 120)

Gonorrhoea	I *Neisseria gonorrhoeae*
	I ♂ Urethritis and urethral discharge
	I ♀ 40% asymptomatic
	I Dysuria and vaginal discharge
	I Conjunctival infection in the newborn
	I Arthritis and rash in systemic disease

| *Investigations* | I Microscopy and culture of urethral or vaginal swabs |

| *Management* | I Amoxicillin and probenecid |
| | I Ciprofloxacin |

Chlamydia	I *Chlamydia trachomatis*
	I ♂ Urethritis with discharge
	I ♀ Acute salpingitis → subfertility
	I Ophthalmic trachoma → blindness
	I Reiter's syndrome – oral ulcers, arthritis, conjunctivitis, urethritis (see page 290)

Investigations	▌ Serology (IgM) or antigen detection
Management	▌ Tetracycline or erythromycin
Syphilis	▌ See page 128
HIV	▌ See page 132
Human papilloma virus (HPV)	▌ Sexual transmission ▌ Results in cervical dysplasia ▌ Cervical carcinoma

Notifiable diseases

▌ See Table 7.6

Table 7.6   Diseases notifiable under the Public Health (Infectious Diseases) Regulations 1988

Acute encephalitis	Ophthalmia neonatorum
Acute poliomyelitis	Paratyphoid fever
Anthrax	Plague
Cholera	Rabies
Diphtheria	Relapsing fever
Dysentery	Rubella
Food poisoning	Scarlet fever
Leptospirosis	Smallpox
Malaria	Tetanus
Measles	Tuberculosis
Meningitis	Typhoid fever
Meningococcal	Typhus fever
Pneumococcal	Viral haemorrhagic fever
Haemophilus influenzae	Viral hepatitis A, B, C
Viral	Whooping cough
Unspecified	Yellow fever
Mumps	

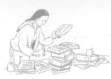

Self-assessment questions

Multiple choice questions

1. The following diseases are paired with their correct mode of transmission:
   A. Leishmaniasis – sandfly bites
   B. Hepatitis A – intravenous drug use
   C. Giardiasis – faecal–oral spread
   D. *Taenia solium* – infected meat products
   E. *Neisseria gonorrhoeae* – sexual intercourse

2. The following antibiotics act by disrupting bacterial cell wall synthesis:
   A. Amoxicillin
   B. Metronidazole
   C. Cefuroxime
   D. Ciprofloxacin
   F. Gentamicin

3. The following are live attenuated vaccines:
   A. Oral polio vaccine
   B. Tetanus
   C. Bacille Calmette–Guérin (BCG)
   D. *Haemophilus influenzae b*
   E. Hepatitis B vaccine

4. The following are recognized side-effects of the named antibiotic:
   A. Ampicillin – Rash in infectious mononucleosis
   B. Gentamicin – renal toxicity
   C. Flucloxacillin – ototoxicity
   D. Sulphonamides – erythema multiforme
   E. Fusidic acid – seronegative arthropathy

5. The following may result in atypical lymphocytes on a blood film:
   A. Epstein–Barr virus
   B. Cytomegalovirus
   C. Influenza A
   D. Toxoplasmosis
   E. Salmonellosis

6. The following are Gram-positive organisms:
   A. *Staphylococcus aureus*
   B. *Escherichia coli*
   C. *Helicobacter pylori*
   D. *Salmonella typhi*
   E. *Giardia lamblia*

7. The following are manifestations of staphylococcal disease:
   A. Osteomyelitis
   B. Scarlet fever
   C. Impetigo
   D. Infective endocarditis
   E. Cerebral abscesses

8. The following are true of *Mycobacterium tuberculosis*:
   A. It may cause a terminal ileitis
   B. Tuberculous meningitis results in a low protein and glucose in CSF
   C. Pyrazinamide is useful in eradicating organisms in macrophages
   D. Infection may cause lupus vulgaris
   E. Miliary infection results from haematogenous spread

9. The following organisms release a neurotoxin:
   A. *Clostridium botulinum*
   B. *Clostridium difficile*
   C. *Clostridium tetani*
   D. *Corynebacterium diphtheriae*
   E. *Yersinia*

10. The following belong to the herpesvirus family:
    A. Cytomegalovirus
    B. Epstein–Barr virus
    C. Coxsackievirus
    D. Varicella zoster virus
    E. Rhabdovirus

11. The following are causes of an acute hepatitic illness:
    A. Epstein–Barr virus
    B. Parvovirus B19
    C. Togaviruses
    D. Dane particle
    E. Rhabdovirus

12. The following are of use in chronic viral hepatitis:
    A. Lamivudine
    B. Azathioprine
    C. Ribavirin
    D. Interferon-α
    E. Zidovudine

13. In the following diseases animal vectors constitute an important mode of transmission:
    A. Yellow fever (togavirus)
    B. Fifth disease (parvovirus B19)
    C. Rabies (rhabdovirus)
    D. Hand, foot and mouth disease (paramyxovirus)
    E. Molluscum contagiosum (pox virus)

14. The following are recognized complications of the named infection:
    A. Measles virus – subacute sclerosing panencephalitis
    B. Rabies – aerophobia
    C. Varicella – pneumonia
    D. Cytomegalovirus – retinitis
    E. Parvovirus B19 – aplastic anaemia

15. Concerning HIV infection:
    A. *Pneumocystis carinii* pneumonia is an AIDS-defining illness
    B. The CD4-positive lymphocyte count is a poor marker of immune status
    C. The median duration of infection prior to the development of AIDS is 2 years
    D. HIV dementia is due to a parvovirus infection
    E. Kaposi's sarcoma is an indication of adenovirus infection

16. The following are causes of abnormal liver function tests in HIV infection:
    A. Zidovudine
    B. Lamivudine
    C. Sclerosing cholangitis
    D. Cytomegalovirus infection
    E. *Mycobacterium avium intracellulare*

17. The following drugs are paired with the appropriate mechanism of action:
    A. Ritonavir – protease inhibitor
    B. Zidovudine – nucleoside analogue

C. Nevirapine – viral RNA inhibitor

D. Lamivudine – inhibition of cell wall synthesis

E. Saquinavir – protease inhibitor

18. The following increase the risk of systemic candidiasis:
    A. Diabetes mellitus
    B. Oral prednisolone
    C. Chronic renal failure
    D. Acute viral hepatitis
    E. Intravenous cephalosporin therapy

19. The following are not features of falciparum malaria:
    A. Thrombocytopenia
    B. Intravascular haemolysis
    C. Bronchospasm
    D. Hyposplenism
    E. Hypoglycaemia

20. The following are indicators of severe malaria:
    A. Fever > 38°C
    B. Parasitaemia > 2%
    C. Dark urine
    D. Glucose-6-phosphate deficiency
    E. Convulsions

21. The following may cause conjunctivitis in the newborn babies of infected mothers:
    A. Syphilis
    B. Chlamydia
    C. Gonorrhoea
    D. HIV
    E. Rubella

22. The following are true of syphilis infection:
    A. Acute infection usually presents as a painless ulcer
    B. A rash involving the palms of the hands suggests a secondary streptococcal infection
    C. Neurological signs may be due to intracerebral abscesses
    D. Syphilis meningitis may complicate tertiary syphilis
    E. Congenital infection results in an internuclear ophthalmoplegia

23. The following are true of sexually transmitted disease:
    A. The incidence of non-specific urethritis is falling
    B. Gonorrhoea infection is asymptomatic in 90% of infections in males
    C. Chlamydia is an important cause of male infertility
    D. Gonorrhoea may result in a pustular rash
    E. Reactive arthritis is not associated with chlamydia infection

25. The following may result in oral ulceration:
    A. Syphilis
    B. Ulcerative colitis
    C. Behçet's syndrome
    D. Mumps infection
    E. Toxoplasma gondii

Extended matching questions

Question 1 *Theme: fever of unknown origin*

A. Acute bronchopulmonary aspergillosis
B. *Pneumocystis carinii*
C. Staphylococcal pulmonary abscess
D. Aspergilloma
E. *Mycobacterium tuberculosis*
F. Falciparum malaria
G. Leishmaniasis
H. Liver abscess
I. Acute hepatitis A
J. *Streptococcus pneumoniae* pneumonia
K. *Mycoplasma* pneumonia
L. Schistosomiasis

For each of the following questions, select the best answer from the list above:

I. A 42-year-old Ugandan woman with known HIV infection and a CD4 lymphocyte count of 86 is admitted with a cough, haemoptysis, weight loss and cervical lymphadenopathy. A chest X-ray reveals diffuse apical shadowing of the left lung.
What is the most likely diagnosis?

II. An 18-year-old man is admitted with a cough with rust-coloured sputum, anorexia, a temperature of 38.6°C and marked shortness of breath. On examination he is noted to have perioral herpes and coarse crackles at the right upper zone with some bronchial breathing.
What is the most likely diagnosis?

III. A 28-year-old woman is admitted with a fever and jaundice. She has recently returned from India after visiting her family. She has a moderately enlarged liver and spleen. On full blood count she is noted to have a platelet count of 76.
What is the most likely diagnosis?

Question 2 *Theme: Investigation of pyrexia*

A. Full blood count
B. Thick and thin blood film
C. Urea and electrolytes
D. Liver function tests
E. Serum calcium
F. Blood glucose
G. Blood cultures
H. Urine microscopy and culture
I. Sputum culture
J. Chest X-ray
K. Abdominal X-ray
L. Ultrasound of the liver
M. CT scan of the head
N. CT scan of the liver and pancreas
O. Endoscopic retrograde cholangiopancreatogram

For each of the following questions, select the best answer from the list above:

I. A 57-year-old woman is admitted with right upper quadrant pain, jaundice and a fever. On examination, she is tender in the right hypochondrium.
What single investigation would be most useful in reaching a diagnosis?

II. A 28-year-old man returns from a trip to Kenya. He has a fever and is jaundiced. He has moderate splenomegaly.
What single investigation would you choose to make the diagnosis?

III. A 76-year-old man develops a fever and cough with white frothy sputum a week after a mitral valve replacement. On examination he has fine crackles in both lung bases and a pansystolic murmur.
Which investigation will be of most use in guiding treatment?

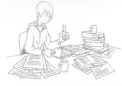

Short answer questions

1. Write short notes on the antimicrobial treatment of the following:
   A. Chronic hepatitis C
   B. Osteomyelitis
   C. Infective endocarditis

2. Outline the mechanisms of pathology caused by:
   A. *Mycobacterium leprae*
   B. *Clostridium tetani*
   C. *Salmonella typhi*

3. Write short notes on the following:
   A. Management of acute malaria
   B. Insect vectors in human disease
   C. Non-pharmacological prevention of malaria

4. Outline the importance of the following in the management of HIV and AIDS:
   A. Combination antiretroviral treatment
   B. CD4 lymphocyte count and HIV DNA measurement
   C. Screening for opportunistic infections

Essay questions

1. With reference to specific organisms, discuss the causes, investigations and immediate therapies used in the management of acute meningitis.

2. Outline the causes, investigations and management of pneumonia, including the clinical features in the history and examination.

3. Outline the possible causes, appropriate investigations and management of a 21-year-old man presenting with urethral discharge and discomfort.

4. A 34-year-old man with known HIV is admitted with drowsiness and convulsions. Outline the management of such a patient, mentioning specific diseases and their treatment in your answer.

5. Outline the classification of immunizations, giving examples of each type and their role in the management of disease.

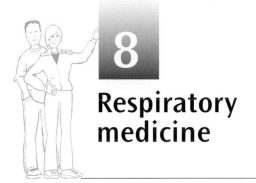

8

Respiratory medicine

If you need more detailed explanation refer to Kumar & Clark, Clinical Medicine, Chapter 14.

EXAMINING THE RESPIRATORY SYSTEM (K&C, p. 844)

Examination should contain all of the following and be done in roughly this order:

Look for
- Clues around the bed
  - Oxygen
  - Inhalers
  - Nebulizers
  - Peak flow meter

Expose the chest
- Maintain the dignity of the patient
- Act professionally (e.g. avoid showing embarrassment about exposing the breasts in female patients)
- Look for:
  - Cyanosis
  - Breathlessness/use of accessory muscles
  - Weight loss
  - Chest wall scars or deformity
  - Prominent veins on the chest wall (suggesting superior vena cava (SVC) obstruction)

Hands
- Flapping tremor of CO_2 retention – hold arms outstretched with wrists fully extended and fingers splayed and watch for movements of fingertips

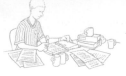

Table 8.1 Some common causes of finger clubbing

Respiratory	Cardiovascular
Lung cancer	Cyanotic heart disease
Fibrosis, e.g. cryptogenic	Infective endocarditis
fibrosing alveolitis (CFA)	**Gastrointestinal**
Chronic lung sepsis	Cirrhosis
Bronchiectasis	Inflammatory bowel disease
Lung abscess	(IBD)
Empyema	**Others**
Mesothelioma	Congenital

▌ Clubbing (Table 8.1)
▌ Peripheral cyanosis
▌ Nicotine staining

Face   ▌ Anaemia
▌ Central cyanosis

Neck   ▌ Examine JVP (remember a fixed distended JVP suggests SVC obstruction)
▌ Check for lymphadenopathy

Thorax (Table 8.2)   ▌ Locate tracheal position and apex beat
▌ Check for lymphadenopathy (axilla)

Assess chest expansion

Anterior   ▌ Place hands on upper aspect of chest either side of sternum
▌ Ask patient to breathe in and out and watch your thumbs move laterally
▌ Do they move symmetrically?
▌ Repeat with your hands over lateral lower aspect of chest

Posterior   ▌ Place hands over lateral lower aspect of chest and repeat the above

Percussion   ▌ Hand firmly on chest wall
▌ Compare left with right anteriorly and posteriorly
▌ Don't forget apices and under arms
▌ Tap distal i.p. joint with middle finger

Table 8.2 Physical signs of respiratory disease

Pathology	Chest wall movement	Tracheal deviation	Percussion note	Breath sounds	Vocal resonance	Added sounds
Consolidation (pneumonia)	Reduced on affected side	None	Dull	Bronchial	Increased	Crackles
Collapse (main or bronchus)	Reduced on affected side	Towards lesion	Dull	Diminished/absent	Reduced/absent	None
Fibrosis (generalized)	Reduced	None	Normal	Vesicular	Increased	Crackles
Pleural effusion (> 500 mL)	Reduced	Away if massive	Stony dull	Diminished/absent	Reduced/absent	None
Pneumothorax (large)	Reduced	Away from lesion	Normal or hyper-resonant	Diminished/absent	Reduced/absent	None
Chronic obstructive pulmonary disease (COPD)	Reduced	None	Normal	Prolonged expiration	Normal	Expiratory wheeze
Asthma	Reduced	None	Normal	Prolonged expiration	Normal	Expiratory wheeze Crackles

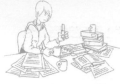

Table 8.3 Abnormal breath sounds

Pathogenic process	Description of breath sounds	Auscultatory features
Airways obstruction	Wheezes	High-pitched end-expiratory 'squeaking' noises Monophonic = single airway obstruction Polyphonic = many small airways obstruction
Consolidation	Bronchial breathing	Breath sounds with prolonged expiratory phase (similar to breath sounds heard over trachea)
Fibrosis	Fine crackles	Short-lived end-inspiratory high-pitched added sounds 'like bubbles popping'
Fluid in alveoli (pulmonary oedema)	Fine crackles	Short-lived end-inspiratory high-pitched added sounds 'like bubbles popping'
Pleural inflammation	Pleural rub	Localized creaking/groaning added sounds

Listen to breath sounds
I Use diaphragm of stethoscope and again compare left with right
I Listen for added sounds (wheeze, crackles) (Table 8.3)

Check for vocal resonance and fremitus
I Ask patient to say 99 and listen with stethoscope (resonance) or palpate (vocal fremitus)

Measure peak flow
I Normal values
— 40-year-old 175 cm tall ♂ = 620 L/min
— 40-year-old 155 cm tall ♀ = 460 L/min

> **PEAK FLOW**
> The patient's lips should be tight around the mouthpiece
> Ask the patient to take a deep breath and then blow out as hard and as fast as possible
> Remember to assess the best of three measurements

Investigations in lung disease

Radiology
I Chest X-ray (see Chapter 5)
I CT scan of the chest
— Mass lesions
— Interstitial lung disease
— Bronchiectasis

I Ventilation perfusion (V/Q) scan
— Diagnosis of pulmonary embolus

Endoscopy I Bronchoscopy
— Allows direct visualization of bronchi
— Biopsies and cytology

Measuring respiratory function (K&C, p. 849)

Peak flow rate I See above
I ↓ in airflow limitation

Blood gas analysis (Table 8.4) (K&C, p. 945)
I Arterial blood sample (usually radial artery) measures partial pressure of O_2 and CO_2
I Essential to manage acute severe asthma and respiratory failure

Pulse oximetry I Measures the difference in absorption of light by oxyhaemoglobin and deoxyhaemoglobin
I Used to assess and monitor arterial oxygen saturation

Spirometry (K&C, p. 849)
I Measures maximum inspiration then forced expiration using a vitalograph
I Forced expiratory volume in 1 second (FEV_1) = volume of air expired in first second
I Forced vital capacity (FVC) = maximum volume of air expired
I FEV_1: FVC ratio ↓ in airflow limitation, e.g. asthma
I FEV_1 and FVC ↓ in restrictive diseases, e.g. fibrosis

Table 8.4   Abnormalities of blood gases in respiratory failure

	Pao_2	$Paco_2$	pH	HCO_3
Type I e.g. Severe asthma, pneumonia, acute respiratory distress syndrome (ARDS)	↓	↓ or →	↑ or →	→ or ↓
Type II e.g. COPD, CNS depression (opiates), respiratory muscle weakness	↓	↑	↓	↑

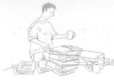

Transfer factor
- Measures diffusing capacity of the lungs
- Decreased in alveolar disease
  — Fibrosing alveolitis
  — Sarcoidosis
  — Asbestosis
- Decreased in alveolar loss
  — Emphysema
- Increased in pulmonary haemorrhage

Sampling lung tissue

Pleural biospy
- Pleural lesions
  — Malignancy
  — Tuberculosis

Pleural aspirate
- Removing pleural effusion fluid
- Microscopy and culture in infection
- Protein content (transudate vs exudates)
- Cytology (malignancy)

Pulmonary infection (K&C, p. 885)

Pneumonia
- Inflammation of the substance of the lung

Aetiology
(Table 8.5)
- Bacterial
- Viral
- Opportunistic organisms
- Chemical

Clinical features
- Cough
- +/– Purulent sputum
- Fever
- Pleuritic chest pain
- Breathlessness

Specific features

Mycoplasma
- Cold agglutinins occur in 50%
- Abnormal liver function
- Diarrhoea

Staphylococcus aureus
- Abscesses – in lung and elsewhere

Table 8.5 Aetiology of pneumonia in the UK

Infecting agent	%	Clinical circumstance
Streptococcus pneumoniae	50	Community pneumonia patients usually previously fit
Mycoplasma pneumoniae	6	As above
Influenza A	5	As above
Haemophilus influenzae	5	Pre-existing lung disease, e.g. COPD
Chlamydia pneumoniae	5	Community-acquired in institutions/families
Chlamydia psittaci	3	Contact with birds (not inevitable)
Staphylococcus aureus	2	Children/i.v. drug users/flu outbreaks
Legionella pneumophila	2	Institutional outbreaks (hospitals/hotels)
Coxiella burnetii	1	Abattoir and hide workers
Pseudomonas aeruginosa	< 1	Cystic fibrosis
Pneumocystis carinii *Actinomyces israelii* *Nocardia asteroides* *Cytomegalovirus* *Aspergillus fumigatus*	< 1	AIDS/lymphomas/leukaemias/use of immunosuppressant drugs
Anaerobic organisms	< 1	Inhalation pneumonia/alcohol excess/postoperative
None isolated	20	

Coxiella burnetii
▌ Multiple lesions on chest X-ray

Strep. pneumoniae
▌ Rust-coloured sputum
▌ Peri-oral HSV

Investigations ▌ Chest X-ray
▌ Arterial blood gases or oxygen saturation
▌ Blood/sputum culture
▌ Serology for atypical organisms

Management ▌ Antibiotics
— typical: amoxycillin
— atypical: amoxycillin + erythromycin
▌ Oxygen
▌ Correct/prevent dehydration

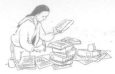

Complications
- Respiratory failure
  — Type 1 – low Pao_2, low/normal $Paco_2$
- Lung abscess
  — Particularly aspiration pneumonia, staphylococcal or *Klebsiella* infection, bronchial obstruction (cancer or foreign body)
- Empyema
  — Pus in the pleural space

Tuberculosis
(*K&C*, p. 892)
- Caseating granulomatous infection due to *Mycobacterium* tuberculosis in the lung
- TB is a notifiable disease and contact tracing is important

Patients at risk
- Those from developing countries (including contacts)
- Immunosuppressed patients
- HIV, steroids, malignancy
- Alcoholics/homeless

Clinical features
- See Fig. 8.1
- May be none
- Malaise and lethargy
- Anorexia/weight loss
- Fever
- Cough
- Haemoptysis
- Signs of
  — Pleural effusion
  — Pneumonia
  — Fibrosis

Investigations
- Chest X-ray
  — Affects upper zones particularly
  — +/– Calcification
  — +/– Cavitation
- Sputum microscopy (Ziehl–Nielsen stain)
- Bronchoscopy and washings

Management
- 6 months of combination of antibiotics, usually
  — Isoniazid
  — + Rifampicin
  — + Pyrazinamide for first 2 months
- Compliance is vital

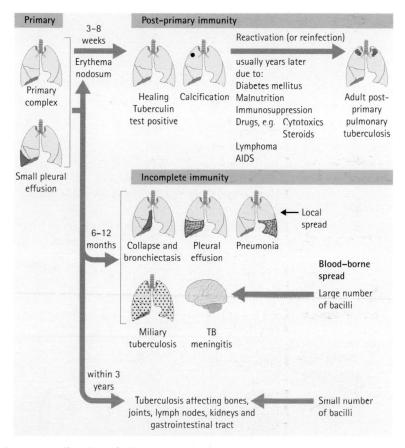

Fig. 8.1   Manifestations of primary and post-primary tuberculosis.

▌ Multi-resistant TB does occur, particularly in HIV, and may require more antibiotics (according to sensitivities) over a longer period

Side-effects of anti-TB drugs

Rifampicin
▌ Liver dysfunction
▌ Discoloration of body fluids
▌ Reduced effectiveness of oral contraceptives and other drugs

Isoniazid
▌ High doses cause polyneuropathy
▌ Pyridoxine is added to prevent this

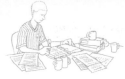

Pyrazinamide
▌ Liver dysfunction

Ethambutol
▌ Retrobulbar neuritis (patients need ophthalmology monitoring)

Streptomycin
▌ Vestibular nerve damage

Other mycobacteria   *M. kansasii*
▌ Usually less severe disease than *M. tuberculosis*
▌ Particularly middle-aged men
▌ COPD and working in dusty conditions (e.g. miners)

M. avium intracellulare (MAI)
▌ Immunosuppressed patients, e.g. HIV

Pulmonary malignancy (K&C, p. 911)

Bronchial carcinoma   ▌ Malignant tumour of bronchial tree

Epidemiology   ▌ Most common malignancy (32 000 deaths/year in UK)
▌ Third most common cause of death in UK

Cell types   ▌ Small cell (20–30%)
▌ Non-small cell
— Squamous (40%)
— Large cell (25%)
— Adenocarcinoma (10%)
— Alveolar cell (1–2%)

Aetiology   ▌ Smoking (including passive)
— Squamous
▌ Urban > rural
▌ Occupational
— adenocarcinoma
— asbestos, coal, chromium

Table 8.6   *Frequency of common presenting symptoms of bronchial carcinoma*

Symptom	Frequency (%)
Cough	41
Chest pain	22
Cough and pain	15
Haemoptysis	7
Chest infection	< 5
Others (malaise, breathlessness etc)	< 5

Clinical features

- See Table 8.6
- Often no clinical signs
- Clubbing
- Supraclavicular nodes (small cell)
- Signs of:
  — Pleural effusion or collapse
  — Unresolved chest infection
  — Chronic lung disease (e.g. asbestosis)

Spread of bronchial carcinoma

Direct
- Pleura and ribs
- Erosion of ribs and involvement of lower brachial plexus nerves in apical tumours (Pancoast's tumour)
- Sympathetic ganglion (Horner's syndrome – small pupil and ptosis)
- Recurrent laryngeal nerve palsy with unilateral vocal cord paralysis (hoarseness, bovine cough)
- Spinal cord compression
- Oesophagus (dysphagia)
- SVC obstruction (headache, facial congestion, fixed distended veins)

Metastatic
- Bones
- Liver
- Brain
- Adrenal glands

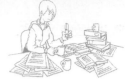

Non-metastatic extrapulmonary manifestations
▌ Ectopic hormone production, adrenocorticotrophic hormone (ACTH) e.g. (small cell)
▌ Neurological, e.g. myasthenic syndrome
▌ Hypertrophic pulmonary osteoarthropathy (HPOA)
▌ Vascular/thrombotic/haematological
▌ Cutaneous, e.g. dermatomyositis

Investigations
▌ Chest X-ray
▌ Blood tests
— hyponatraemia
— polycythaemia
— anaemia
▌ CT scan/MRI for staging
▌ Bronchoscopy

Management

Surgery
▌ Only 20% of cases suitable
▌ For non-small cell

Radiotherapy
▌ Particularly for squamous cell
▌ Can be useful for symptom control
▌ Used for SVC obstruction

Chemotherapy
▌ Combination chemotherapy
— Particularly useful for small cell
— Also used for non-small cell

Prognosis
▌ 20% alive 1 year after diagnosis
▌ 6–8% 5-year survival

Obstructive lung disease

Asthma
(K&C, p. 874)
▌ Chronic inflammatory disease of the airways
▌ Three components
— Reversible airflow limitation
— Airway hyper-responsiveness to stimuli
— Inflammation of the bronchi

Epidemiology	I Prevalence increasing

Aetiology and precipitating factors	I Atopy and allergy
	I Increased airway responsiveness
	I Pollution
	I Occupational, e.g. isocyanates
	I Drugs, e.g. NSAIDs

Clinical features	I Cough
	I Wheeze
	I Breathlessness
	I Chest tightness

Investigations	I Chest X-ray
	I Lung function tests
	I Peak flow charts
	I Skin testing of allergies

Management	I Self-management plan
	I Avoid precipitants
	I β_2-agonists
	I Anticholinergics
	I Corticosteroids
	I Leukotriene antagonists (selected cases)

Chronic obstructive pulmonary disease (COPD) (K&C, p. 863)

I Chronic bronchitis
— Mucoid sputum
— > 3months/year
I Emphysema
— Dilatation and destruction of alveoli
I Airways obstruction which occurs mostly in smokers/ex-smokers
I May have some reversible airway obstruction

Aetiology	I Smoking (> 40 pack years)
	I Rarely, α_1-antitrypsin deficiency

Clinical features	I Cough and sputum
	I Wheeze
	I Breathlessness

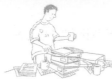

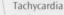

ACUTE SEVERE ASTHMA

Suggested by
Tachycardia
Tachypnoea
Inability to speak in full sentences

Emergency treatment
High-flow oxygen and monitor oximetry
Nebulized salbutamol 5 mg +/- ipratropium bromide 500 μg
i.v. steroids

Initial investigations
Measure arterial blood gases
Chest X-ray to exclude pneumothorax

Second-line therapy
i.v. aminophylline/salbutamol if not responding to repeated
   nebulizers
Ventilation if approaching respiratory failure

▌ Exacerbating factors
  — Upper respiratory tract infection
  — Cold/foggy weather
  — Pollution
▌ Tachypnoea with prolonged expiration
▌ Use of accessory muscles
▌ Intercostal muscle recession on inspiration
▌ Pursed lips on expiration
▌ Reduced chest expansion
▌ Hyperinflation
▌ Cyanosis
▌ Signs of:
  — Right ventricular failure (oedema,
    hepatomegaly, ↑ JVP)
  — CO_2 retention (bounding pulse, peripheral
    vasodilatation, flapping tremor, confusion, coma)

Investigations ▌ Spirometry
▌ Chest X-ray
▌ Blood gases
▌ Sputum examination
▌ ECG (P pulmonale, right branch bundle block, right
  ventricular hypertrophy)

I Haemoglobin and packed cell volume
I White cell count
I α_1-antitrypsin level

Management (acute)

I *Stop smoking*
I β_2-agonists
I Steroids
I Prompt antibiotics if infection present
I Diuretics for right ventricular failure
I Assisted ventilation continuous positive airways pressure – (CPAP)

Management (chronic)

I *Stop smoking*
I Flu and pneumococcal vaccines
I β_2-agonists
I Steroids
I Prompt antibiotics
I Diuretics for right ventricular failure
I Home nebulizers
I Home oxygen if Pao_2 on air < 7.3 kPa on two occasions, 3 weeks apart

Surgery

I Lung volume reduction in carefully selected patients

Prognosis

I 50% of patients with severe breathlessness die within 5 years
I Stopping smoking improves prognosis

Obstructive sleep apnoea (K&C, p. 869)

I Occurs in patients who are overweight

Clinical features

I Snoring/nocturnal choking
I Daytime somnolence
I Poor sleep
I Morning headaches
I Reduced libido
I Ankle swelling

Investigations

I Sleep study (measure oximetry, abdominal/thoracic movement and EEG during sleep)

Management

I CPAP ventilation at night

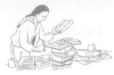

Bronchiectasis (*K&C*, p. 869)

▌ Abnormal and permanently dilated airways

Aetiology ▌ See Table 8.7

Clinical features ▌ Cough and excessive sputum
▌ Recurrent chest infections
▌ Halitosis
▌ Haemoptysis
▌ Clubbing
▌ Coarse crackles in affected areas
▌ Hyperinflation (resonant percussion note, impalpable apex)

Investigations ▌ Chest X-ray
▌ High-resolution CT of the lung
▌ Sputum examination
▌ Immunoglobulins
▌ Sweat electrolytes for cystic fibrosis

Management ▌ Postural drainage
▌ Antibiotics
▌ Bronchodilators if airflow limitation

Table 8.7 Causes of bronchiectasis

Congenital Deficiency of bronchial wall elements Pulmonary sequestration	**Immunological over-response** Allergic bronchopulmonary aspergillosis Post-lung transplant

Mechanical bronchial obstruction
Intrinsic
Foreign body
Inspissated mucus
Post-tuberculous stenosis
Tumour
	Immune deficiency
	Primary
	  Panhypogammaglobulinaemia
	  Selective immunoglobulin deficiencies
	    (IgA and IgG_2)
	Secondary
	  HIV and malignancy

Extrinsic
Lymph node
Tumour
	Mucociliary clearance defects
	Genetic
	  Primary ciliary dyskinesia (Kartagener's
	    syndrome with dextrocardia and situs
	    inversus)

Postinfective bronchial damage
Bacterial and viral pneumonia, including
  pertussis, measles and aspiration
  pneumonia
	Cystic fibrosis
	Acquired
	  Young's syndrome – azospermia
	    sinusitis

Granuloma and fibrosis Tuberculosis, sarcoidosis and fibrosing alveolitis	

    ❚ Steroids
    ❚ Heart/lung transplant

Prognosis ❚ Life expectancy ≈ 55 years

Cystic fibrosis (K&C, p. 871)

❚ Autosomal recessive disorder of the cystic fibrosis transmembrane conductance regulator (CFTR) which induces low salt and chloride excretion into airways leading to increased viscosity of airway secretions

Clinical features *Respiratory*
    ❚ Recurrent chest infections
    ❚ Clubbing
    ❚ Sinusitis
    ❚ Haemoptysis
    ❚ Nasal polyps
    ❚ Spontaneous pneumothorax
    ❚ Respiratory failure
    ❚ Right ventricular failure

Gastrointestinal
    ❚ Steatorrhoea (pancreatic insufficiency)
    ❚ Meconium ileus
    ❚ Gallstones
    ❚ Cirrhosis

Investigations ❚ Sweat electrolyte test
    ❚ DNA analysis for genotype

Management ❚ Antibiotics
    ❚ Pancreatic/nutritional supplements
    ❚ CFTR gene therapy
    ❚ Lung transplant

Prognosis ❚ Median survival 40 years

Occupational lung disease (K&C, p. 907)

Exposure to dusts, gases, vapours and fumes at work can lead to
❚ Acute bronchitis and pulmonary oedema from irritants, e.g. SO_2, chlorine

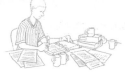

I Pulmonary fibrosis due to mineral dust, e.g. coal
I Occupational asthma
I Extrinsic allergic bronchiolar alveolitis
I Bronchial carcinoma due to industrial agents, e.g. asbestos, radon

Coal-worker's pneumoconiosis (K&C, p. 908)

I Patients may qualify for industrial injuries benefit

Aetiology I Deposition of dust particles in small airways

Clinical features I Breathlessness
I Cough +/– black sputum

Investigations I Chest X-ray – fine micronodular shadowing
I Spirometry – mixed restrictive and obstructive pattern with reduced gas transfer

Complications I Progressive massive fibrosis
— Large round masses in upper lobes
— May have necrotic centres
— May be associated with rheumatoid factor and antinuclear factor
— Respiratory failure

Silicosis (K&C, p. 908)

I Sand blasting, pottery, ceramics and foundry workers

Aetiology I Inhaled silica dust induces fibrosis

Clinical featues I Breathlessness
I Cough

Investigations I Chest X-ray
— Fibrosis
— Large round masses in upper lobes
— Eggshell calcification of hilar nodes

Complications I Respiratory failure

Asbestosis (K&C, p. 908)

I Ubiquitous use of asbestos put many at risk
I Particular problems with roofers, shipyard workers, those making gas masks in World War II

Aetiology ▌ Deposition of inhaled blue fibres in airways
▌ Synergistic effect of smoking

Clinical features ▌ Breathlessness
▌ Cough
▌ Chest pain

Investigations ▌ Chest X-ray
— Fine reticulonodular shadowing
— Honeycomb lung
— Pleural plaques/effusion
▌ Spirometry – restrictive +/– ↓ gas transfer

Diseases caused ▌ Pleural plaques
by asbestos ▌ Pleural effusion
▌ Bilateral diffuse pleural thickening*
▌ Mesothelioma*
▌ Asbestosis (restrictive fibrotic lung disease)*
▌ Carcinoma of the bronchus*

* Patients eligible for industrial injuries benefit

Pulmonary inflammation and fibrosis

Sarcoid (K&C, p. 897)

▌ A multisystem granulomatous disorder presenting usually as
— Bilateral hilar lymphadenopathy
— Pulmonary infiltration
— Skin/eye lesions

Epidemiology ▌ 19 in 100 000
▌ Female > male
▌ More severe in blacks than whites

Aetiology ▌ Unknown

Clinical features ▌ Commonly presents in third or fourth decade
(Table 8.8)

Extrapulmonary ▌ Skin
features — Erythema nodosum
— Lupus pernio

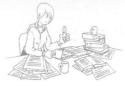

Table 8.8   Presenting symptoms of sarcoid

Presentation	%
Respiratory symptoms/abnormal chest X-ray	50
Fatigue or weight loss	5
Peripheral lymphadenopathy	5
Fever	4
Normal chest X-ray	20

❚ Eye
— Uveitis
— Conjunctivitis
— Keratoconjunctivitis sicca
❚ Face
— Parotitis
— Facial nerve palsy
❚ Metabolic
— Hypercalcaemia (10%)
❚ CNS
— Meningoencephalitis
— Spinal cord disease
— Myopathy
— Polyneuropathy
❚ Gastrointestinal
— Hepatosplenomegaly
❚ Cardiovascular
— Cardiomyopathy

Investigations ❚ Chest X-ray
❚ CT chest
❚ Blood tests
— FBC (normocytic anaemia)
— ↑ ESR
— ↑ Ca^{++}
— ↑ Serum angiotensin-converting enzyme (ACE)
❚ Transbronchial biopsy
❚ Spirometry
— Restrictive defect
— ↓ Gas transfer

Management ❚ Steroids

Pulmonary involvement in systemic diseases

Rheumatoid ▍ Rheumatoid factor always present
arthritis (Fig 8.2) ▍ Lung features may precede arthropathy

Systemic lupus ▍ Pleurisy/pleural effusion
erythematosus

Systemic sclerosis ▍ Pulmonary fibrosis/honeycomb lung

Wegener's ▍ Granulomatous vasculitis of small arteries
granulomatosis ▍ Rhinorrhoea
▍ Nasal ulceration
▍ Nodular masses (+/− cavitation)
▍ Migratory pulmonary infiltrates
▍ Associated with antineutrophil cytoplasmic
antibodies (ANCA)
▍ Treated with cyclophosphamide

Churg–Strauss ▍ Systemic vasculitis
syndrome ▍ Asthma
▍ Rhinitis

Cricoarytenoid arthritis

Rheumatoid pneumoconiosis (Caplan's syndrome)

Nodules and cavities

Small airway disease

Obliterative bronchiolitis

Diffuse fibrosing alveolitis

Small unilateral pleural effusion

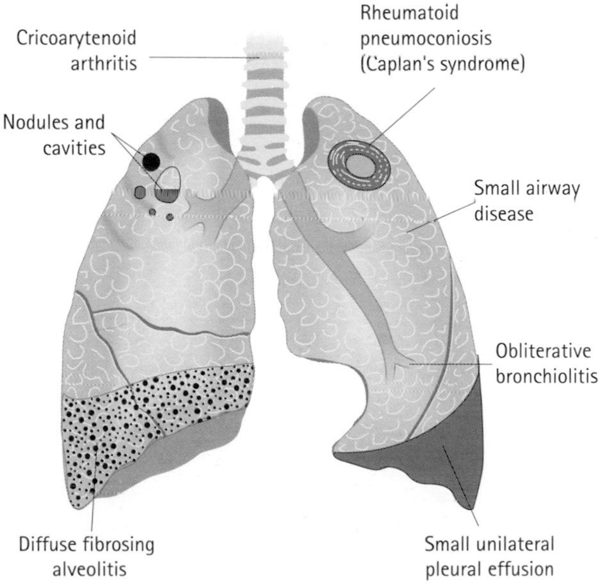

Fig. 8.2 Respiratory manifestations of rheumatoid disease.

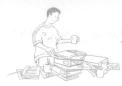

▌ Eosinophilia
▌ Associated with ANCA
▌ Treated with steroids

Goodpasture's ▌ Disease associated with anti-glomerular basement
syndrome membrane (GBM) antibodies which cross-react with
the glomerulus and the lung
▌ Cough
▌ Haemoptysis (can be massive)
▌ Intrapulmonary haemorrhage
▌ Glomerulonephritis
▌ Treated with steroids

Pulmonary fibrosis and honeycomb lung
▌ See Table 8.9

Cryptogenic fibrosing alveolitis *(K&C, p. 904)*
Clinical features ▌ Breathlessness
▌ Cyanosis
▌ Clubbing
▌ Bilateral fine inspiratory crackles
▌ Signs of:
— Respiratory failure
— Pulmonary hypertension
— Right heart failure

Disease associations ▌ Coeliac disease
▌ Ulcerative colitis
▌ Renal tubular acidosis

Investigations ▌ Chest X-ray – reticulonodular shadowing
▌ High-resolution CT
▌ Spirometry
— Restrictive pattern
— ↓ Gas transfer

Table 8.9   The main causes of honeycomb lung

Localized	Diffuse
Systemic sclerosis	Crytogenic fibrosing alveolitis
Sarcoidosis	Rheumatoid lung
Tuberculosis	Langerhans' cell histiocytosis
Asbestosis	Tuberous sclerosis
Berylliosis	Neurofibromatosis

I Bronchoalveolar lavage – hypercellular
I Transbronchial biopsy

Management   I Oxygen
I Steroids
I Immunosuppressants

Complications   I Respiratory failure

Prognosis   I Median survival 5 years

Extrinsic allergic alveolitis (K&C, p. 905)
Aetiology   I See Table 8.10
I Hypersensitivity reaction

Clinical features   I Fever
I Malaise
I Breathlessness
I Cough
I Tachypnoea
I Coarse inspiratory crackles
I Wheeze

Table 8.10   *Extrinsic allergic (bronchiolar) alveolitis – some causes*

Disease	Situation	Antigens
Farmer's lung	Forking mouldy hay or any other mouldy vegetable material	Thermophilic actinomycetes and *Micropolyspora faeni*
Bird fancier's lung	Handling pigeons, cleaning lofts or budgerigar cages	Proteins present in the 'bloom' on the feathers and in excreta
Maltworker's lung	Turning germinating barley	*Asperigillus clavatus*
Humidifier fever	Contaminated humidifying systems in air conditioners or humidifiers in factories (especially in printing works)	Possibly a variety of bacteria or amoeba (e.g. *Naegleria gruberi*)
Mushroom workers	Turning mushroom compost	Thermophilic actinomycetes

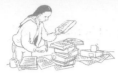

Investigations
- Chest X-ray – fluffy nodular shadowing
- Precipitating antibodies (e.g. pigeon protein)
- Spirometry
  — restrictive pattern
  — ↓ gas transfer
- Bronchoalveolar lavage – hypercellular

Management
- Avoid precipitant
- Steroids

Pneumothorax (*K&C*, p. 917)

- Air in the pleural space leading to lung deflation

Aetiology
- Spontaneous
- Chest trauma
- Intubation and ventilation

Clinical features
- See Table 8.2
- Pleuritic chest pain
- Breathlessness

Specific features
- Young patients: ♂ > ♀ 6:1, often tall and thin
- > 40 years usually associated with COPD
- Rarely caused by asthma
- If severe can present as tension pneumothorax (mediastinal shift and respiratory compromise)

Investigations
- Chest X-ray

Management
- Simple aspiration (second intercostal space mid-clavicular line)
- Intercostal drain if recurs after aspiration
- BTS guidelines (Fig. 8.3)
- Surgery for recurrent pneumothorax

Complications
- Bronchopleural fistula

TENSION PNEUMOTHORAX

Oxygen
Cannula into pleura (second intercostal space anteriorly)
Then manage as in Figure 8.3

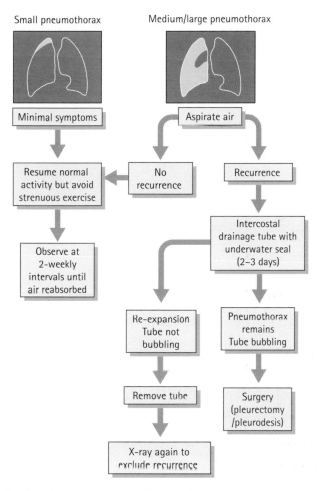

Fig. 8.3 Algorithm for the management of pneumothorax.

Carbon monoxide poisoning (K&C, p. 981)

▍ Carbon monoxide combines readily with haemoglobin and prevents the formation of oxyhaemoglobin

Aetiology ▍ Gas appliances with poor ventilation

Clinical features ▍ Mental impairment
▍ Nausea and vomiting

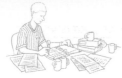

■ Headache
■ Hallucinations
■ Fits
■ Drowsiness and coma
■ Mild–moderate toxicity
— Tachycardia
— Tachypnoea
■ Severe toxicity
— Hypotension
— Bradycardia
— Myocardial damage
— Respiratory distress

Investigations   ■ Blood carboxyhaemoglobin level

Management   ■ Remove the source
■ High-flow oxygen
■ Hyperbaric oxygen if
— Coma
— Carboxyhaemoglobin level > 10%

Self-assessment questions

Multiple choice questions

1. The following are causes of clubbing:
   A. Empyema
   B. Asthma
   C. Ventricular septal defect
   D. Diverticular disease
   E. Mesothelioma

2. In pleural effusion the following signs may be found:
   A. Hyper-resonant percussion note
   B. Reduced breath sounds
   C. Reduced chest expansion
   D. Increased vocal resonance
   E. Tracheal deviation

3. In asthma:
   A. Peak flow rate is low
   B. The patient may have reduced air entry on chest auscultation
   C. FEV_1: FVC ratio is normal
   D. FVC is low
   E. JVP is elevated

4. In pneumonia:
   A. *Strep. pneumoniae* is the commonest cause
   B. *Haemophilus influenzae* pneumonia usually occurs in patients with normal lungs
   C. Pneumonia is only caused by bacteria

D. *Pneumocystis carinii* pneumonia occurs in patients who are immunosuppressed

E. *Staph. aureus* may present with extrapulmonary abscesses

5. In pneumonia:

A. *Chlamydia psittaci* is associated with contact with birds

B. Cold agglutinins are rare in *Mycoplasma* pneumonia

C. Patients can be dehydrated

D. *Mycobacterium kansasii* usually presents in young adults

F. *Staph. aureus* is associated with recent influenza infection

6. In tuberculosis:

A. Treatment is with combination antibiotics

B. Presentation can be with erythema nodosum

C. Mycobacteria are identified by haematoxylin and eosin stain

D. Pneumonia usually affects the lower zones of the lungs

E. Treatment with isoniazid causes eye problems

7. Lung cancer:

A. Is the most common cause of malignancy-related death in the UK

B. Most commonly is an adenocarcinoma

C. Can present with a pleural effusion

D. Patients frequently present with cough

E. Patients may have no clinical signs

8. In lung cancer:

A. A Pancoast's tumour presents with pain in the arm

B. A right recurrent laryngeal nerve palsy may occur

C. Horner's syndrome is associated with ptosis and a dilated pupil

D. Spread to bone is common

E. Dermatomyositis may occur

9. In the treatment of lung cancer:

A. Surgery can cure in some cases

B. Radiotherapy is used for SVC obstruction

C. Chemotherapy is most successful in small cell cancer

D. A 20% 5-year survival is the norm

E. Prednisolone is used in palliative care

10. In asthma:

A. Airway hyper-responsiveness is a major feature

B. Exacerbations can be precipitated by particular weather conditions

C. Attacks can be precipitated by use of paracetamol

D. Peak flow measurements can help in management

E. Intravenous aminophylline may be useful in severe cases

11. In COPD:

A. A common cause is α_1-antitrypsin deficiency

B. Disease occurs in smokers

C. A bounding pulse suggests CO_2 retention

D. Stopping smoking can improve prognosis

E. Home oxygen is used in patients with $Pao_2 < 10$ kPa

12. Obstructive sleep apnoea:

A. Is treated with inhaled steroids

B. Can present with morning headaches

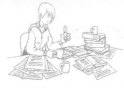

C. Is diagnosed by a sleep study
D. Commonly occurs in thin patients
E. Is treated with CPAP

13. Pneumothorax:

A. Can be a complication of mechanical ventilation
B. Leads to a hyper-resonant percussion note on the affected side
C. Can resolve spontaneously
D. Always requires chest drain insertion
E. Usually presents with haemoptysis

14. In cryptogenic fibrosing alveolitis:

A. Coarse crackles are heard on auscultation
B. Spirometry shows a reduced FVC

C. There is a good prognosis
D. Clubbing is common
E. There is an association with coeliac disease

15. Regarding occupational lung disease:

A. In coal-worker's pneumoconiosis the sputum may be black
B. Patients may qualify for industrial injury benefits
C. Eggshell calcification occurs in asbestosis
D. The risk of lung cancer may be increased
E. Cigarette smoking in patients exposed to asbestosis only slightly increases the risk of bronchial adenocarcinoma

Extended matching questions

Question 1 *Theme: breathlessness*

A. Adenocarcinoma of the lung
B. Asthma
C. Chronic obstructive pulmonary disease
D. Extrinsic allergic alveolitis
E. Cryptogenic fibrosing alveolitis
F. Mesothelioma
G. Heart failure
H. Iron deficiency anaemia
I. Pneumothorax

For each of the following questions, select the best answer from the list above:

I. A 23-year-old female has intermittent episodes of breathlessness and cough. She has a past history of eczema and her FEV_1:FVC ratio is reduced. What is the most likely diagnosis?

II. A 50-year-old male smoker who works on a farm presents with progressive increasing breathlessness and weight loss over 6 months. He has finger clubbing. What is the most likely diagnosis?

III. An 80-year-old female presents with episodes of breathlessness on exertion. She takes ibuprofen for joint pains and nifedipine for hypertension. She has normal pulmonary function tests and the PA chest X-ray is also normal. What is the most likely diagnosis?

Question 2 *Theme: pneumonia*

A. *Streptococcus pneumoniae*
B. *Mycobacterium tuberculosis*
C. *Haemophilus influenzae*
D. *Mycoplasma pneumoniae*
E. *Pneumocystis pneumonia*
F. *Staphylococcus aureus*
G. *Chlamydia psittaci*
H. *Legionella pneumophila*
I. *Coxiella burnetii*
J. *Influenza A*

For each of the following questions, select the best answer from the list above:

I. A-28-year old female who has previously been well and takes the oral contraceptive pill presents with a fever and a cough productive of rust-coloured sputum. A chest X-ray reveals a right middle lobe pneumonia. What is the most likely microbiological causal agent?

II. A 50-year-old male who is known to have HIV with a low CD4 count presents with a history of fever and breathlessness. The chest X-ray looks normal and there are few clinical findings apart from marked hypoxia. What is the most likely microbiological causal agent?

III. An 80-year-old female presents with fever and cough. She lives in an old people's home where there has recently been a flu outbreak. A chest X-ray shows right lower zone shadowing with an area suggesting a cavity. What is the most likely microbiological causal agent?

Short answer questions

1. Write short notes on the following:
   A. Symptoms and signs of pneumothorax
   B. Changes in lung function tests in patients with cryptogenic fibrosing alveolitis
   C. Superior vena cava obstruction
   D. Empyema

2. Write short notes on the following:
   A. Symptoms and signs of pneumonia
   B. Complications of pneumonia
   C. Side-effects of anti-TB drugs

3. Write short notes on the following:
   A. Cell types of bronchial carcinoma
   B. Presenting symptoms of lung cancer
   C. Bronchoscopy

4. Write short notes on the following:
   A. Presenting symptoms of sleep apnoea syndrome
   B. Clinical signs in COPD
   C. Cystic fibrosis
   D. Treatment of bronchiectasis

5. Write short notes on the following:
   A. Management of pneumothorax
   B. Asbestosis
   C. Extrinsic allergic alveolitis
   D. Goodpasture's syndrome

Essay questions

1. Outline the investigations you would consider in the investigation of a 50-year-old smoker with breathlessness.

2. Discuss the role of lung function tests.

3. Outline the investigations of a patient presenting with cough and a fever.

4. Discuss the treatment of community-acquired pneumonia.

5. Outline the investigations of a patient presenting with haemoptysis.

6. Discuss the presenting symptoms and signs of lung cancer.

7. Outline the assessment and management of a patient presenting with acute severe asthma.

8. Discuss the long-term treatment of patients with COPD.

9. Discuss the causes of pulmonary fibrosis.

10. Outline the investigations you would carry out in a patient presenting with hilar lymphadenopathy on a chest X-ray.

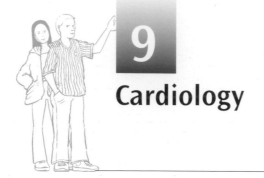

9

Cardiology

Examining the cardiovascular system (*K&C*, p. 709)

Examination should contain all of the following and be done in roughly this order:

- ❚ Position the patient at 30–45° to the horizontal with the chest and upper body exposed

General inspection
- ❚ Look for central cyanosis
- ❚ Note breathlessness
- ❚ Count the respiratory rate

Hands
- ❚ Peripheral cyanosis
- ❚ Nicotine stains
- ❚ Clubbing (congenital cyanotic heart disease, infective endocarditis)
- ❚ Splinter haemorrhages and nail fold infarcts (infective endocarditis)

Face
- ❚ Central cyanosis (blue lips and tongue)
- ❚ Malar flush (mitral valve disease)
- ❚ Pallor

Chest
- ❚ Scars (sternotomy, pacemaker, mitral valvotomy)
- ❚ Visible pulsations

Radial pulse
(Table 9.1)
Rate
- ❚ Time it with the minute hand on a watch or clock
- ❚ Record the rate as beats per minute (be exact)
- ❚ Feel both radial pulses

Table 9.1   The radial pulse

Character of radial pulse	Cause
Low volume	Low BP Aortic stenosis
Collapsing pulse	Aortic regurgitation
Pulsus alternans	Variable volume due to cardiac failure
Pulsus paradoxus	Volume reduces on inspiration in acute asthma

COLLAPSING PULSE

With the flats of your fingers over the radial pulse, raise the patient's arm above the level of the heart (without causing discomfort)

Normally there is no change or there is a reduction in the impulse

If the pulse is collapsing you will feel a strong, fast impulse which falls away immediately

Rhythm   ❙ Regular or irregular
— Atrial fibrillation
— Multiple ventricular ectopics

Radiofemoral delay   ❙ Coarctation of the aorta

Blood pressure   ❙ See information box

BLOOD PRESSURE

Use an appropriately sized cuff

Apply the cuff 25 mm above the antecubital fossa and palpate brachial artery. Inflate cuff until pulsation not palpable, place the diaphragm of the stethoscope over the artery, then deflate at a rate of 2–5 mmHg/second

When a sound is heard with each pulse (Korotkoff 1) this is the systolic pressure

The point at which the sound disappears (Korotkoff 5) represents the diastolic pressure

Record each to the nearest 2 mmHg

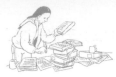

Carotid pulse   ❙ Feel each carotid artery separately
❙ Character (slow rising in aortic stenosis, collapsing in aortic regurgitation)

Jugular venous pulse (JVP) (*K&C*, p. 711)

❙ See Fig. 9.1 and Tables 9.2 and 9.3

Fig. 9.1
The jugular venous pulse.

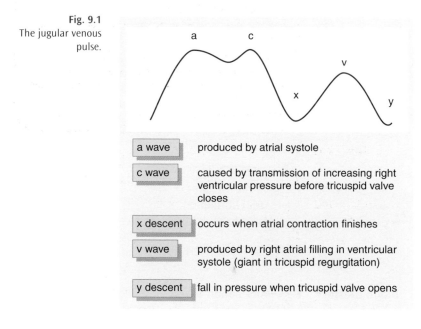

a wave	produced by atrial systole
c wave	caused by transmission of increasing right ventricular pressure before tricuspid valve closes
x descent	occurs when atrial contraction finishes
v wave	produced by right atrial filling in ventricular systole (giant in tricuspid regurgitation)
y descent	fall in pressure when tricuspid valve opens

Table 9.2   Features which differentiate the jugular venous pulse from the carotid pulse

JVP has double impulse
JVP not seen on sitting up and inspiration, when normal
JVP is impalpable
JVP fills from above if the internal jugular vein is occluded by light pressure at the base of the neck
Hepatojugular reflux – if pressure is put on the abdomen it increases venous return from the liver and the JVP becomes more prominent

Table 9.3   Causes of an abnormal jugular venous pressure

Right ventricular failure
Fluid overload
Tricuspid regurgitation (large v wave)
Pericardial effusion or restrictive pericarditis (pulsus paradoxus)
Complete heart block (giant a waves due to atrial contraction
   against a closed tricuspid valve)
Superior vena caval obstruction (non-pulsatile)

JUGULAR VENOUS PULSE

With the patient at 45° turn the face to the left to relax the neck strap muscles

Assess the internal jugular venous pulsation

The height of the JVP is measured vertically from the sternal angle. Use a ruler or finger breadths to measure the height accurately

The upper limit of normal is 4 cm

Apex beat
(Table 9.4)

I Position in terms of intercostal space and mid-clavicular line
I Most lateral and inferior position of palpable beat

Reasons for failure to locate the apex beat

I Fat or muscular chest wall
I Left pneumothorax or pleural effusion
I Emphysema
I Pericardial effusion
I Dextrocardia

Precordium

I Palpate over each valvular area with the palm of the hand for thrills (palpable murmurs)

Table 9.4   The apex beat

Quality	Haemodynamics	Causes
Hyperdynamic (thrusting)	Volume overload	Aortic regurgitation Mitral regurgitation
Sustained (heaving)	Pressure overload	Aortic stenosis Hypertension
Tapping	Palpable first heart sound	Mitral stenosis
Dyskinetic segment		Left ventricular aneurysm

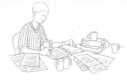

❚ Right ventricular hypertrophy may cause a sustained impulse (heave) at the left sternal edge

Auscultation
(Table 9.5 and Fig. 9.2)

❚ Listen with both the bell and the diaphragm to each valvular area
❚ Time any abnormal sounds with the carotid pulse

Mitral area

❚ After the apex, listen in the left axilla for radiation of mitral murmurs
❚ Turn the patient on to the left side and listen to the apex and axilla again in held expiration to accentuate difficult-to-detect murmurs, especially the 'rumbling' mid-diastolic murmur of mitral stenosis

Table 9.5   Cardiac auscultation

High-pitched sounds (diaphragm)
S_1 and S_2
Opening snap
Ejection murmurs
Early diastolic murmur of aortic regurgitation

Low-pitched sounds (bell)
S_3 and S_4
Mid-diastolic murmur of mitral stenosis

Fig. 9.2
Valvular areas.

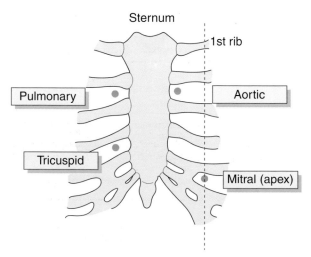

Aortic area   ▮ When listening at the left sternal edge sit the patient forward in held expiration to accentuate the early diastolic murmur of aortic regurgitation
▮ Listen for radiation of aortic murmurs to the carotids with the diaphragm followed by the bell for carotid bruits

Lung bases   ▮ While the patient is sitting forward examine the lung bases for crackles indicating pulmonary oedema

Abdomen   ▮ Liver enlargement in right ventricular failure
▮ Pulsation of liver in tricuspid regurgitation
▮ Abdominal aortic aneurysm
▮ Aortic and renal bruits

Peripheral pulses   ▮ Examine all of them and listen for femoral bruits

Peripheral oedema   ▮ Check for dependent pitting oedema at ankles and sacrum

NORMAL AND ABNORMAL SIGNS IN CARDIOVASCULAR EXAMINATION

Heart sounds   ▮ See Figure 9.3

S_1 ▮ Closure of mitral valve and tricuspid at the onset of systole

$S_2 (A_2 P_2)$ ▮ Closure of the aortic and pulmonary valves at the end of systole

S_3 ▮ Occurs in early diastole and is due to rapid ventricular filling

Heart sounds

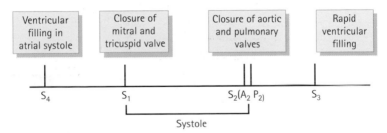

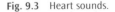

Fig. 9.3 Heart sounds.

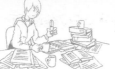
I Normal in young people, or if the left ventricle is stiff
I Volume overload in mitral regurgitation

S_4 I Occurs in late diastole due to ventricular filling in
atrial systole
I Always abnormal due to reduced ventricular
distensibility, e.g. aortic stenosis, acute myocardial
infarction (MI)

Fig. 9.4
Common murmurs.
EC: Ejection click.
OS: opening snap

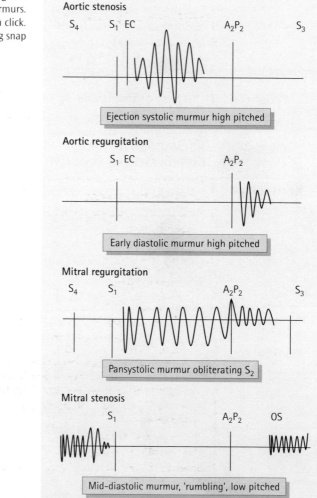

Aortic stenosis

S_4 S_1 EC A_2P_2 S_3

Ejection systolic murmur high pitched

Aortic regurgitation

S_1 EC A_2P_2

Early diastolic murmur high pitched

Mitral regurgitation

S_4 S_1 A_2P_2 S_3

Pansystolic murmur obliterating S_2

Mitral stenosis

S_1 A_2P_2 OS

Mid-diastolic murmur, 'rumbling', low pitched

Prosthetic valve sounds ❙ Mechanical valves make loud heart sounds often audible without a stethoscope

Common murmurs ❙ See Figure 9.4

Investigations in cardiology (K&C, p. 716)

CHEST X-RAY (see Ch. 5)

❙ Heart size and shape
❙ Lung fields

ELECTROCARDIOGRAPHY (K&C, p. 719)

❙ The electrocardiogram (ECG) is a recording of the electrical activity of the heart
❙ It is the vector sum of all the depolarization and repolarization potentials of all the myocardial cells

Limb leads ❙ Six of the leads are obtained by recording from the limbs (Fig. 9.5).

PERFORMING AN ECG

Connect the ECG machine to a power point and switch on

Connect the leads

    Limb leads
        Red to right arm
        Yellow to left arm
        Green to left leg
        Black (neutral) to right leg

    Chest leads
        V_1 Fourth intercostal space just to right of sternum
        V_2 Fourth intercostal space just to left of sternum
        V_3 Halfway between V_2 and V_4
        V_4 Fifth intercostal space left of mid-clavicular line
        V_5 On same horizontal as V_4 in anterior axillary line
        V_6 On same horizontal as V_4 in mid-axillary line

Check that there is paper and that the paper speed is correct (25 mm/s)

Ask the patient to keep still

Press record/acquire ECG

Label the ECG with the patient's name, and the date and time

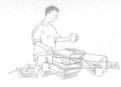

Chest leads ▌ The other six leads record potentials between points on the chest wall (Fig. 9.5) and an average of the three limbs

Aspects of the heart (Fig. 9.5)
▌ V_1 and V_2 – right ventricle
▌ V_3 and V_4 – interventricular septum

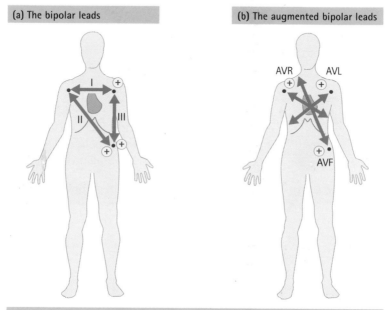

(a) The bipolar leads

(b) The augmented bipolar leads

AVR   AVL

AVF

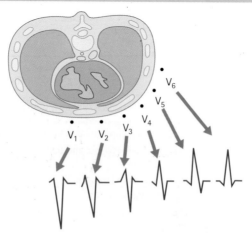

(c) The chest (unipolar) leads

V_6

V_5

V_4

V_3

V_1 V_2

Fig. 9.5   The connections or directions that comprise the 12-lead ECG.

I V_5 and V_6 – left ventricle
I Leads II, III and AVF – inferior aspect
I Leads I and AVL – lateral left ventricle

ECG paper I The standard paper speed is 25 mm/s
I This means each small square = 0.04 s
I Each large square = 0.2 s

Normal ECG   I P wave is atrial depolarization
waveform (Fig. 9.6)   I QRS is ventricular depolarization
I T wave is ventricular repolarization

Normal ECG   I P wave duration ≤ 0.12 s
intervals   I PR interval 0.12–0.22 s
I QRS complex duration ≥ 0.1 s

Axis   I The normal axis of the heart is –30° and +90°
I Axis deviation can be identified by looking at the
positive and negative deflections in leads I, II and
III (Fig. 9.7)

The normal 12-lead   I See Fig. 9.8
ECG

The exercise ECG

I Assesses cardiac response to exercise
I Detects myocardial ischaemia (ST depression and
T wave changes) during exertion

Fig. 9.6
Waves and intervals of
the normal ECG.

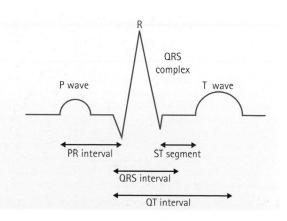

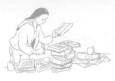

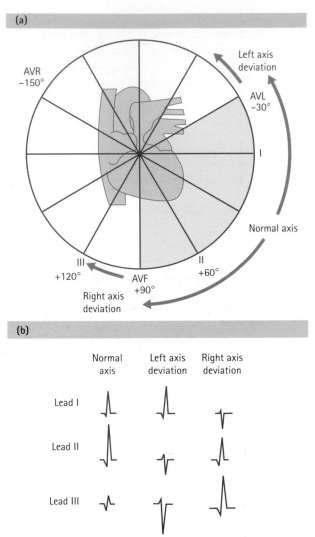

(a)

Left axis
deviation

AVR
−150°

AVL
−30°

I

Normal axis

III
+120°

II
+60°

AVF
+90°

Right axis
deviation

(b)

	Normal axis	Left axis deviation	Right axis deviation
Lead I			
Lead II			
Lead III			

Fig. 9.7 The cardiac axis. A. The hexaxial reference system, illustrating the six leads in the frontal plane, e.g. lead I is 0°, lead II is +60°, lead III is +120°. B. Calculating the direction of the cardiac vector. In the first column the QRS complex with zero net amplitude (i.e. when the positive and negative deflections are equal) is seen in lead III. The mean QRS vector is therefore perpendicular to lead III and is either −150° or +30°. Lead I is positive, so the axis must be +30°, which is normal. In left axis deviation (second column) the main deflection is positive (R wave) in lead I and negative (S wave) in lead III. In right axis deviation (third column) the main deflection is negative (S wave) in lead I and positive (R wave) in lead III. The frontal plane QRS axis is normal only if the QRS complexes in leads I and II are predominantly positive.

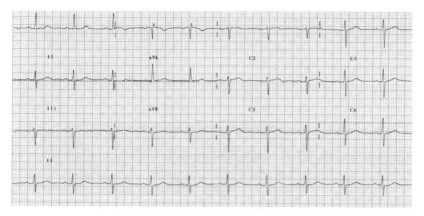

Fig. 9.8 The normal 12-lead ECG.

PROCEDURE FOR EXERCISE ECG

Continuous recording of pulse rate and 12 lead ECG and intermittent BP recordings (every 60 seconds)

The patient walks on a treadmill, slowly on the flat at first then graduating to high-speed walking (or running) on a gradient until a predesignated target heart rate (according to age) is reached or until symptoms or ECG abnormalities prevent further exertion

The ECG is analysed for ischaemic changes

Indications
- Investigation of chest pain
- Risk assessment after MI

Contraindications
- Recent MI (within 1 week)
- Unstable angina
- Aortic stenosis
- Hypertrophic obstructive cardiomyopathy

24-hour ambulatory taped ECG (K&C, p. 722)

- 24-hour recording of ECG via a portable recorder
- Records transient changes, e.g. paroxysmal tachycardias or rhythm pauses
- Event recording can link symptoms to changes in the ECG

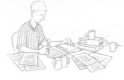

Echocardiography (K&C, p. 722)

- Non-invasive ultrasound examination of the heart
- Records dynamic anatomy of the four chambers and the valves
- Doppler echo gives information about
  — Blood flow
  — Ejection fraction
  — Pressure gradients

Abnormalities detected on echocardiography

- Valve stenosis
- Valve regurgitation
- Aortic root dissection
- Valve vegetations
- Cardiac failure (reduced ejection fraction)
- Cardiomyopathies
- Pericardial effusion
- Masses in heart chambers, e.g. thrombus, myxoma
- Left ventricular aneurysm
- Congenital heart disease

NUCLEAR IMAGING (E.G. THALLIUM SCAN) (K&C, p. 727)

- Used to measure myocardial function and perfusion defects and position
- Detects reversible ischaemia, e.g. resting or stress-induced, and irreversible ischaemia, e.g. MI

CARDIAC CATHETERIZATION (Table 9.6) (K&C, p. 728)

- Uses intraluminal catheter inserted via peripheral blood vessel to perform pressure measurements and contrast imaging from within the heart chambers, great vessels and coronary arteries

CORONARY ANGIOGRAPHY

- X-ray contrast medium is injected directly into the main coronary arteries via an intracardiac catheter

Indications
- Angina refractory to medical therapy
- Strongly positive exercise test
- Unstable angina
- Angina after MI

Table 9.6   Cardiac catheterization

Functions of cardiac catheter	Chambers and vessels examined
Direct pressure measurements	Right atrium Aorta Right ventricle Left ventricle Pulmonary artery
Indirect pressure measurements	Left atrium using pulmonary capillary wedge pressure
Blood sampling for P_aO_2	From all chambers to detect right to left shunts

▌ Young patients with angina or MI
▌ Uncertain diagnosis

Valvular heart disease (K&C, p. 783)

Investigations
▌ Chest X-Ray
▌ ECG
▌ Echocardiogram
▌ Cardiac catheterization

Management
▌ Antibiotic prophylaxis
  Required for patients with congenital abnormalities of heart or great vessels or valve disease for procedures which may cause a significant bacteraemia
  Example regime: gentamicin 160 mg plus amoxicillin 1 g
▌ Medical
▌ Surgical

Mitral stenosis

Aetiology
▌ Rheumatic fever

Clinical features
▌ Progressive breathlessness
▌ Paroxysmal nocturnal dyspnoea   ⎫ Secondary to
▌ Orthopnoea   ⎬ pulmonary venous
▌ Haemoptysis   ⎪ hypertension
▌ Recurrent bronchitis   ⎭

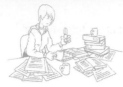
I Mitral facies (malar flush – a cyanotic purple discoloration over the upper cheeks)
I Small-volume pulse
I Atrial fibrillation
I Tapping apex beat
I Loud first heart sound
I Opening snap (OS)
I 'Rumbling' mid-diastolic murmur at apex with presystolic accentuation (if in sinus rhythm)
I Signs of right ventricular failure

Investigations I Chest X-Ray
— Large left atrium (widened carina)
— Convex left heart border
I ECG
— Bifid P wave or atrial fibrillation
— Right ventricular hypertrophy
— Right axis deviation
I Echocardiogram

Management *Medical*
I Diuretics
I Digoxin
I Anticoagulation for atrial fibrillation

Surgery
I For non-responsive or severe disease
I Balloon valvotomy
I Closed valvotomy
I Open valvotomy
I Mitral valve replacement

Complications I Atrial fibrillation
I Systemic embolization
I Pulmonary hypertension
I Pulmonary infarction
I Chest infections
I Tricuspid regurgitation
I Right ventricular failure

Mitral regurgitation (K&C, p. 786)

Aetiology
- Mitral valve prolapse
- Rheumatic fever
- Ischaemic heart disease
- Dilated cardiomyopathy
- Infective endocarditis

Clinical features
- Palpitations
- Exertional breathlessness
- Fatigue
- Cardiac failure
- Apex (laterally displaced, hyperdynamic, systolic thrill)

Heart sounds
- Soft first heart sound
- Loud pansystolic murmur at apex radiating to axilla
- Third heart sound
- Signs of cardiac failure

Investigations
- Chest X-ray
- Echocardiography
- Cardiac catheterization

Management
- Surgery (valve replacement)
- Symptomatic
  — ACE inhibitors, diuretics

Aortic stenosis (K&C, p. 788)

Aetiology
- Congenital
- Rheumatic fever
- Calcific

Clinical features
- Often no symptoms
- Exercise-induced angina, syncope, breathlessness
- Sudden death
- Small-volume slow-rising pulse
- Sustained apex beat
- Systolic thrill in aortic area

Heart sounds
- Ejection murmur in aortic area radiating to carotids
- Ejection click
- Soft second heart sound
- Fourth heart sound

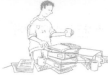

Investigations ▌ ECG – left ventricular hypertrophy/strain

Management ▌ Avoid exercise
▌ Avoid vasodilators
▌ β-blockers for angina
▌ Surgery – aortic valve replacement

Aortic regurgitation (*K&C*, p. 791)

Aetiology ▌ Rheumatic fever
▌ Marfan's syndrome
▌ Syphilitic aortitis
▌ Connective tissue disorders

Clinical features ▌ No symptoms
▌ Palpitations
▌ Angina
▌ Left ventricular failure
▌ Collapsing pulse
▌ Pistol shot femorals
▌ Wide pulse pressure

Heart sounds ▌ Apex (displaced, diffuse, hyperdynamic)
▌ Soft high-pitched early diastolic murmur at left sternal edge
▌ Maybe systolic aortic flow murmur
▌ Visible carotid or head nodding

Management ▌ Medical – treat heart failure
▌ Surgery – valve replacement

Tricuspid regurgitation (*K&C*, p. 792)

Aetiology ▌ Dilatation of right ventricle
▌ Chronic lung disease
▌ Pulmonary hypertension
▌ Infective endocarditis in intravenous drug users

Clinical features ▌ Exertional breathlessness
▌ Gastrointestinal upset secondary to congestion
▌ Elevated JVP with giant v wave
▌ Enlarged pulsatile liver
▌ Peripheral oedema
▌ Ascites
▌ Pleural effusions
▌ Right ventricular impulse at left sternal edge

Heart sounds ▌ Pansystolic murmur at lower left sternal edge, louder in inspiration

Management ▌ Medical – treat right ventricular failure
▌ Surgical valve resection – for infective endocarditis

Ischaemic heart disease (*K&C*, p. 766)

Aetiology ▌ Occlusive coronary artery disease
▌ Atheroma
▌ Thrombosis
▌ Spasm

Risk factors
for atheroma ▌ Age
▌ Male sex
▌ Family history
▌ Hyperlipidaemia
▌ Smoking
▌ Hypertension
▌ Diabetes mellitus

Angina (*K&C*, p. 769)

Clinical features ▌ Chest pain – heavy, tight, gripping
▌ Central, radiates to arms and jaw ⎫ Exertional
▌ Breathlessness   ⎬ – relieved
▌ Usually no signs   ⎭ by rest

Investigations ▌ Resting ECG (normal or signs of previous MI)
▌ Exercise ECG (ST depression > 1 mm during exercise which reverts to normal – Fig. 9.9)
▌ Thallium scans
▌ Coronary angiography

Management ▌ Eliminate risk factors
— Patient should stop smoking
— Treat hypertension
— Optimize diabetes treatment
— Treat hyperlipidaemia
▌ Aspirin

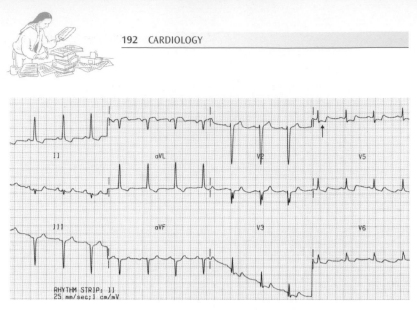

Fig. 9.9   Twelve-lead ECG in angina showing ST depression and T wave inversion.

UNSTABLE ANGINA

Clinical features
Pain at rest
'Crescendo' angina

Management
Admission for bed rest
High-flow oxygen
Aspirin 300 mg chewed stat then 75–150 mg daily
Pain relief
    Diamorphine 2.5–5 mg i.v. (plus antiemetic)
Heparin
    Low molecular weight heparin subcutaneously to full
        anticoagulant dose, e.g. enoxaparin 1 mg/kg/day
Standard medical anti-anginal therapy
    β-blockers unless contraindicated
    Atenolol 50 mg orally
Nitrates
    GTN i.v. infusion titrated to pain
    Isosorbide mononitrate 60 mg orally daily
Glycoprotein IIb/IIIa receptor inhibitors
Prompt angiography and revascularization

❙ Nitrates, e.g. glyceryl trinitrate (GTN), isosorbide
mononitrate
❙ β-blockers, e.g. atenolol
❙ Calcium channel blockers, e.g. amlodipine
❙ Potassium channel blockers, e.g. nicorandil

❚ Revascularization
— Percutaneous transluminal coronary angioplasty (PTCA)
— Intracoronary stents
— Coronary artery bypass grafting (CABG)

Myocardial infarction (K&C, p. 774)

Aetiology   ❚ Coronary atheroma

Clinical features   ❚ Chest pain
— Severe
— Sudden onset at rest
— Persists several hours
❚ 'Silent' in 20%
❚ Sweating
❚ Breathlessness
❚ Nausea and vomiting
❚ Patient is pale, sweaty and grey
❚ Tachycardia
❚ Heart failure

Diagnostic criteria   ❚ Two out of three of
— History of ischaemic-type chest pain
— Evolving ECG changes
— Rise and fall in cardiac enzymes

Investigations   *ECG*
❚ See Figures 9.10–9.12 and Table 9.7

Table 9.7   Assessment of infarct site

Full-thickness infarct
Q waves
> 1 mm broad and 2 mm deep
Negative deflection at start
of QRS complex
Normal in AVR and V_1
ST elevation
T wave inversion

Non-Q wave (subendocardial) infarct
No Q waves
Deep ST depression
T wave inversion

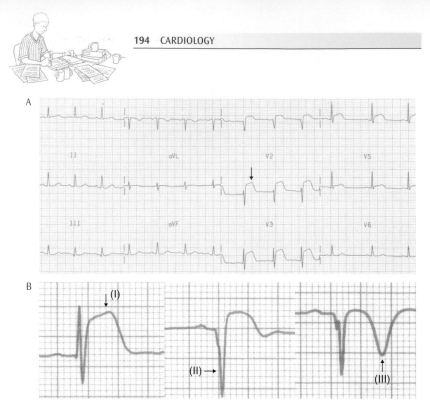

Fig. 9.10 Myocardial infarction. A. Twelve-lead ECG showing full-thickness anterior MI with S–T elevation B. Progressive ECG changes with time during an acute MI. ST elevation (i); Q waves (ii); T inversion (iii).

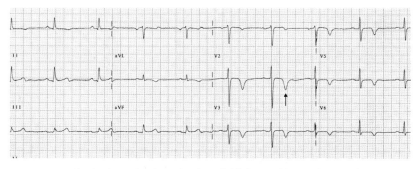

Fig. 9.11 Twelve-lead ECG showing subendocardial infarct. Widespread T wave inversion, no Q waves.

Cardiac enzymes

❙ Creatine kinase (CK) peaks 24 hours after MI
❙ Cardiac-specific troponins (very high specificity for myocardial ischaemia) rise early (2–4 hours, also raised in unstable angina)

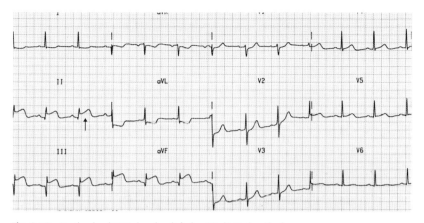

Fig. 9.12 Twelve-lead ECG showing inferior MI. (S–T elevation)

▎ Aspartate aminotransferase (AST) and
lactate dehydrogenase (LDH) rise 2–5 days
after MI

Assessment of
infarct site ▎ See Table 9.8

Acute management ▎ See information box (p. 196)

Aftercare *Ongoing pain after thrombolysis*
▎ I.v. β-blocker or nitrate
▎ Emergency angiography and revascularization

Table 9.8 Typical ECG changes in acute MI

Infarct site	Leads showing main changes
Anterior	V_2–V_5
Antero-septal	V_1–V_3
Antero-lateral	V_4–V_6, I and AVL
Lateral	I, II and AVL
Inferior	II, III and AVF
Posterior	V_1 and V_2 (reciprocal)
Subendocardial	Any

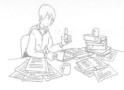

ACUTE MANAGEMENT OF SUSPECTED MI

Clinical features
Chest pain
Sweating
Breathlessness
Vomiting
Pale, sweaty, grey

ECG
See Figure 9.10

Immediate treatment
Fast Track through A&E
Oxygen 60%
Diamorphine 2.5–5 mg i.v.
Metoclopramide 10 mg i.v.
Aspirin 300 mg chewed

No contraindications to thrombolysis
Aim for rapid 'door to needle time'
Streptokinase 1.5 million units i.v. over 1 hour
Or
Recombinant tissue plasminogen activator (rtPA) accelerated protocol

With contraindications to thrombolysis
Emergency primary PTCA

Follow up with
Coronary care and monitoring for 48 hours

Pain-free with signs of heart failure
❙ Nitrate +/– diuretic
❙ ACE inhibitor long-term

Pain-free with no complications
❙ β-blocker long-term
❙ Return to work in 2–3 months

All patients
❙ Aspirin 75–150 mg/day
❙ β-blocker if no contraindications
❙ Risk factor stratification
❙ Exercise ECG +/– angiography
❙ Structured rehabilitation
❙ No driving for 1 month

Complications   *Early*
I Arrhythmias
I Sudden death
I Pericarditis
I Cardiac failure
I Cardiogenic shock
I Ruptured papillary muscle or chordae tendinae
I Ventricular septal defect (VSD)
I Cardiac rupture

Late
I Deep venous thrombosis (DVT), pulmonary embolism (PE)
I Mural thrombus
I Cardiac aneurysm
I Dressler's syndrome (fever, chest pain, pericarditis secondary to autoimmune carditis)

Sudden cardiac death   I See Figures 9.13 and 9.14

Prognosis   I 50% die acutely
I 10 % die in hospital
I 20% die within 2 years

Cardiac failure (K&C, p. 755)

I Occurs when the heart is unable to maintain sufficient cardiac output to meet the demands of the body despite adequate venous filling pressures

Aetiology   I See Table 9.9

Left ventricular failure (K&C, p. 757)
Aetiology   I Ischaemic heart disease
I Hypertension
I Mitral valve and aortic valve disease
I Cardiomyopathy

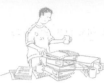

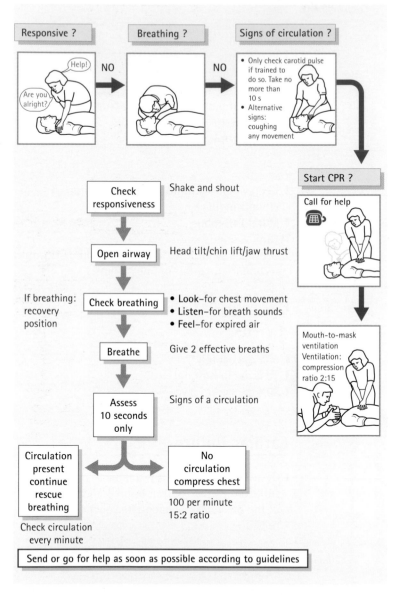

Fig. 9.13 Basic life support.

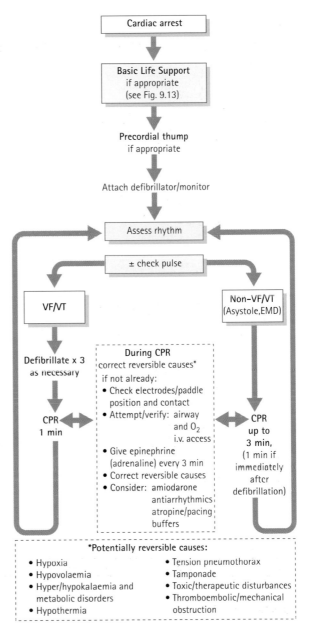

Fig. 9.14 Universal advanced life support algorithm. Reproduced by permission of the European Resuscitation Council and Laerdal Medical Ltd. CPR: Cardiopulmonary resuscitation. EMD: Electromechanical dissociation. VF/VT: Ventricular fibrillation/Ventricular tachycardia.

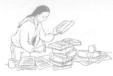

Table 9.9   Causes of cardiac failure

Myocardial dysfunction	High cardiac output
Ischaemic heart disease	Thyrotoxicosis
Cardiomyopathy	Anaemia
Hypertension	Paget's disease
Volume overload	Left to right shunts
Valve disease	**Compromised ventricular filling**
Fluid overload	
Obstruction to flow	Constrictive pericarditis
Aortic stenosis	Pericardial tamponade
Chronic lung disease	**Altered rhythm**
	Atrial fibrillation

Clinical features
- Fatigue
- Exertional breathlessness
- Orthopnoea
- Paroxysmal nocturnal dyspnoea (PND)
- Pulmonary oedema pink frothy sputum
- Distress
- Tachycardia
- Enlarged heart
- Gallop rhythm (triple fast rhythm due to third or fourth heart sound)
- Fine crackles at lung bases

Right ventricular failure (K&C, p. 757)

Aetiology
- Chronic lung disease = cor pulmonale
- Pulmonary emboli
- Pulmonary hypertension
- Left to right shunts
- Tricuspid regurgitation

Clinical features
- Tiredness
- Anorexia, nausea
- Gastrointestinal upset
- Raised JVP
- Dependent pitting oedema
- Pleural effusions
- Hepatic enlargement
- Ascites
- Functional tricuspid regurgitation

ACUTE PULMONARY OEDEMA

Clinical features
Extreme breathlessness (often in middle of night)
Wheeze
Anxiety
Cold sweat
Cough with frothy pink sputum
Grey and/or cyanosed
Tachypnoea
Peripherally shut down and cold
Raised JVP
Gallop rhythm
Crackles and wheeze throughout chest
Hypotension

Immediate investigations
Chest X-ray – exclude pneumothorax
Arterial blood gases – low Po_2, $\pm$ high Pco_2
ECG – arrhythmia

Immediate management
Sit up
High-flow oxygen
I.v. furosemide (frusemide) 40–80 mg
I.v. diamorphine 2.5–5 mg (not if BP < 80 systolic)
I.v. metoclopramide 10 mg
I.v. GTN (if not hypotensive)
Nebulized salbutamol 2.5 mg if bronchospasm

Investigation and treatment of cardiac failure (K&C, p. 758)

Investigations
I Chest X-ray
I ECG
I Echocardiogram
— left ventricular ejection fraction < 45%

Management
I Identify and treat causes or aggravating factors
I Drugs ·
— Diuretics (spironolactone, furosemide (frusemide))
— ACE inhibitors
— β-blockers
— Digoxin
— Nitrates
— Anticoagulation

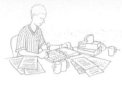

I Surgery
— CABG
— Valve replacement
— Pacemaker
— Heart transplant

Hypertension (*K&C*, p. 819)

I See Figure 9.15

Primary 'essential' hypertension
Aetiology I Genetic
I Obesity
I Alcohol
I Sodium intake
I Stress

Secondary hypertension
Aetiology *Renal*
I Diabetic nephropathy
I Renovascular disease
I Adult polycystic disease
I Chronic glomerulonephritis

Endocrine
I Conn's syndrome
I Adrenal hyperplasia
I Phaeochromocytoma
I Cushing's syndrome
I Acromegaly

Cardiovascular
I Coarctation of the aorta

Drugs
I Oral contraceptive pill
I Steroids
I Carbenoxolone

Pregnancy
I Second half of pregnancy
I Pre-eclampsia
I Hypertension and proteinuria

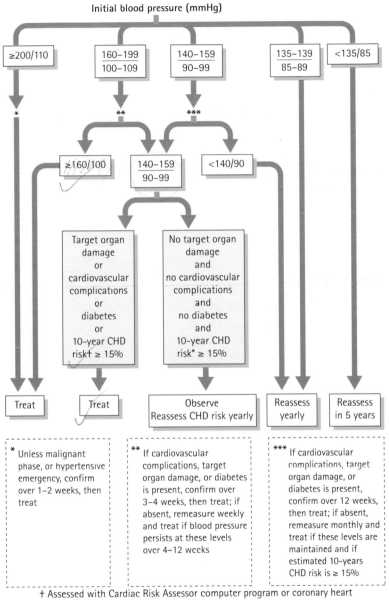

Fig. 9.15   Blood pressure thresholds and drug treatment in hypertension. From Ramsay LE et al. (1999) British Medical Journal 309: 630.

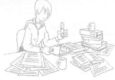

Clinical features
▌ Usually no symptoms
▌ Features of underlying cause
▌ Headaches
▌ Nose bleeds
▌ Nocturia
▌ Complications (see below)
▌ Elevated blood pressure
▌ Renal artery bruit
▌ Radiofemoral delay (coarctation of the aorta)
▌ Left ventricular hypertrophy

Retinal changes
▌ Grade 1 – tortuosity of retinal arteries and 'silver wiring'
▌ Grade 2 – grade 1 plus arteriovenous nipping
▌ Grade 3 – grade 2 plus flame haemorrhages and soft 'cotton wool' exudates
▌ Grade 4 – grade 3 plus papilloedema

Investigations
▌ Chest X-ray
▌ ECG (left ventricular hypertrophy and strain)
▌ Echocardiogram (left ventricular hypertrophy)
▌ Urinalysis for casts, protein and red cells
▌ Fasting blood glucose and lipids
▌ Serum urea, creatinine and electrolytes

Complications
▌ Cerebrovascular disease
▌ Coronary artery disease
▌ Retinopathy
▌ Renal disease

Management
General measures
▌ Weight loss
▌ Alcohol reduction
▌ Salt restriction
▌ Exercise

Drug therapy
▌ See Table 9.10

Malignant hypertension (K&C, p. 826)
Clinical features
▌ Diastolic BP > 140 mmHg
▌ Progressive renal failure, proteinuria and haematuria

Table 9.10   Drug treatment of secondary hypertension

Class	Example	Side-effects
Thiazide diuretics	Bendroflumethiazide (bendrofluazide)	Hypokalaemia
β-blockers	Atenolol	Bronchospasm Nightmares Cold peripheries Impotence
ACE inhibitors	Enalapril	Dry cough Profound first-dose hypotension Renal function deterioration
ACE II receptor antagonists	Losartan	
Calcium channel blockers	Amlodipine	Impotence Hypotension
α-blockers	Doxazosin	Hypotension

▌ Cerebral oedema or haemorrhage
▌ Grade 4 retinopathy
▌ Hypertensive encephalopathy

Management ▌ Aim to reduce diastolic BP to 100–110 mmHg over 24–48 hours
▌ Oral treatment is usual
▌ In urgent situations, e.g. aortic dissection,
▌ i.v. sodium nitroprusside or β-blockers

Congenital heart disease (K&C, p. 797)

▌ Affects 1% of live births

Disease ▌ Maternal rubella infection
associations ▌ Maternal alcohol abuse
▌ Chromosomal abnormalities, e.g.
  — Down's syndrome
  — Turner's syndrome

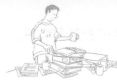

ACYANOTIC – LEFT TO RIGHT SHUNT (*K&C*, p. 799)

Ventricular septal defect (VSD)
- 1:500 live births

Clinical features
- Often no symptoms
- Fatigue
- Dyspnoea
- Loud pansystolic murmur at lower left sternal edge
- Thrill at lower left sternal edge
- Pulmonary hypertension

Management
- Antibiotic prophylaxis for procedures
- Surgical closure

Complications
- Pulmonary hypertension
- Reversal of shunt
- Eisenmenger's syndrome
  — Blood bypasses the lungs

Atrial septal defect (ASD)
Clinical features
- Usually none until adulthood
- Breathlessness
- Fatigue
- Right ventricular heave
- Loud pulmonary second sound
- Fixed splitting of second heart sound (A_2–P_2)
- Mid-diastolic murmur at left sternal edge

Management
- Antibiotic prophylaxis
- Surgical closure

Complications
- Pulmonary hypertension

Persistent ductus arteriosus
- Continuous aorta to pulmonary artery shunt

Aetiology
- Idiopathic
- Prematurity

Clinical features
- Left heart failure
- Congestive heart failure
- Infective endocarditis
- Continuous 'machinery' murmur

Management
- Surgical closure
- Aspirin

CYANOTIC – RIGHT TO LEFT SHUNT

Fallot's tetralogy (*K&C*, p. 802)
- VSD
- Overriding aorta
- Right ventricular outflow obstruction
- Right ventricular hypertrophy

Clinical features
- Breathlessness
- Fatigue
- Hypoxia on exertion – cyanosis +/– syncope
- Squatting – to improve venous return and reduce shunt
- Right parasternal heave
- Systolic ejection murmur
- Central cyanosis
- Finger clubbing
- Polycythaemia

Management
- Surgical correction

Eisenmenger's syndrome
- Reversal of shunt in large VSD due to secondary pulmonary hypertension giving right to left shunt and cyanosis

NO SHUNT

Coarctation of the aorta (*K&C*, p. 801)
- ♂ > ♀
- Turner's syndrome
- Associated with bicuspid aortic valve and aortic stenosis

Clinical features
- Hypertension in upper limbs
- Radiofemoral delay
- Mid- to late systolic murmur over the back

Investigations
- CXR
  — Dilated aorta
  — Rib notching (due to large collateral arteries eroding ribs)

Management
- Surgical excision

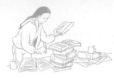

Inflammatory and infective diseases of the heart

Acute pericarditis (K&C, p. 815)

Aetiology
- Viral (Coxsackie virus)
- Post-MI (acute in 20% of full-thickness anterior MI)
- Dressler's syndrome (type 3 hypersensitivity about 3 weeks after MI)
- Uraemic
- Tuberculous
- Malignant

Clinical features
- Chest pain
  — Substernal
  — Sharp
  — Worse on breathing
  — Relieved by sitting forward
  — Worse on lying flat
- Fever
- Malaise
- Pericardial friction rub (sounds like 'walking on snow')

Investigations
- ECG (widespread 'saddle-shaped' ST elevation)

Management
- Anti-inflammatory drugs
- Rest
- Treat underlying cause

Pericardial effusion (K&C, p. 817)

Clinical features
- Raised JVP
- Kussmaul's sign (JVP elevates during inspiration)
- Pulsus paradoxus
- Failure to locate apex beat
- Quiet heart sounds

Investigations
- ECG (low-voltage complexes)
- Chest X-ray (large globular heart)
- Echocardiogram
- Pericardiocentesis for diagnosis and to treat incipient tamponade

Myocarditis (K&C, p. 810)

Aetiology
- Viral
  — Coxsackie
  — Influenza
  — Rubella
  — Polio
- Protozoal
  — *Trypanosoma cruzi* (Chagas disease)
  — *Toxoplasma gondii*
- Toxins
  — Lead poisoning
  — Radiation injury
- Bacterial infection
  — Diphtheria
  — Q fever
  — *Coxiella burneti*

Clinical features
- Autoimmune disease
- Acute cardiac failure
- Fever

Investigations
- Chest X-ray
- ECG
  ST and T wave abnormalities
  — Arrhythmias
- Cardiac enzymes
- Echocardiography
- Endomyocardial biopsy
- Viral antibody titres

Management
- Treat heart failure
- Treat underlying cause

Rheumatic fever (K&C, p. 79)

Aetiology
- Group A streptococcal infection

Clinical features
(Table 9.11)
- General
  — Fever
  — Malaise

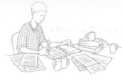

Table 9.11   Duckett Jones diagnostic criteria in rheumatic fever

Two or more major *or* one major plus two or more minor *plus* evidence of recent streptococcal infection

Major
Carditis
Polyarthritis
Chorea
Erythema marginatum
Subcutaneous nodules

Minor
Fever
Arthralgia
Previous rheumatic fever
Raised erythrocyte sedimentation rate (ESR)/C-reactive protein (CRP)
Raised white cell count
Prolonged PR interval

▌ Carditis
 — New or changing murmurs
 — Cardiac failure
 — Pericardial effusion
▌ Arthritis
 — Fleeting polyarthritis of large joints
▌ Sydenham's chorea (St Vitus' dance)
 — Choreoathetoid movements
▌ Skin
 — Erythema marginatum
 — Subcutaneous nodules (painless)

Investigations ▌ Throat swab
▌ Antistreptolysin-O titre
▌ ESR
▌ CRP

Management ▌ Penicillin to eradicate streptococci
▌ Bed rest
▌ High-dose aspirin
▌ Corticosteroids (prednisolone 60–120 mg/day)

Infective endocarditis (K&C, p. 793)

  ▌ Most commonly affects rheumatic or congenitally abnormal valves, VSD or patent ductus
  ▌ Prosthetic valves may also be affected

Aetiology
  ▌ *Streptococcus viridans* (50% of cases)
  ▌ *Enterococcus faecalis*
  ▌ *Staphylococcus aureus*
  — Often acute
  — Associated with central venous catheters, temporary pacing wires and in i.v. drug users
  — Poor prognosis
  ▌ *Staphylococcus epidermidis*
  — I.v. drug users
  — Alcoholics
  ▌ *Coxiella burneti* (Q fever)

Clinical features
  ▌ (* Seen in > 50% of cases)
  ▌ General
  — Malaise*
  — Clubbing
  ▌ Cardiac
  — Murmurs*
  — Cardiac failure*
  ▌ Arthralgia
  ▌ Pyrexia*
  ▌ Skin lesions
  — Osler's nodes
  — Splinter haemorrhages
  — Janeway lesions
  — Petechiae*
  ▌ Eyes
  — Roth spots
  ▌ Splenomegaly
  ▌ Neurological (cerebral emboli)
  — Mycotic aneurysm
  — Renal (haematuria*)

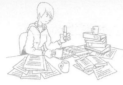

Investigations   *Blood*
- Anaemia
- Raised serum CRP and ESR
- Mildly abnormal liver biochemistry
- Raised total serum immunoglobulins
- Raised total complement and C3

Urinalysis
- Proteinuria with casts
- Microscopic haematuria

Blood cultures
- At least six sets from different veins at different times (positive in 75% of cases)

Echocardiography
- Trans-oesophageal echocardiograpy (TOE) is best for visualizing vegetations and is mandatory in non-native valves

Management   *Antibiotics*
- Bactericidal antibiotics chosen on the basis of blood culture results and sensitivities
- I.v. antibiotics for 2–6 weeks with back-titrations to confirm bactericidal serum levels

Indications for surgery
- Significant extensive valve damage
- Early infection of prosthetic valve
- Persistent infection with negative blood cultures
- Embolization
- Progressive cardiac failure
- Tricuspid valve infection in i.v. drug users

Prophylaxis
- See page 187

Cardiac arrhythmias (K&C, p. 735)

I Bradycardia – heart rate < 60 bpm
I Tachycardia – heart rate > 100 bpm

Sinus arrhythmia

I Due to normal changes in autonomic tone
I Heart rate increases in inspiration and falls in expiration

Sinus bradycardia

Aetiology
I Hypothermia
I Hypothyroidism
I Raised intracranial pressure
I Drugs (β-blockers, digoxin)
I Ischaemia

Sinus tachycardia

Aetiology
I Fever
I Exertion
I Emotion
I Pregnancy
I Anaemia
I Cardiac failure
I Thyrotoxicosis
I Drugs (sympathomimetics)

Sinus node disease (sick sinus syndrome)

Aetiology
I Ischaemia
I Infarction
I Degenerative disease

Clinical features
I Combinations of fast and slow supraventricular rhythms

Investigations
I ECG – long interval between P waves > 2 seconds

Management
I Permanent pacemaker
I Antiarrhythmic drugs to combat tachycardia
I Anticoagulation

Atrioventricular block (K&C, p. 736)

First-degree
I Prolonged PR interval (Fig. 9.16)

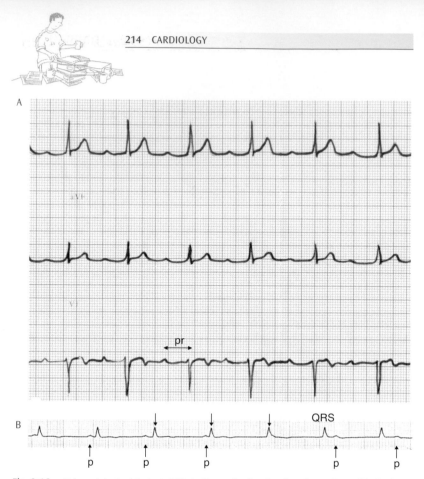

Fig. 9.16 Atrioventricular block. A. ECG rhythm strip showing first-degree heart block with prolongation of the PR interval. B. Complete heart block with dissociation of the P waves and QRS complexes.

Second-degree
- Some P waves conduct to ventricles
- Mobitz type 1 ('Wenckebach' – Fig. 9.17)
  — Progressive elongation of PR interval until failure to conduct
- Mobitz type 2
  — Dropped QRS conduction without progressive PR elongation
- 2:1 or 3:1 block
  — every second or third P wave conducts to ventricles (Fig. 9.18)

Third-degree (complete heart block)
- No P waves conduct
- Ventricular rhythm is maintained by spontaneous escape rhythm from ventricular myocardium with broad complexes

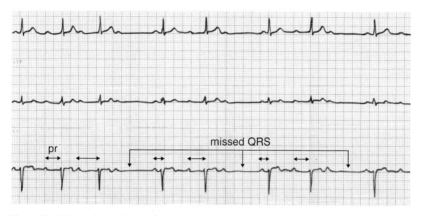

Fig. 9.17 ECG rhythm strip showing second-degree 'Wenckebach' heart block, with prolongation of the PR interval and missed QRS.

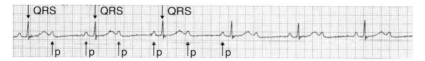

Fig. 9.18 ECG rhythm strip showing second-degree '2:1' heart block.

Clinical features   ▌ Maybe no symptoms (first- and second-degree)
                      ▌ Dizziness
                      ▌ Syncope
                      ▌ Blackouts (Stokes–Adams attacks) (third-degree)
                      ▌ Cannon 'a' waves in JVP in third degree

Management   ▌ Permanent pacemaker for symptomatic
               bradycardias

Intraventricular conductance disturbances (K&C, p. 739)

Aetiology   *Right bundle branch block (RBBB – Fig. 9.19)*
              ▌ Congenital heart disease
              ▌ Cor pulmonale
              ▌ Pulmonary embolus
              ▌ Myocardial infarction
              ▌ Cardiomyopathy
              ▌ Hyperkalaemia
              ▌ Can be normal

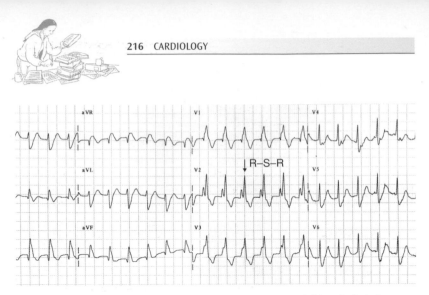

Fig. 9.19 Twelve-lead ECG showing right bundle branch block and right axis deviation.

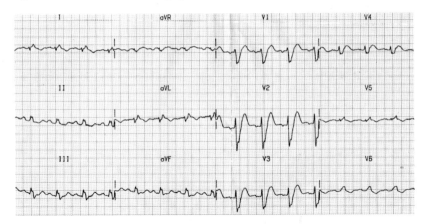

Fig. 9.20 Twelve-lead ECG showing left bundle branch block.

Left bundle branch block (LBBB – Fig. 9.20)
- Aortic stenosis
- Hypertension
- Acute MI
- Severe coronary artery disease
- Cardiomyopathy

Management
- Permanent pacemaker for symptomatic cases

ATRIAL TACHYARRHYTHMIAS (K&C, p. 743)

Aetiology
- Ischaemic heart disease
- Rheumatic heart disease

I Thyrotoxicosis
I Cardiomyopathy
I Wolff–Parkinson–White syndrome
I Pneumonia
I Atrial septal defect
I Pericarditis
I Pulmonary embolus

Atrial flutter I Atrial rate about 300/min with 2:1 or 3:1 AV
conduction

Investigations I ECG (Fig. 9.21) – sawtooth atrial flutter waves
between QRS complexes

Management I Electrical cardioversion
I Class III antiarrhythmic drugs

Atrial fibrillation I Uncoordinated rapid continuous activation of atria
from multiple foci
Aetiology I See above

Clinical features I No symptoms
I Reduced exercise tolerance
I Palpitations
I Heart failure
I Embolic events
I Completely irregular pulse

Investigations I ECG (Fig. 9.22)
— No p waves
— Irregular rapid QRS rhythm

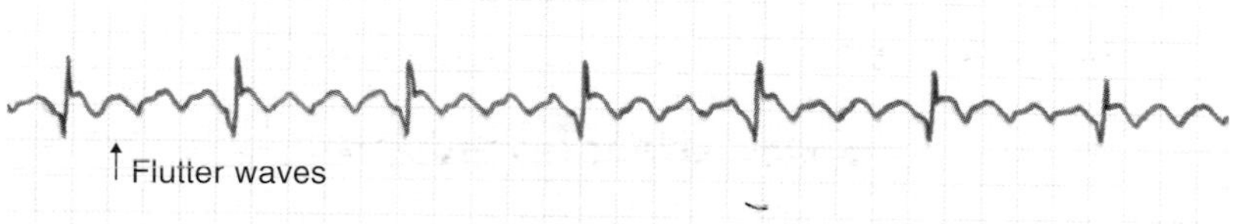

↑ Flutter waves

Fig. 9.21 ECG rhythm strip showing atrial flutter.

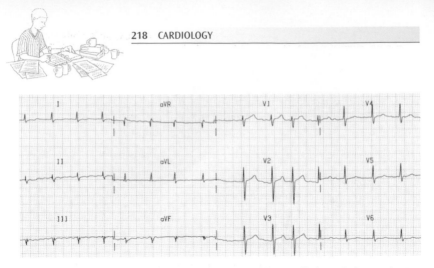

Fig. 9.22   Twelve-lead ECG showing atrial fibrillation with controlled ventricular rate (no P waves).

Management

I Treat the cause
I Control ventricular rate
  — Digoxin
  — β-blockers
  — Verapamil
I Cardioversion
  — Electrical DC cardioversion
  — Drugs (amiodarone, flecainide)
I Prophylaxis against thrombotic events
  — Warfarin

SUPRAVENTRICULAR TACHYCARDIA (K&C, p. 740)

Aetiology

I Provoked by
  — Exertion
  — Caffeine
  — Alcohol
  — β$_2$-agonists
I Congenital
  — Wolff–Parkinson–White syndrome
  — Lown–Ganong–Levine syndrome

Clinical features

I Palpitations
I Chest pain
I Breathlessness
I Syncope
I Polyuria
I Rapid regular pulse 140–280/min

Investigations
(Fig. 9.23)

▌ ECG
— Narrow complex QRS tachycardia
— Occasionally broad complex when associated with interventricular conductance disturbances

Management
(Fig. 9.24)

▌ Vagotonic manoeuvres
▌ Carotid sinus massage
▌ Ocular pressure
▌ Valsalva manoeuvre
▌ Drugs
— adenosine in increasing i.v. doses with continuous rhythm monitoring (avoid in asthma)
▌ Prophylaxis

VENTRICULAR TACHYARRHYTHMIAS (K&C, p. 745)

Ventricular tachycardia

▌ Three or more ventricular beats at 120/min or more

Clinical features

▌ Palpitations
▌ Dizziness
▌ Syncope
▌ Angina

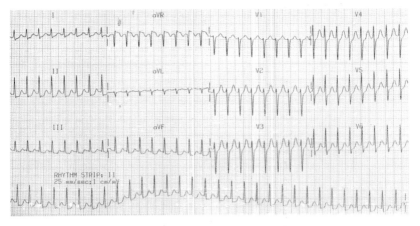

Fig. 9.23 Supraventricular tachycardia.

Fig. 9.24
Management of
supraventricular
tachycardia.

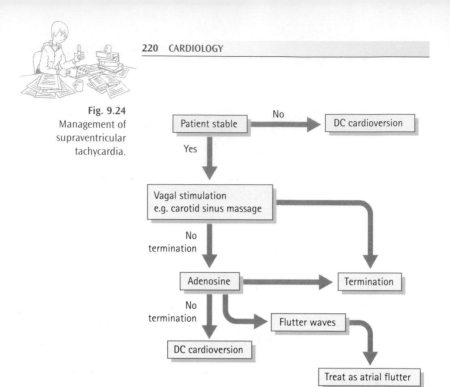

Investigations
(Fig. 9.25)

▌ ECG – broad complex tachycardia

Management

▌ See Figure 9.26

**Ventricular
fibrillation**

▌ See Figure 9.27

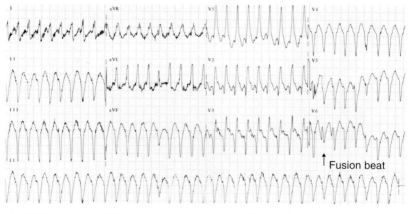

Fig. 9.25   Twelve-lead ECG showing ventricular tachycardia.

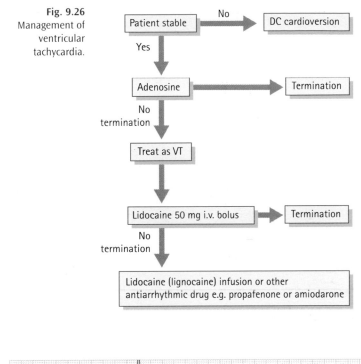

Fig. 9.26 Management of ventricular tachycardia.

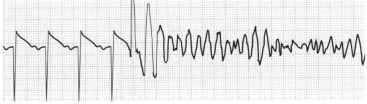

Fig. 9.27 Four beats of sinus rhythm followed by a ventricular ectopic beat that initiates ventricular fibrillation. The ST segment during sinus rhythm is elevated owing to acute MI in this case.

Electromechanical dissociation (EMD)

- See Figure 9.13
- Electrical activity
- No muscle activity

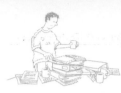

Self-assessment questions

Multiple choice questions

1. The following are features of aortic stenosis:
   A. Collapsing pulse
   B. Ejection systolic murmur
   C. Syncope on exertion
   D. Loud second heart sound
   E. Opening snap

2. The following are features of mitral stenosis:
   A. Atrial fibrillation
   B. Tapping apex beat
   C. Pansystolic murmur
   D. Pulmonary hypertension
   E. Right axis deviation on ECG

3. In mitral regurgitation:
   A. The pulse is characteristically collapsing
   B. There is an apical pansystolic murmur radiating to the axilla
   C. The ECG shows left ventricular hypertrophy
   D. The commonest cause is hypertension
   E. Atrial fibrillation is common

4. In tricuspid regurgitation:
   A. There is a pansystolic murmur radiating to the axilla
   B. Pulmonary hypertension is a cause
   C. There may be pulsatile hepatomegaly
   D. Giant v waves are seen in the jugular venous pulse
   E. Complete heart block is common

5. In acute myocardial infarction:
   A. The ECG shows raised ST segments
   B. The pain is characteristically left-sided and worse on inspiration
   C. Diamorphine is contraindicated
   D. Creatine kinase levels are maximally elevated 12–18 hours after the onset of pain
   E. Treatment with streptokinase reduces mortality

6. The following are signs of congestive cardiac failure:
   A. Raised jugular venous pressure
   B. Gallop rhythm
   C. Splenomegaly
   D. Papilloedema
   E. Splinter haemorrhages

7. In unstable angina:
   A. The most common heart rhythm is atrial fibrillation
   B. The ECG shows ST depression and T wave inversion
   C. Creatine kinase is normal
   D. Treatment of choice is anticoagulation with warfarin
   E. Thirty-day mortality is 50%

8. In systemic hypertension:
   A. The commonest cause is renal artery stenosis
   B. Complications include heart failure and renal failure
   C. Effective treatment reduces the incidence of stroke
   D. There are commonly no symptoms
   E. The first-line treatment is methyldopa

9. The following are features of tetralogy of Fallot:
   A. Episodes of cyanosis
   B. Atrial septal defect
   C. Overriding aorta
   D. Normal life expectancy
   E. Right ventricular hypertrophy

10. The following are features of acute rheumatic fever:
    A. Recent streptococcal throat infection
    B. Clubbing
    C. Roth spots
    D. Sydenham's chorea
    E. Osler's nodes

11. In acute pericarditis:
    A. The chest pain is characteristically crushing and radiates down the right arm
    B. The ECG shows widespread concave ST elevation
    C. There is usually pulsus paradoxus
    D. Viral infections are a common cause
    E. High-dose prednisolone is the treatment of choice

12. The following are features of infective endocarditis:
    A. Spider naevi
    B. Osler's nodes
    C. Splenomegaly
    D. Microscopic haematuria
    E. Clubbing

13. In patients with atrial fibrillation:
    A. The cardiac rhythm becomes more irregular with exertion
    B. Common causes include rheumatoid arthritis and obstructive jaundice
    C. A fourth heart sound is always absent
    D. Digoxin should always be given
    E. Complications include stroke and mesenteric infarction

14. In supraventricular tachycardia:
    A. The onset is characteristically sudden
    B. Symptoms may include angina and breathlessness
    C. Carotid sinus massage causes the heart rate to accelerate
    D. First-line treatment is atropine
    E. There is often no underlying heart disease

15. The following are features of complete heart block:
    A. Syncopal attacks
    B. Cannon waves in the jugular venous pulse
    C. Atrioventricular dissociation on ECG
    D. It responds to an atrial pacemaker
    E. Sudden death

Extended matching questions

Question 1 *Theme: central chest pain*

A. Reflux oesophagitis
B. Angina
C. Myocardial infarction
D. Dissecting thoracic aortic aneurysm
E. Mitral valve prolapse
F. Costochondritis
G. Gallstones
H. Duodenal ulcer
I. Pneumothorax
J. Mesothelioma
K. Pulmonary embolus

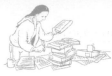

For each of the following questions, select the best answer from the list above:

I. A 20-year-old male with Marfan's syndrome presents with severe chest pain at rest associated with nausea and shortness of breath. Blood pressure is decreased in the right arm compared with the left arm.
What is the most likely diagnosis?

II. A 55-year-old male smoker with diabetes presents with a history of self-limiting central chest pain lasting 5 minutes, associated with nausea and shortness of breath which started while playing football with his grandson.
What is the most likely diagnosis?

III. A 45-year-old obese female smoker presents with episodic burning chest pain, worse at night and after spicy foods.
What is the most likely diagnosis?

Question 2 *Theme: ankle swelling*

A. Left ventricular failure
B. Cardiomyopathy
C. Deep venous thrombosis
D. Nephrotic syndrome
E. Cellulitis
F. Ruptured Baker's cyst
G. Liver failure
H. Gout
I. Charcot's joints

For each of the following questions, select the best answer from the list above:

I. A 60-year-old male alcoholic present with a 3-month history of swelling of the abdomen and ankles, and shortness of breath on exertion. On examination there are no signs of chronic liver disease. His pulse is 120/minute with atrial fibrillation and the apex beat is displaced laterally and inferiorly; he has ascites and ankle oedema.
What is the most likely diagnosis?

II. A 70-year-old female with a history of myocardial infarction 10 years ago, and who returned from Australia 1 week ago, presents with swollen ankles, worse on the right, and shortness of breath on exertion.
What is the most likely diagnosis?

II. A 50-year-old diabetic female on enalapril presents with a painful swollen right ankle which started 10 days ago. Examination reveals erythema and oedema, with a small painless ulcer on the right heel.
What is the most likely diagnosis?

Question 3 *Theme: palpitations*

A. Supraventricular tachycardia
B. Atrial fibrillation
C. Woolf–Parkinson–White syndrome
D. Anxiety
E. Thyrotoxicosis
F. Hypertension
G. Stokes–Adams attacks
H. Digoxin toxicity
I. β_2-agonists
J. Cocaine abuse

For each of the following questions, select the best answer from the list above:

I. A 69-year-old female smoker being investigated for chest pains presents with sudden onset of rapid palpitations associated with dizziness and shortness of breath. Her pulse is irregular, rate 160/minute, and BP is 90/60. The ECG shows no P waves.
What is the most likely diagnosis?

II. A 68-year-old female recently saw her GP for wheeze and shortness of breath, and was prescribed some treatment. She now presents with episodes of dizziness, palpitations and tremor. On examination her pulse is regular, 130/min. The ECG shows a sinus tachycardia.
What is the most likely diagnosis?

III. A 22-year-old law student presents with intermittent episodes of palpitations, shortness of breath and tingling in his fingers and round his lips. Examination is normal. Thyroid function tests a year ago (for similar symptoms) were normal.
What is the most likely diagnosis?

Objective structured clinical examination questions

1. Refer to Figure 9.6 and comment on the following in this order:
   A. Rate
   B. Rhythm
   C. Axis
   D. QRST morphology

Short answers questions

1. What are the complications of the following
   A. Aortic stenosis
   B. Myocardial infarction
   C. Infective endocarditis

2. What are the features of the following
   A. Cardiac failure
   B. Coarctation of the aorta
   C. Stokes Adams attacks

I3. List the causes of the following
   A. Mitral stenosis
   B. Cardiac failure
   C. Atrial fibrillation and the clinical and ECG features which distinguish AF from other tachyarrhythmias

Essay questions

1. How would you investigate and interpret results in a patient with a murmur detected clinically?

2. What are the complications of mitral valve disease?

3. Discuss the therapeutic options available to treat a patient with angina pectoris.

4. Describe the management of a patient presenting with acute severe chest pain at rest.

5. Describe how you would investigate a patient with episodes of syncope.

6. Discuss the differential diagnosis of a patient with possible acute rheumatic fever.

7. Describe the management of a 35-year-old man with a 4-week history of fever, the murmur of aortic regurgitation and splinter haemorrhages.

8. Describe the management of a 60-year-old man presenting acutely with dizziness and a heart rate of 36 beats per minute.

9. A 55-year-old man is brought to hospital unconscious and pulseless. Describe how you would manage him.

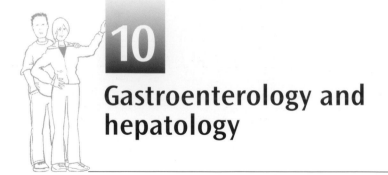

10

Gastroenterology and hepatology

Examining the abdomen (K&C, p. 255)

Examination should include all of the following and be done in roughly this order:

Expose the abdomen
- Xiphisternum to the suprapubic area
- Maintaining the dignity of the patient is vital

Look for
- Jaundice (Table 10.1)
- Weight loss/malnutrition
- Stigmata of chronic liver disease (Table 10.2)
- Shape of the abdomen and signs of distension
- Stomas
  — Bowel: ileostomy or colostomy
  — Urinary: ileal conduit
- Operation scars

Table 10.1   Causes of jaundice

Pre-hepatic	Post-hepatic
Haemolytic anaemia	Cholangiocarcinoma
Hepatic	Pancreatic carcinoma
Abnormal bilirubin	Sclerosing cholangitis
metabolism	Gallstones
Viral hepatitis	
Drugs → hepatitis or	
cholestasis	
Malignancy	
Chronic liver disease	

Table 10.2 Stigmata of chronic liver disease

Skin	Abdomen
Jaundice	Ascites
Spider naevi	Hepatomegaly
Palmar erythema	Splenomegaly
Dupuytren's contractures	
Caput medusae	**Hands**
Bruising	Liver flap
Xanthelasma	
Mouth	**Eyes**
Fetor hepatis	Anaemia
Bleeding gums	Jaundice

Hands
- Anaemia
- Clubbing
- Palmar erythema
- Dupuytren's contractures
- Liver flap
- Koilonychia — iron deficiency anaemia
- Leuconychia — hypoalbuminaemia

Face
- Anaemia
- Jaundice
- Fetor hepatis
- Spider naevi

Thorax
- Spider naevi – demonstrate filling from the central arteriole by pressing in the centre
- Lymphadenopathy – supraclavicular fossae (a node in the left fossa may indicate oesophageal or gastric cancer)

Abdomen
- Obvious masses
- Visible peristalsis
- Scratch marks due to obstructive jaundice
- Stretch marks
- Caput medusae
- Scars
- Hernias (periumbilical, inguinal and femoral)

Palpation
- Ask if the abdomen is tender and, if so, where
- Start palpating away from this point

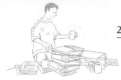

Fig. 10.1
Anatomical regions of
the abdomen.
EP: Epigastrium
SC: Subcostal
LN: Loin
UM: Umbilical
F: Flank
SP: Suprapubic
IF: Iliac fossa

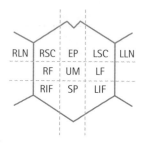

I Start gently, with the flat of the fingers, eliciting tenderness and obvious masses
I Then palpate more deeply in an ordered way around the abdomen looking for deep masses
I Describe the location of findings as per the regions shown in Figure 10.1

Liver
(Tables 10.3 and 10.4)

I The normal liver is only just palpable in slim people on inspiration
I Start from the right inguinal ligament
I Use the pulps of the finger or the side of the index finger (with the hand flat)
I Ask the patient to take deep breaths in and out
I As the patient breathes in, the diaphragm flattens, pushing the liver down on to your fingers. Note the position of the lowest palpable point

Table 10.3   Causes of hepatomegaly

Infective	**Metabolic**
Acute viral hepatitis	Haemochromatosis
Epstein–Barr virus	
Malaria	**Malignant**
Kala-azar	Hepatocellular cancer
	Chronic leukaemia
Inflammatory	Secondary malignancy
Alcoholic liver disease	
Primary biliary cirrhosis	**Cardiovascular**
	Right ventricular failure
Infiltration	Tricuspid regurgitation
Amyloid	

Table 10.4   Causes of hepatosplenomegaly

Hepatic
Chronic liver disease with portal hypertension

Malignancy
Leukaemia
Lymphoma

Infection
Viral hepatitis
Epstein–Barr infection

Infiltration
Amyloid
Sarcoid

▮ The upper limit is defined by percussing in the mid-clavicular line from the nipple and noting the boundary between resonance and dullness (normally the sixth intercostal space)
▮ Note any tenderness or palpable texture

Spleen
(Tables 10.4 and 10.5)

▮ Start from the right inguinal region
▮ Palpate towards the left hypochondrium
▮ The normal spleen is not palpable
▮ If it is, ask the patient to roll on to his or her right side to bring the spleen forward, making it easier to feel
▮ You will not be able to feel the upper margin
▮ You may just feel the splenic notch in the anterior aspect and the spleen is dull to percussion

Kidneys
(Table 10.6)

▮ Place your hand under the loin just below the level of the costal margin

Table 10.5   Causes of splenomegaly

Malignancy	Infective
Myelofibrosis	Malaria
Lymphoma	Kala-azar
Chronic myeloid leukaemia	**Chronic liver disease**
Infiltration	Portal hypertension
Gaucher's disease	
Amyloid	

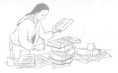

Table 10.6   Causes of enlarged kidneys

Bilateral	Unilateral
Polycystic kidney disease	Renal carcinoma
Hydronephrosis	Hydronephrosis
Amyloid	Large renal cyst

I Use this hand to push the kidney up towards your other hand (balloting)
I If you are able to feel the kidney, just below the hypochondrium, it is enlarged
I You should be able to feel the upper pole of an enlarged kidney
I Always check for a transplanted kidney, usually in the right iliac fossa
I Check for an arteriovenous fistula (for haemodialysis) on the forearm

Ascites
(Table 10.7)

I Eliciting shifting dullness is the easiest and most appropriate test

Shifting dullness

I Percuss the abdomen from the umbilicus laterally until the boundary between resonance and dullness is apparent
I Position your hand so that this boundary is between the middle and ring fingers of your splayed hand
I Ask the patient to roll towards you keeping your hand on the abdomen
I Allow the fluid to settle (at least 15–20 seconds), then percuss again to demonstrate that the boundary has moved

Table 10.7   Causes of ascites

Hepatic	Hypoalbuminaemia
Chronic liver disease	Nephrotic syndrome
(Portal hypertension)	Protein-losing enteropathy
	Protein malnutrition
Peritoneal	
Peritoneal malignancy	
	Vascular
Infection	Hepatic vein thrombosis
Tuberculosis	Budd-Chiari syndrome

Fluid thrill ▌ (Do not do this in an exam unless asked to by the examiner)
▌ Ask the examiner or the patient to place the lateral aspect of his or her hand firmly on the abdomen in the midline, then flick or tap the lateral aspect of the abdomen with one hand
▌ The other hand is placed on the opposite side to detect the vibration

Hernial orifices ▌ Palpate the hernial orifices
▌ Ask the patient to cough and feel for an impulse
▌ Repeat with the patient standing
▌ Tell the examiner that you would like to examine the genitalia and carry out a rectal exam

Gastrointestinal investigations (K&C, p. 256)

RADIOLOGY

Plain abdominal film ▌ See Chapter 5

Barium swallow ▌ Outlines the oesophagus

Strictures ▌ Smooth < 2 cm = peptic
▌ Rough > 2 cm = malignant
▌ Distal 'rat's tail' = achalasia

Pouches ▌ Pharyngeal pouch

Barium meal ▌ Outlines the stomach

Ulcers ▌ 'Circles of barium'

Masses ▌ Usually malignant

Barium follow-through ▌ Outlines the small bowel

Strictures ▌ e.g. Crohn's disease

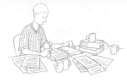

Obstruction

Barium enema
- Outlines the colon
- Air + barium introduced (double contrast)

Strictures
- Apple core lesion (cancer)

Diverticulae
- Pockets outside the bowel

Colitis
- Smooth, no folds ± ulcers

Ultrasound
- Images the liver, gallbladder, pancreas, spleen and kidneys

Stones
- Gallbladder and kidney

Masses
- Liver cyst/tumour
- Pancreatic cancer

CT
- Intra-abdominal organs
- Lymphadenopathy

MRI
- Pancreas
- Biliary tree
- Perianal sepsis

ENDOSCOPY

Gastroscopy
- Examines the oesophagus, stomach and parts one and two of the duodenum
- Allows macroscopic diagnosis
- Biopsies for histology
- Therapeutic procedures
  — Dilatation of strictures
  — Injection of bleeding ulcers

Endoscopic retrograde cholangiopancreatography (ERCP)
- Outlines the pancreatic duct and biliary tree

Stones
- Gallbladder or bile duct

Strictures
- Carcinoma of the pancreas
- Cholangiocarcinoma
- Sclerosing cholangitis

Stents
- Tubes inside the bile duct, used to bypass obstructions

Colonoscopy	▌ Examines the colon and terminal ileum
	▌ Allows biopsies and therapeutic procedures, e.g. polypectomy
	▌ Screening for colorectal cancer
Sigmoidoscopy	▌ Examines the rectum and sigmoid colon
	▌ Investigation of rectal bleeding
Proctoscopy	▌ Examines the anus
	▌ Haemorrhoids
	▌ Anal fissure

BREATH TESTS

^{13}C urea breath test	▌ Diagnosis of *Helicobacter pylori* infection
	▌ Urea split by *H. pylori* → ammonia + $^{13}CO_2$
	▌ $^{13}CO_2$ exhaled and detected in breath
	▌ Sensitivity 98%; specificity 99%
H_2 breath test	▌ Diagnosis of bacterial overgrowth
	▌ Lactulose meal
	▌ Bacteria ferment carbohydrate, releasing hydrogen
	▌ Breath hydrogen peaking at < 2 hours indicates overgrowth

STOOL TESTS

Microscopy and culture	
	▌ Infections
Blood	▌ Malignancy

Oesophageal disease

Hiatus hernia (Fig. 10.2) *(K&C, p. 263)*	▌ Herniation of the stomach into the thorax
	▌ Sliding: gastro-oesophageal junction above diaphragm
	▌ Rolling: fundus herniates beside oesophagus
	▌ Disrupts lower oesophageal sphincter → gastro-oesophageal reflux
Clinical features	▌ Usually none
	▌ Heartburn due to reflux
Management	▌ Treat reflux (see below)
	▌ Surgery for large hernias/severe reflux

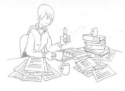

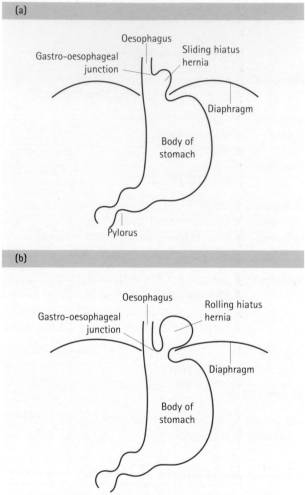

Fig. 10.2 Rolling and sliding hernias. A. The sliding hernia displaces the gastro-oesophageal junction proximally. B. The rolling hernia does not.

Gastro-oesophageal reflux disease (GORD) (K&C, p. 263)

❚ Passage of gastric contents into the oesophagus due to relaxation of the lower oesophageal sphincter

❚ Acid or bile causes mucosal irritation

Aetiology	I Ineffective lower oesophageal sphincter
	I Hiatus hernia
	I Obesity
	I Alcohol (increased acid secretion)
	I Oesophageal dysmotility
	I Pregnancy
	I Drugs: nifedipine/isosorbide mononitrate

Clinical features	I Retrosternal burning pain (heartburn)
	I Often during the night or when bending over
	I Associated bitter taste in the mouth
	I Sore throat
	I Excessive salivation (water-brash)
	I Nocturnal cough or bronchospasm (aspiration)
	I Dysphagia (difficulty in swallowing)
	I Peptic strictures

Investigations	I Trial of antacid/proton pump inhibitor
	I Upper GI endoscopy
	I Oesophageal pH studies

Management	I Lifestyle changes: reduce smoking/alcohol
	I Lose weight
	I Antacids
	I Histamine$_2$-receptor blockers, e.g. ranitidine
	I Proton Pump inhibitors, e.g. omeprazole
	I (Laparoscopic) Nissen fundoplication

Complications	I Peptic oesophageal strictures
	I Barrett's oesophagus
	I Oesophageal adenocarcinoma

Barrett's oesophagus (*K&C*, p. 265)	I Columnar epithelium with intestinal metaplasia replaces normal squamous mucosa
	I Increased risk of adenocarcinoma ($\male \gg \female$)
	I Associated with gastro-oesophageal reflux

Oesophageal carcinoma (*K&C*, p. 269)	I 55% squamous cell carcinomas
	I 45% adenocarcinomas
	I Prevalence: 10–15/100 000 and increasing

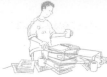

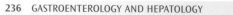

Clinical features
- Dysphagia
- Progressive: solids then liquids
- Weight loss
- Anorexia

Investigations
- Upper GI endoscopy and biopsy
- Barium swallow
- CT to stage tumour

Management
- 10% 5-year survival
- Squamous cell cancer
  — Radiotherapy
  — Surgery
- Palliation: oesophageal stents reduce dysphagia

Achalasia
(*K&C*, p. 266)
- Rare:1/100 000/year
- Failure of relaxation of lower oesophageal sphincter
- → Dysphagia (intermittent to solids and liquids)

Investigations
- Barium swallow – rat's tail appearance
- Endoscopy – to exclude malignancy
- Oesophageal manometry
  — Measurement of sphincter pressure (raised)
  — Aperistaltic oesophagus

Management
- Endoscopic balloon dilatation of sphincter
- Injection of Botulinum toxin into sphincter
- Surgery (Heller's procedure: division of muscle)

The stomach

Dyspepsia
- Symptoms referable to the upper gastrointestinal tract

Epidemiology
- 75–90% of population get symptoms
- 4% of all GP consultations

Aetiology
- Non-ulcer (functional) dyspepsia
- GORD
- Gastritis
- Peptic ulcer disease
- Gastric malignancy
- NSAIDs

Clinical features   ▋ Heartburn
▋ Epigastric pain
▋ Pain, discomfort or 'fullness' after eating
▋ Nausea
▋ Bloating

Alarm signals   ▋ Weight loss
▋ Vomiting
▋ Haematemesis, melaena or anaemia
▋ Dysphagia
▋ Previous gastric ulcer or gastric surgery
▋ Non-steroidal anti inflammatory drugs (NSAIDs)

Investigations   ▋ ^{13}C urea breath test for *H. pylori*
▋ *H. pylori* serology
▋ Upper GI endoscopy if over 45 years old

Management   ▋ Depends on cause
▋ Consider a trial of proton pump inhibitors if no alarm signals and age < 50

Peptic ulceration   ▋ Breaches in the mucosa in the stomach or
(*K&C*, p. 272)   duodenum

Aetiology   ▋ Gastric ulcers
— *H. pylori* (60%)
— NSAIDs
— Adenocarcinoma
— Lymphoma
— Steroids
— Bisphosphonates
— Selective COX II inhibitors
— Chronic renal failure
— Hypercalcaemia
▋ Duodenal ulcers
— *H. pylori* (98%)
— NSAIDs
— Zollinger–Ellison syndrome

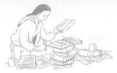

Clinical features
- Pain
- Pain at night often related to food
- Nausea
- GI haemorrhage (haematemesis or melaena)
- Anaemia
- Tender abdomen

Investigations
- Upper GI endoscopy
- Barium meal
- Urease test at endoscopy
- Biopsy for histology

Management
- *H. pylori* eradication therapy (proton pump inhibitor and two antibiotics for 7 days)
- Stop NSAIDs
- Proton pump inhibitors for 8 weeks

Complications
- Haemorrhage → haematemesis/melaena
- Perforation → peritonism and air under diaphragm on chest X-ray
- Gastric outlet obstruction

Gastritis
(*K&C*, p. 276)
- Inflammation of the gastric mucosa
- Often asymptomatic

Aetiology
- *H. pylori*
- NSAIDs
- Autoimmune (pernicious anaemia)

Management
- *H. pylori* eradication
- Avoid NSAIDs

Upper GI bleeding (*K&C*, p. 282)

Aetiology
- Oesophageal causes
  - Varices
  - Ulceration
  - Reflux disease → erosions
  - Mallory–Weiss tear (associated with vomiting)
  - Malignancy
- Gastric causes
  - Ulcers
  - Erosions
  - Malignancy

▌ Duodenal causes
— Ulceration

Clinical features   ▌ Nausea
▌ Haematemesis
▌ Melaena
▌ Dizziness due to hypovolaemia
▌ Hypotension
▌ Tachycardia
▌ Stigmata of chronic liver disease
— Splenomegaly
— Ascites   } Portal hypertension
— Spider naevi
— Caput medusae

Investigations   ▌ Full blood count – low haemoglobin, high platelets
▌ Urea and electrolytes – high urea
▌ Liver biochemistry – abnormal in liver disease
▌ Coagulation – elevated prothrombin time
▌ Upper GI endoscopy to identify and treat cause

Management   ▌ See 'Medical emergencies' box
▌ 80% will stop spontaneously
▌ Upper GI endoscopy
▌ Therapy depends on cause (see below)

Varices
▌ Endoscopic therapy
— Inject sclerosant
— Elasticated band around varix
▌ Non-endoscopic therapy
— Vasopressin analogues
— Sengstaken tube
— Transjugular intrahepatic portosystemic shunt (TIPS)

Ulcers
▌ Adrenaline (epinephrine) injection
▌ Sclerosant injection
▌ Heat coagulation

Surgery
▌ Required for uncontrollable bleeding

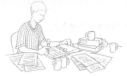

UPPER GASTROINTESTINAL HAEMORRHAGE

Haematemesis and/or melaena is indicative of gastrointestinal bleeding:

   I.v. access: two large bore lines in big veins
   Measure blood pressure and pulse
   Immediate fluid resuscitation with colloid
Blood for full blood count/urea and electrolytes/coagulation
Immediate blood group and cross-match
Request senior review
Assess for evidence of perforation
Assess medical risk – age/heart disease/diabetes
Assess causal factors – NSAIDs/liver disease
Fluid-resuscitate with blood once available
Consider endoscopy or surgical intervention

GASTRIC TUMOURS (*K&C*, p. 277)

Benign tumours
- Leiomyoma
- May ulcerate → bleeding

Adenocarcinoma

Epidemiology
- Fourth most common cause of cancer-related death
- 15/100 000 men/year
- Wide geographical variation, e.g. common in Japan

Aetiology
- *H. pylori*
- Low dietary vitamin C and β-carotene
- Smoking
- Family history
- Pernicious anaemia
- Previous gastric surgery

Clinical features
- Abdominal pain
- Early satiety
- Weight loss
- Nausea and vomiting
- Upper GI bleeding
- Palpable epigastric mass
- Left supraclavicular lymph node (Virchow's)
- Enlarged liver due to metastases

Investigations
- Upper GI endoscopy or
- Barium swallow and meal

▌ CT   ⎫ To stage
▌ Endoscopic ultrasound   ⎬ tumour
                              ⎭

Management ▌ Surgery for low-stage tumours
              ▌ Palliation for high-stage tumours
              ▌ Poor response to chemotherapy/radiotherapy
              ▌ 10% 5-year survival

MALT lymphoma ▌ Mucosa-associated lymphoid tissue lymphoma
(K&C, p. 280)   ▌ Associated with *H.pylori*
                   ▌ 80% are cured by eradication of the infection

Small bowel disease

Coeliac disease ▌ Hypersensitivity to gliadin in wheat, barley, rye
(K&C, p. 291)   → small intestinal disease

Epidemiology ▌ England 1:1000; Ireland 1:300
                ▌ Caucasians mainly
                ▌ Positive family history

Pathology ▌ → Subtotal villous atrophy (Table 10.8)
             — Loss of villi
             — Crypt hyperplasia
             ▌ → Malabsorption (see Table 10.9)

Clinical features ▌ Abdominal pain
                     ▌ Diarrhoea
                     ▌ Steatorrhoea/malabsorption
                     ▌ Weight loss

Table 10.8   Causes of villous atrophy

Coeliac disease
Whipple's disease
Small bowel lymphoma
Primary hypogammaglobulinaemia
Infection enteritis in children
Kwashiorkor
Cow's milk protein intolerance
Zollinger–Ellison syndrome

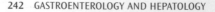

Table 10.9   Causes of small bowel malabsorption

Coeliac disease
Dermatitis herpetiformis
Tropical sprue
Bacterial overgrowth
Intestinal resection
Crohn's disease
Whipple's disease
Radiation enteritis
Giardia intestinalis
Lymphoma

I Symptoms of anaemia
I Mouth ulceration
I Anaemia → pale conjunctivae
I Dermatitis herpetiformis (blistering rash on extensor surfaces)

Investigations   I Anti-endomysial antibodies   } Negative after
I Tissue transglutaminase   } gluten-free diet
I Antigliadin antibodies
I Antireticulin antibodies
I Endoscopy and duodenal biopsy
I Full blood count
— Anaemia (macrocytic or microcytic)
— Hyposplenism, Howell–Jolly bodies

Disease   I Thyroid disease/diabetes
associations   I Primary biliary cirrhosis
I Autoimmune hepatitis

Complications   I Ulcerative jejunitis
I Small bowel lymphoma
I Oesophageal carcinoma
I Osteomalacia

Management   I Gluten-free diet
I Iron/folate supplementation

Bacterial   I Bacterial colonization of the small bowel
overgrowth   I Commonly *Escherichia* or *Bacteroides*
(*K&C*, p. 294)   I → Bacterial consumption of vitamin B_{12}

$\rightarrow$ Breakdown of bile salts
$\rightarrow$ Bacterial synthesis of folate

Aetiology   ▌ Small bowel structural abnormalities
▌ Strictures

Clinical features   ▌ Diarrhoea
▌ Steatorrhoea

Investigations   ▌ Lactulose breath tests
▌ Low vitamin B_{12}
▌ High folate

Management   ▌ Correct structural cause
▌ Tetracyclines
▌ Ciprofloxacin
▌ Metronidazole

Whipple's   ▌ Due to *Tropheryma whippeii*
disease   ▌ $\rightarrow$ Villous atrophy
(K&C, p. 295)   ▌ Diarrhoea and steatorrhoea
▌ Rare

Management   ▌ Antibiotics

Small bowel   ▌ Lymphomas
tumours   ▌ Adenocarcinomas (rare)
(K&C, p. 298)   ▌ Carcinoids

Carcinoid   ▌ Associated with metastatic carcinoid tumours
syndrome   ▌ Due to serotonin (5-hydroxytryptamine, 5-HT),
(K&C, p. 299)   bradykinin and histamine secretion by metastases
▌ Only symptomatic after hepatic involvement

Clinical features   ▌ Flushing
▌ Diarrhoea
▌ Right heart failure
▌ Hepatomegaly
▌ Pulmonary valve stenosis
▌ Tricuspid regurgitation

Investigations   ▌ 24-hour urinary 5-hydroxyindoleacetic acid (5-HIAA)
▌ CT or ultrasound of liver
▌ Octreotide-labelled scan

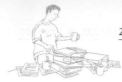

Management ❚ Octreotide to reduce symptoms
❚ Embolization of hepatic secondaries

Inflammatory bowel disease (K&C, p. 300)

Inflammatory diseases of the GI tract, of unknown aetiology. Both Crohn's disease and ulcerative colitis demonstrate uncontrolled inflammation.

Crohn's disease

Epidemiology ❚ 50–60/100 000
❚ More common in Caucasian races
❚ Familial association
❚ Genetic predisposition

Pathology ❚ Any part of gut from mouth to anus
❚ Skip lesions – patchy disease with normal mucosa in between
❚ Commonly terminal ileum and ascending colon
❚ → Ulceration, abscesses and fistulae
❚ Full bowel wall thickness involved
❚ Inflammatory infiltrates
❚ Non-caseating granulomata

Clinical features ❚ Depend on the area of bowel involved
❚ Mouth ulcers
❚ Diarrhoea
❚ Abdominal pain – colicky
❚ Nausea/vomiting
❚ Low-grade pyrexia
❚ Generally unwell, lethargy, weight loss
❚ Cutaneous fistulae (often perianal)

Disease associations ❚ Small joint arthritis
(Fig. 10.3) ❚ Sacroiliitis
❚ Ankylosing spondylitis
❚ Iritis/uveitis/conjunctivitis
❚ Erythema nodosum – tender lower leg lesions
❚ Pyoderma gangrenosum – skin ulceration
❚ Sclerosing cholangitis

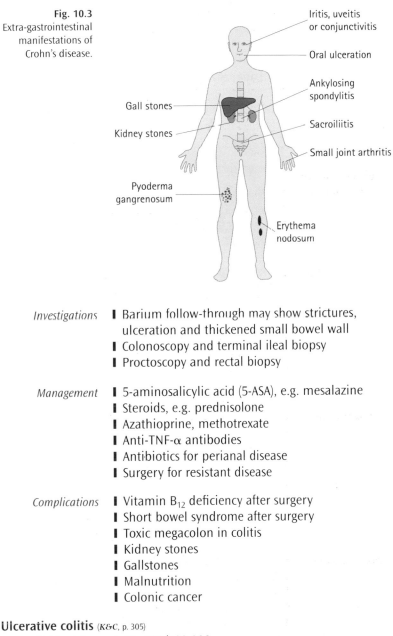

Fig. 10.3
Extra-gastrointestinal
manifestations of
Crohn's disease.

Iritis, uveitis
or conjunctivitis

Oral ulceration

Ankylosing
spondylitis

Gall stones

Sacroiliitis

Kidney stones

Small joint arthritis

Pyoderma
gangrenosum

Erythema
nodosum

Investigations
I Barium follow-through may show strictures, ulceration and thickened small bowel wall
I Colonoscopy and terminal ileal biopsy
I Proctoscopy and rectal biopsy

Management
I 5-aminosalicylic acid (5-ASA), e.g. mesalazine
I Steroids, e.g. prednisolone
I Azathioprine, methotrexate
I Anti-TNF-α antibodies
I Antibiotics for perianal disease
I Surgery for resistant disease

Complications
I Vitamin B_{12} deficiency after surgery
I Short bowel syndrome after surgery
I Toxic megacolon in colitis
I Kidney stones
I Gallstones
I Malnutrition
I Colonic cancer

Ulcerative colitis (*K&C*, p. 305)

Epidemiology
I 80–120/100 000
I Uncommon in smokers

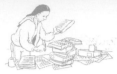

Pathology
- Limited to colon
- Inflammation spreads proximally from the rectum
- Mucosal inflammation
- → erythema, oedema and ulceration
- Inflammatory infiltrate
- Crypt abscesses
- Goblet cell depletion

Clinical features
- Diarrhoea
- Blood or mucus per rectum
- Mouth ulcers

Disease associations
- Uveitis/iritis/conjunctivitis
- Erythema nodosum/pyoderma gangrenosum
- Arthritis/sacroiliitis/ankylosing spondylitis
- Sclerosing cholangitis

Investigations
- Sigmoidoscopy and rectal biopsy
- Colonoscopy and biopsy
- Barium enema

Indicators of acute severe colitis urgent treatment
- > Six stools per day
- Fever > 37.5°C
- Tachycardia > 90 bpm
- ESR > 30 mm/hr

TOXIC MEGACOLON

Dilatation of the (transverse) colon with a high risk of perforation
Signs: fever, abdominal pain, bloody diarrhoea, tachycardia, hypotension

I.v. access and fluid resuscitation
Plain abdominal film to monitor colon diameter
Erect chest X-ray to rule out perforation
I.v. steroids and s.c. heparin
Early surgical involvement

Daily plain abdominal film
Maximum of 5 days of steroids
Consider i.v. ciclosporin

If poor response to treatment → colectomy

	I Haemoglobin < 10 g/dL
	I Albumin < 30 g/L
Management	I 5-ASA, e.g. mesalazine
	I Steroids, e.g. prednisolone
	I Azathioprine
	I Ciclosporin
	I Topical 5-ASA or steroids (enemas)
Complications	I Toxic megacolon
	I Iron deficiency anaemia
	I Increased risk of colorectal cancer

Colonic disease

Colorectal cancer (*K&C*, p. 316)

Epidemiology	I 1 in 27 of the population
	I Associated with 'Western' diet
	I Risk reduced by taking aspirin
	I 10% are familial
Aetiology	I Genetic predisposition
	— *apc* gene mutation
	— *p53* gene mutation
	— Microsatellite instability (failure of DNA repair)
Pathology	*Adenomatous polyps → dysplastic mucosa →*
	adenocarcinoma
	I Most commonly in sigmoid colon or rectum
	Microsatellite instability tumours
	I Not associated with polyp formation
	I More common in ascending colon and caecum
Familial cancers	*Familial adenomatous polyposis (FAP)*
	I *apc* gene mutation
	I → Multiple adenomatous polyps
	I → Very high risk of malignant change
	Hereditary non-polyposis colorectal cancer (HNPCC)
	I Associated with microsatellite instability

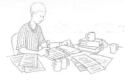

I Associated increased risk of upper GI and gynaecological cancers

Clinical features   **I** Change in bowel habit to diarrhoea
I Rectal blood/mucus
I Weight loss

Investigations   **I** Full blood count – iron deficiency anaemia
I Colonoscopy or
I Barium enema
I CT to stage the cancer (Table 10.10)

Management   **I** Surgical resection
I Adjuvant chemotherapy

Complications   **I** Bowel obstruction
I Iron deficiency anaemia
I Hepatic metastases

Screening   **I** Not yet introduced in the UK
— Faecal occult blood
— Sigmoidoscopy at 55 years

Table 10.10   Staging and survival of colorectal cancers

TNM classification	Modified Dukes' classification	5-Year survival (%)
Stage 0 — carcinoma in situ		
Stage I — no nodal involvement no metastases: tumour invades submucosa (T1,N0,M0); tumour invades muscularis propria (T2,N0,M0)	A	90–100
Stage II — no nodal involvement, no metastases: tumour invades into subserosa (T3,N0,M0); tumour invades other organs (T4,N0,M0)	B	75–85
Stage III — regional lymph nodes involved (any T,N1,M0)	C	30–40
Stage IV — distant metastases (any T, any N)	D	< 5

Diverticular disease *(K&C, p. 312)*	❚ Presence of mucosal pouches protruding outside the bowel ❚ Very common: 50% of those > 50 years old
Clinical features	❚ 90% asymptomatic ❚ Change in bowel habit ❚ Left iliac fossa pain (diverticulitis)
Investigations	❚ Barium enema ❚ Colonoscopy ❚ CT scan
Management	❚ High-fibre diet ❚ Antibiotics for diverticulitis
Complications	❚ Diverticulitis – inflammation/infection ❚ Diverticular abscess ❚ Lower GI bleeding ❚ Perforation
Functional bowel disease *(K&C, p. 326)*	❚ Irritable bowel syndrome ❚ GI symptoms without an identified pathology
Clinical features	❚ Left iliac fossa pain ❚ Alternating diarrhoea and constipation ❚ Bloating ❚ Rabbit pellet stools ❚ Sensation of incomplete evacuation
Investigations	❚ Normal physical examination ❚ Rule out gynaecological problems ❚ Sigmoidoscopy/colonoscopy
Management	❚ Reassurance ❚ Antispasmodics ❚ Dietary changes (e.g. increased fibre) ❚ Antidepressants may help

Changes in bowel habit

DIARRHOEA (Fig. 10.4) *(K&C, p. 320)*

An increase in stool weight to > 300 g per day, usually associated with an increase in stool frequency.

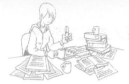

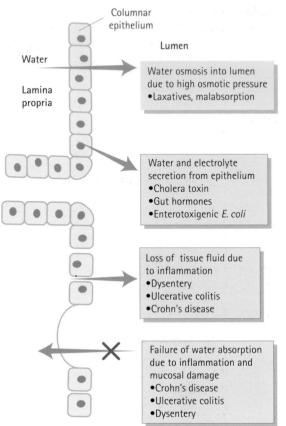

Fig. 10.4   Mechanisms of diarrhoea.

Osmotic diarrhoea	▌ Non-absorbable hypertonic substances in the bowel lumen → Osmotic pressure draws water into the bowel
Aetiology	▌ Purgatives, e.g. magnesium sulphate ▌ Malabsorption → solutes in the bowel, e.g. glucose ▌ Absorptive defects, e.g. glucose-galactose deficiency ▌ Diarrhoea stops when the patient stops eating or taking the purgative
Secretory diarrhoea	▌ Increased secretion and decreased absorption of fluid and electrolytes

Aetiology
- Cholera toxin
- *E.coli* heat-labile and stable toxins
- Hormones, e.g. vasoactive intestinal peptides
- Bile salts following terminal ileal resection
- Some laxatives

Inflammatory diarrhoea
- Mucosal inflammation → loss of fluid and blood
- May also → absorptive failure
- e.g. Ulcerative colitis, Crohn's disease, dysentery due to *Shigella*

INCREASED STOOL FREQUENCY

Abnormal GI tract motility
- Post-vagotomy
- Diabetic autonomic neuropathy
- Hyperthyroidism

Structural abnormalities
- Diverticular disease
- Colorectal carcinoma

Other
- Faecal impaction and overflow

CONSTIPATION (*K&C*, p. 309)

Aetiology
- Old age
- Immobility
- Low-volume/fibre diets
- Intestinal obstruction
- Colonic disease, e.g. colorectal carcinoma
- Hypothyroidism
- Hypocalcaemia
- Depression
- Drugs
  - — Opiates
  - — Iron
  - — Antidepressants
  - — Aluminium antacids

Management
- Bulking laxatives – fibre/bran
- Stimulants – anthraquinones (senna), bisacodyl
- Osmotics – magnesium sulphate
- Suppositories – bisacodyl
- Enemas – phosphate

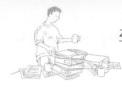

Gastrointestinal infections (K&C, p. 70)

A very common cause of morbidity and mortality, notably in the developing world.

VIRAL INFECTIONS

Aetiology
- Rotavirus → epidemic diarrhoea in children
- Enteric adenovirus types 40 and 41
- Calicivirus, e.g. Norwalk virus
- Astrovirus → watery diarrhoea and vomiting
- Small round structured viruses (SRSV)

Management
- Supportive

BACTERIAL INFECTIONS

Cholera·
(*K&C*, p. 87)
- *Vibrio cholerae*
- Faecal–oral transmission
- 'Ricewater' high-volume stools
- Secretory diarrhoea due to cAMP activation
- Treat with oral rehydration therapy
- Tetracycline or ciprofloxacin if severe

Salmonella
(*K&C*, p. 71)
- *Salmonella enteritidis* and *typhimurium*
- Eggs and poultry products
- 2–3 days of diarrhoea and malaise
- Rarely bloody diarrhoea
- Treat with oral rehydration

Staphylococcus
- *Staphylococcus aureus*
- Toxin-related gastroenteritis
- Short-lived diarrhoea and vomiting
- Treat dehydration

Escherichia coli
(*K&C*, p. 72)
- ETEC (enterotoxigenic) → watery diarrhoea
- EIEC (enteroinvasive) → dysentery
- EPEC (enteropathogenic) → diarrhoea
- EAEC (enteroadherent) → diarrhoea
- EHEC (enterohaemorrhagic) → haemorrhagic colitis ± haemolytic uraemic syndrome, associated with serotype O157:H7
- Treat symptoms; if severe, ciprofloxacin

Yersinia
- *Yersina enterocolitica* and *paratuberculosis*
- Enterocolitis, terminal ileitis
- → Fever, diarrhoea and abdominal pain
- May → arthritis and Reiter's syndrome

Campylobacter
(K&C, p. 71)
- *Campylobacter jejuni*
- Mucosal ulcer and inflammation, colitis
- → Diarrhoea ± blood, fever
- Cramping abdominal pains
- Management: supportive only

Complications
- Cholecystitis (salmonella)
- Arthritis (yersinia)
- Guillian-Barré syndrome (campylobacter)
- Haemolytic uraemic syndrome (EHEC 0157:47)

Shigellosis
(K&C, p. 71)
- *Shigella dysenteriae, flexneri, sonnei, boydii*
- Usually affects children
  → Fever, abdominal pain, watery diarrhoea
  → Bloody diarrhoea and abdominal cramps
- Treat symptoms; ciprofloxacin for severe cases

Bacillus cereus
- Toxin-mediated
- Short-lived vomiting
- Often contaminates rice

Clostridium
- *Clostridium perfringens*
- Spores in food
- Watery diarrhoea and pain
- Treat symptoms

Pseudo-membranous colitis
- *Clostridium difficile* A and B toxins
- After antibiotic therapy, e.g. cephalosporins
- → Colitis with ulceration and grey membrane
- → Bloody diarrhoea
- Treat by stopping antibiotics; oral metronidazole or vancomycin

Botulism
- *Clostridium botulinum*
- Preserved canned food
- → Nausea, vomiting and diarrhoea
- Neurotoxin → progressive paralysis

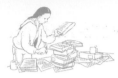

I Supportive treatment and antitoxin
I 50–70% mortality

PROTOZOAL INFECTION (K&C, pp. 106–109)

Amoeba
I *Entamoeba histolytica*
I → Dysentery and colitis, liver abscess
I Treat with metronidazole

Giardia
I *Giardia intestinalis (lamblia)*
I Diarrhoea and malabsorption
I Treat with metronidazole

Cryptosporidium
I *Cryptosporidium parvum*
I Water-borne
I Fever and diarrhoea

HELMINTHS (K&C, p. 112)

Nematodes
I *Strongyloides stercoralis*
I Hookworm *(Ancylostoma duodenale)*
I Roundworm *(Ascaris lumbricoides)*
I Threadworm *(Enterobius vermicularis)*

Cestodes
I Tapeworms *(Taenia saginata/solium)*

Pancreatic disease

Acute pancreatitis (K&C, p. 397)
I Acute inflammation of the pancreas

Aetiology
I Alcohol
I Gallstones
I Trauma
I ERCP
I Drugs
— Azathioprine
— Steroids
— Oral contraceptive
I Infections
— Mumps virus

— Coxsackie
— *Klebsiella*
❚ Metabolic
— Hypercalcaemia
— Hyperlipidaemia
— Renal failure
❚ Other
— Hypothermia
— Malnutrition
— Scorpion bites

Clinical features
❚ Abdominal pain
❚ Nausea and vomiting
❚ Anorexia
❚ Abdominal tenderness and guarding
❚ Flank bruising (Grey–Turner sign)
❚ Basal pulmonary crackles

Investigations
❚ Plain abdominal X-ray – pancreatic calcification
❚ Blood count – elevated neutrophils
❚ Urea and electrolytes – renal failure
❚ Calcium
❚ Amylase – elevated (Table 10.11)
❚ Blood gases – hypoxia and acidosis
❚ Liver function tests
❚ Ultrasound – gallstones
❚ CT – for complications

Table 10.11   Causes of a raised amylase

Pancreatic	Salivary
Acute/chronic pancreatitis	Adenitis, tumours, mumps
Pseudocysts	**Others**
Carcinoma	Diabetic ketoacidosis
Abdominal	Alcohol
Perforation, duodenal ulcer	Anorexia
Ectopic pregnancy	Burns
Ovarian tumours	
Hepatic	
Gallstones	
Acute hepatitis	

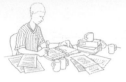

Management	❙ Oxygen
	❙ I.v. access and fluids
	❙ Supportive management
	❙ Analgesia
	❙ Early ERCP for obstructing gallstones
	❙ High-dependency nursing
Complications	❙ Hypoxia (respiratory distress syndrome)
	❙ Hypocalcaemia (fat saponification)
	❙ Renal failure
	❙ Pseudocyst formation
	❙ Sepsis
Prognosis	❙ See Table 10.12

Chronic pancreatitis (*K&C*, p. 400)

❙ Long-standing or repeated attacks of pancreatitis resulting in fibrosis

Aetiology	❙ Alcohol
	❙ Gallstones
Clinical features	❙ Chronic abdominal pain
	❙ Weight loss
	❙ Steatorrhoea
Investigations	❙ Plain abdominal X-ray shows pancreatic calcification
	❙ Amylase is often normal
	❙ Ultrasound – calcification
	❙ Pancreatic function – reduced

Table 10.12 Poor prognostic indicators in acute pancreatitis in the first 48 hours

Age	> 55 years
WCC	> 15 × 10^9/mL
Glucose	> 10 mmol/L
Urea	> 16 mmol/L
Albumin	< 30 g/L
ALT	> 200 IU
Calcium	< 2 mmol/L
LDH	> 600 IU
P_aO_2	< 8 kPa

■ Blood sugar – elevated due to diabetes
■ CT scan

Management ■ Pancreatic supplements
■ Analgesia

Pancreatic malignancy
(*K&C*, p. 402)
■ Majority are adenocarcinomas
■ Often present late
■ Poor prognosis

Clinical features ■ Painless jaundice – bile duct compression
■ Anorexia
■ Weight loss
■ Periumbilical lymphadenopathy

Investigations ■ Ultrasound/CT/MRI to identify primary
■ ERCP

Management ■ ERCP stenting to relieve jaundice
■ Surgical resection of primary (rarely possible)
■ Palliative care

Pancreatic endocrine tumours
■ Gastrinomas and rarely other hormone-secreting tumours (e.g. insulinomas)
■ Symptoms depend on hormone secreted

Zollinger–Ellison syndrome
■ Gastrin-secreting tumour
■ → High gastric acid secretion
■ → Multiple gastroduodenal ulcers
■ Diarrhoea

Jaundice (Table 10.13 and Fig. 10.5) (*K&C*, p. 346)

PRE-HEPATIC

Increased red cell breakdown ■ Haemolytic anaemia

HEPATIC

Failure of bilirubin metabolism or excretion
Congenital defects ■ Gilbert's syndrome
■ Crigler–Najjar syndrome

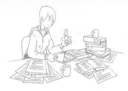

Table 10.13   Classification of hyperbilirubinaemia

Unconjugated	Conjugated
Water-insoluble	Water-soluble
Not excreted by kidney	Renal excretion
Pre-hepatic jaundice	Post-hepatic jaundice
Gilbert's syndrome	Some inherited jaundice
Crigler–Najjar syndrome	Hepatitis and cirrhosis

Fig. 10.5
Bilirubin metabolism.

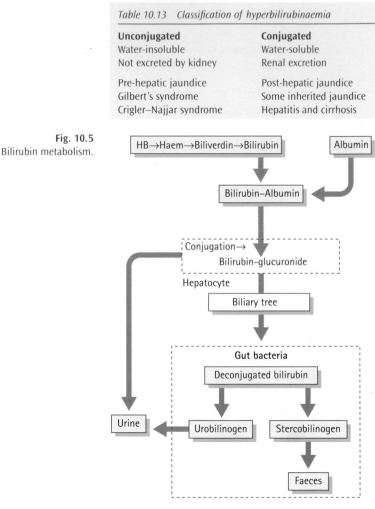

Hepatic inflammation (hepatitis)
- Viral hepatitis
- Drugs (see Table 10.10)
- Autoimmune hepatitis
- Alcohol
- Haemochromatosis
- Wilson's disease

Cirrhosis
- Alcohol
- Chronic hepatitis
- Metabolic disorders

Hepatic tumours   ▌ Hepatocellular carcinoma
▌ Hepatic metastases

POST-HEPATIC

Biliary obstruction   ▌ Gallstones
▌ Cholangiocarcinoma
▌ Pancreatic carcinoma
▌ Primary biliary cirrhosis
▌ Sclerosing cholangitis

Hepatitis (Table 10.14) (K&C, p. 350)

Acute hepatocyte breakdown leading to release of aminotransferases (ALT, AST) and jaundice. Prolonged or severe damage results in synthetic failure, leading to a reduction in the synthesis of albumin and clotting factors (causing an elevated prothrombin time).

VIRAL HEPATITIS (K&C, p. 351)

Hepatitis A (HAV)   ▌ RNA virus
▌ Faecal–oral spread (e.g. shellfish)
▌ Incubation 2–3 weeks
▌ No progression → chronic liver disease

Clinical features   ▌ Nausea
▌ Anorexia
▌ Jaundice ± hepatomegaly/rash

Investigations   ▌ Anti-HAV IgM
▌ Elevated ALT/aspartate aminotransferase (AST)
▌ Elevated bilirubin (may be subclinical)

Table 10.14   Causes of chronic hepatitis

Viruses	Hereditary
Hepatitis B ± D	α_1-antitrypsin disease
Hepatitis C	Wilson's disease
Autoimmune hepatitis	**Others**
Drugs	Ulcerative colitis
Methyldopa	Alcohol (rare)
Isoniazid	

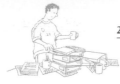

Management	▌ Supportive

Hepatitis B (HBV)
(*K&C*, p. 353)

▌ DNA virus
▌ Blood/saliva/sexual/vertical spread
▌ Incubation 1–5 months
▌ 10–15% carriage in Africa and Far East

Clinical features

▌ Jaundice/malaise ± rash
▌ May be asymptomatic

Investigations
(Fig. 10.6)

▌ Liver biochemistry – ALT elevated first then bilirubin

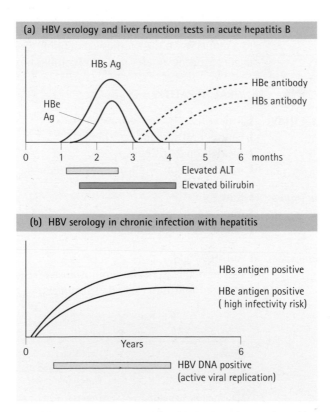

Fig. 10.6   Hepatitis B. A. HBV serology and liver biochemistry in acute hepatitis B. B. HBV serology in chronic infection with hepatitis.

Acute infection
❚ Surface antigen (HBsAg) first marker
❚ e antigen (HBeAg)

Seroconversion
❚ Anti-HBs antibody
❚ Anti-HBe antibody
❚ Anti-HBc antibody (IgM)

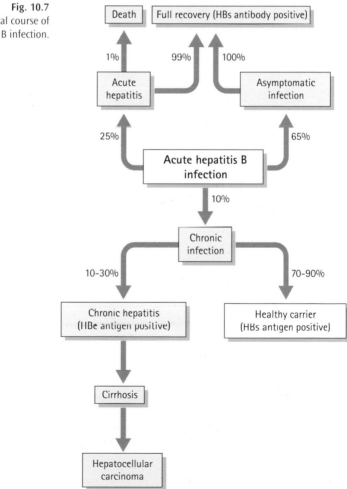

Fig. 10.7
Clinical course of
hepatitis B infection.

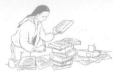

Successful clearance of virus or post vaccine
❚ Anti-HBs antibody

Chronic carrier state
❚ HBs antigen (chronic infection)
❚ HBe antigen (infectious carrier)
❚ Positive HBV DNA (active viral replication)

Management ❚ Treat symptoms
❚ Interferon and lamivudine for chronic infection

Complications ❚ Chronic infection → chronic liver disease
❚ Hepatocellular carcinoma
❚ 1% → fulminant hepatitis → death

Hepatitis D ❚ Only causes hepatitis when it coinfects with
hepatitis B
❚ Commonest in i.v. drug abusers
❚ Diagnosis by detection of specific antibodies

Hepatitis C ❚ RNA virus
(HCV; Fig. 10.8) ❚ Blood spread (rarely sex/saliva)
(*K&C*, p. 356) ❚ Acute infection often asymptomatic
❚ 50% → chronic liver disease
❚ 30% of these → cirrhosis
❚ 5% of these → hepatocellular carcinoma

Investigations ❚ Anti-HCV antibodies
❚ HCV RNA in blood
❚ Abnormal liver function in chronic infection
❚ Ultrasound and α-fetoprotein to detect
hepatocellular carcinoma

Management ❚ Interferon and ribavirin give the best chance of
clearance of the virus (in 60–70%)

Others ❚ Hepatitis E (1–2% mortality in pregnancy)
❚ Epstein–Barr virus (EBV)
❚ Cytomegalovirus (CMV)
❚ Yellow fever

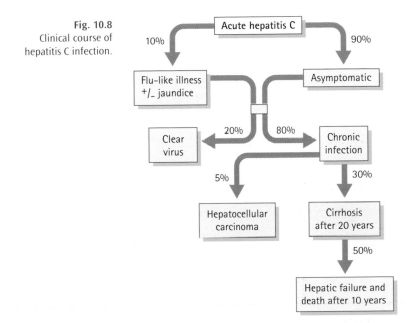

Fig. 10.8
Clinical course of
hepatitis C infection.

AUTOIMMUNE HEPATITIS (K&C, p. 362)

Epidemiology
❙ ♀ > ♂
❙ Associated with other autoimmune disease

Clinical features
❙ May be asymptomatic
❙ Jaundice
❙ Bruising
❙ Signs of acute or chronic liver disease

Investigations
❙ Antinuclear antibodies ⎫
❙ Anti-smooth muscle antibodies ⎬ Type I
❙ Antimitochondrial antibodies ⎭

❙ Anti-liver/kidney microsomal antibodies ⎫ Type II
❙ Anti-liver cytosol antibodies ⎭

Management
❙ Steroids/azathioprine

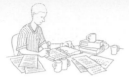

FULMINANT HEPATIC FAILURE (K&C, p. 357)

Aetiology
- Hepatitis A/D/E
- Drugs
  — Paracetamol
  — Volatile liquid anaesthetics
  — Isoniazid
  — Ecstasy
- Wilson's disease
- Pregnancy
- Reye's syndrome

Clinical features
- Jaundice
- Encephalopathy
- Drowsiness → coma
- Hypoglycaemia
- Low potassium or calcium
- Haemorrhage

Management
- Treat on a specialist unit
- Supportive therapy
- Liver transplant

Cirrhosis (K&C, p. 363)

Liver cell necrosis followed by nodular regeneration and fibrosis, resulting in increased resistance to blood flow and deranged liver function.

Aetiology
- Alcohol
- Hepatitis B or C
- Biliary cirrhosis
- Autoimmune hepatitis
- Haemochromatosis
- Wilson's disease
- α_1-antitrypsin disease
- Cystic fibrosis
- Non-alcoholic fatty liver disease (NAFLD)

Clinical features

Chronic liver dysfunction
▮ Jaundice
▮ Anaemia
▮ Bruising
▮ Palmar erythema
▮ Dupuytren's contracture

Portal hypertension
▮ Splenomegaly
▮ Ascites
▮ Spider naevi
▮ Caput medusae
▮ Oesophageal/rectal varices

Investigations
(Table 10.15)
▮ ALT/AST may be high or normal
▮ Alkaline phosphatase is usually high
▮ Bilirubin is usually high
▮ Albumin falls as cirrhosis worsens
▮ Prothrombin time often prolonged
▮ Sodium low in severe disease
▮ α-fetoprotein – hepatocellular carcinoma
▮ Ultrasound – liver may be large, normal or small; splenomegaly
▮ Endoscopy for oesophageal varices

Management
▮ Stop drinking
▮ Treat complications
▮ Transplantation

Table 10.15   Liver function tests

Hepatocellular damage (hepatitis)
Aminotransferases (ALT/AST)
γ-Glutamyl transpeptidase (γ-GT)

Cholestasis (bile ducts)
Bilirubin
Alkaline phosphatase

Synthetic function
Albumin
Prothrombin time

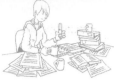

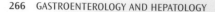

Complications
(Table 10.16)

Ascites (Table 10.17)
❚ Transudate (protein < 30 g/L in fluid)
❚ Treatment
— Water and salt restriction
— Spironolactone + loop diuretics
— Ascitic drainage

Serum–ascites albumin gradient
❚ > 11 g suggests transudate
❚ More sensitive than absolute protein

Spontaneous bacterial peritonitis
❚ → Worsening of clinical state
❚ Diagnosis: ascitic tap
❚ Treatment: parenteral antibiotics

Variceal bleeding
❚ See page 238

Table 10.16   Indicators of poor prognosis in cirrhosis

Albumin < 25 g/L
Sodium < 120 mmol/L
Prolonged prothrombin time
Persistent jaundice
Ascites
Variceal bleeding

Table 10.17   Causes of ascites

Transudate (protein < 30 g/L)	**Exudate (protein > 30 g/L)**
Portal hypertension	Infections
Cirrhosis of the liver	Peritoneal tuberculosis
Portal vein thrombosis	Malignancy
Low serum protein	Ovarian carcinoma
Liver disease	Peritoneal metastases
Nephrotic syndrome	Inflammatory
Malnutrition	Pancreatitis
Others	
Right ventricular failure	
Myxoedema	

Encephalopathy
I See page 270

Hepatorenal syndrome
I Advanced cirrhosis with ascites and jaundice
I Low urine volume
I Low urinary sodium
I Hepatocellular carcinoma

SPECIFIC CAUSES OF CIRRHOSIS

Primary biliary cirrhosis (K&C, p. 373)
I Chronic destruction of bile ducts
I ♀ > ♂

Clinical features
I Jaundice
I Itching
I Xanthelasma
I Hepatosplenomegaly

Investigations
I Antimitochondrial (M2) antibodies
I High alkaline phosphatase
I Relatively normal ALT
I Ultrasound
I Liver biopsy

Management
I Ursodeoxycholic acid may normalize liver biochemistry
I Supplement fat-soluble vitamins (A, D, E, K)
I Colestyramine for itching
I Liver transplant when bilirubin > 100 μmol/L

Hereditary haemochromatosis (K&C, p. 375)
I Autosomal recessive
I 1:400 homozygous
I → Abnormalities of iron transportation
I → Accumulation of iron in epithelial cells
I ♂ = ♀ but women less severely affected due to menstruation

Clinical features
I Cardiomyopathy: cardiac myocytes
I Diabetes: pancreas

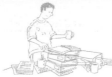

■ Hypogonadism: pituitary
■ Hepatitis and cirrhosis: liver
■ Pigmentation: skin

Investigations
■ Ferritin > 500 μg/L
■ Serum iron > 30 μmol/L
■ Transferrin saturation > 60%
■ Liver biopsy
■ Screen family for genetic mutation (HFe gene)

Management
■ Venesection to normalize ferritin

Wilson's disease
(K&C, p. 376)
■ Autosomal recessive
■ Defect of copper transport
■ → Failure of biliary copper excretion

Clinical features
■ Liver: chronic hepatitis → cirrhosis
■ Basal ganglia: tremor, dysarthria, dementia
■ Kidneys: tubular degeneration
■ Eyes: Kayser–Fleischer rings

Investigations
■ Reduced serum copper and caeruloplasmin
■ Elevated urinary copper
■ Liver biopsy

Management
■ Penicillamine – chelates copper

α_1-antitrypsin deficiency *(K&C, p. 377)*
■ Inherited deficiency of α_1-antitrypsin
■ Autosomal dominant
■ Liver cirrhosis
■ Early emphysema in smokers

ALCOHOL-RELATED LIVER DISEASE AND ALCOHOLISM *(K&C, p. 378)*

Pathology
■ Fatty change
■ Alcoholic hepatitis
■ Cirrhosis

Clinical features
■ Those of the stage of liver disease (see above)

Investigations   ❚ Abnormal liver function
❚ γ-GT elevation
❚ Liver biopsy
❚ Ultrasound
❚ α-fetoprotein for hepatocellular carcinoma
❚ CAGE questionnaire
— Are you **C**oncerned about your alcohol intake?
— Are others **A**nxious about your drinking?
— Do you feel **G**uilty about drinking?
— Do you need an '**E**ye opener' to avoid withdrawal?

Management   ❚ Cessation of alcohol consumption
❚ Support during physical withdrawal (Table 10.18)
❚ Psychological support

Complications   ❚ Hepatocellular carcinoma (10–15%)
❚ End-stage liver disease
❚ Wernicke–Korsakoff syndrome (see below)
❚ Encephalopathy
❚ Dementia
❚ Epilepsy (5–10%)

Wernicke–Korsakoff syndrome
❚ Thiamin deficiency
❚ → Acute Wernicke's syndrome
— Nystagmus, ataxia, confusion
❚ → Chronic Korsakoff's syndrome
— Dementia, chronic amnesia, confabulation
❚ Investigations: red cell transketolase
❚ Management: parenteral thiamine

Table 10.18   Alcohol withdrawal

Clinical features
Morning shakes
Tremor
Delirium tremens: tremor, hallucinations
Convulsions

Management
Benzodiazepines to help with symptoms
Nutritional support

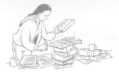

HEPATIC ENCEPHALOPATHY

I Reversible neuropsychiatric deficit

Clinical features
I Flapping tremor of hands
I Decreased level of consciousness
I Personality changes
I Intellectual deterioration
I Slow, slurred speech
I Constructional apraxia – unable to copy a drawn five-pointed star

Worsened by
I Sepsis
I Constipation, diarrhoea or vomiting
I Diuretics
I GI bleeding
I Alcohol withdrawal

Investigations
I Urea and electrolytes
I Full blood count

ASSESSING HEPATIC ENCEPHALOPATHY

Presence of 'liver flap'
Straight arms and hyperextended wrist with fingers splayed
Slow wrist flexion

Assessment of conscious level
Glasgow coma score

Assessment of cognition
Mini-mental test

Assessment of apraxia
Ask patient to copy a five-pointed star

Repeat on a daily basis to demonstrate changes in encephalopathy

I Liver function tests
I EEG
I Blood cultures to detect sepsis
I Ascitic tap for spontaneous bacterial peritonitis

Management I Laxatives to reduce constipation
I Treat sepsis
I Careful fluid balance
I Supportive treatment

Other diseases of the liver

Liver abscess I Single or multiple abscesses
(*K&C*, p. 381) I *E. coli*
I *Enterococcus faecalis*
I *Staphylococcus aureus*
I *Entamoeba histolytica* (amoeba)
I → Fever, rigors, vomiting, weight loss, shock

Investigations I Blood count – anaemia and leucocytosis
I Blood cultures
I Amoeba serology
I Ultrasound

Management I Broad-spectrum antibiotics
I Ultrasound-guided drainage

Budd Chiari syndrome (*K&C*, p. 379)
I Hepatic vein thrombosis
I → Hepatic failure
I Clinical ascites, abdominal pain and vomiting
I Hepatomegaly

Pregnancy related liver disease (*K&C*, p. 382)
I Fatty liver
I Hepatitis
I Cholestasis
I Eclampsia → hepatic necrosis
I HELLP syndrome (haemolysis, elevated liver
enzymes, low platelets)

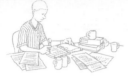

Hepatocellular carcinoma *(K&C, p. 384)*

- Common worldwide
- Alcohol, hepatitis B or C-related
- Investigations: ultrasound and α-fetoprotein
- Local treatment or transplantation

Hepatic metastases
- Commonest hepatic tumours
- GI tract, breast and lung carcinomas

Hepatic steatosis

- 'Fatty liver'
- ALT usually elevated
- Commonly asymptomatic
- Commonly associated with alcohol
- Hyperlipidaemia
- Obesity
- Diabetes mellitus

NASH
- Non-alcoholic steatohepatitis
- Fat deposition and inflammation in the liver

NAFLD
- Non-alcoholic fatty liver disease
- Fat deposition
- Does not require inflammation for the diagnosis
- Excludes alcohol as a cause

Diseases of the biliary tree

Gallstones (Table 10.19) *(K&C, p. 387)*
- 10–20% of the population
- Often an incidental finding at ultrasound

Types
- Cholesterol stones
- Bile pigment stones

Clinical features
- 80% asymptomatic
- Acute cholecystitis – impacted stone leading to inflammation → right hypochondrial and shoulder tip pain, fever, vomiting ± jaundice

Table 10.19   Risk factors for gallstones

Increasing age
♀ > ♂
Multiparity
Obesity
Diet high in animal fat
Weight loss
Contraceptive pill
Ileal resection/disease
Diabetes

| Biliary obstruction by a gallstone → pain and jaundice; ERCP may be required to remove stone

Complications | Pancreatitis
| Biliary – enteric fistula
| Gallstone ileus

Cholangio-carcinoma (K&C, p. 384)

| Primary tumour of bile ducts
| → Obstructive jaundice

Primary sclerosing cholangitis (K&C, p. 393)

| Multiple bile duct strictures
| Associated with ulcerative colitis
| Increased risk of cholangiocarcinoma
| Investigations: ERCP

Drugs and the liver (K&C, p. 385)

The liver is responsible for the initial metabolism of oral drugs (first-pass metabolism) prior to the drug reaching the systemic circulation. Many drugs are also metabolized or excreted by the liver after reaching the systemic circulation. As a result, drugs can be responsible for hepatic disease (Table 10.20 and Fig. 10.9).

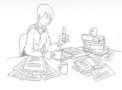
Table 10.20   Drugs and the liver

Drugs causing hepatitis	Penicillins
Isoniazid	Amoxicillin
Methyldopa	Flucloxacillin
Enalapril	NSAIDs
Nifedipine	Salicylates
Ketoconazole	Diclofenac
Volatile anaesthetics	Allopurinol
Rifampicin	Phenytoin
Atenolol	Diltiazem
Verapamil	Antithyroid
Amiodarone	Carbimazole
Cytotoxics	Propylthiouracil
Drugs causing cholestasis	**Miscellaneous**
Oestrogens	*Necrosis*
Ciclosporin	Carbon tetrachloride
Chlorpromazine	Paracetamol
Cimetidine	Salicylates
Erythromycin	Cocaine
Imipramine	*Fibrosis*
Azathioprine	Methotrexate
Haloperidol	Retinoids
Ranitidine	*Tumours*
Nitrofurantoin	High-oestrogen OCP
Hypoglycaemics	*Chronic hepatitis*
Hypersensitivity-mediated damage	Methyldopa
	Isoniazid
Sulphonamides	Nitrofurantoin

Fig. 10.9
Paracetamol
metabolism.

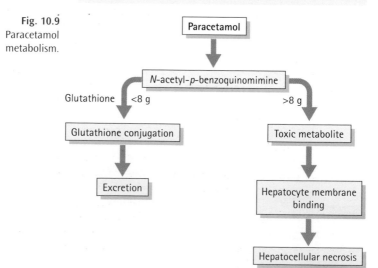

Self-assessment questions

Multiple choice questions

1. The following are causes of jaundice
   A. Cancer of the head of the pancreas
   B. Sulphonamide antibiotics
   C. Malaria
   D. Iron deficiency anaemia
   E. Epstein–Barr virus

2. Ascites may be due to:
   A. Ovarian cancer
   B. Alcohol abuse
   C. Anaemia
   D. Coeliac disease
   E. Hypoalbuminaemia

3. The following may be used to diagnose *Helicobacter pylori* infection:
   A. Blood urease test
   B. Endoscopy and biopsy
   C. *H. pylori* antigen in stool
   D. ^{13}C urea breath test
   E. Serum *H. pylori* antibodies

4. The following are causes of hepatosplenomegaly:
   A. Portal hypertension
   B. Carcinoma of the head of the pancreas
   C. Non-Hodgkin's lymphoma
   D. Amyloidosis
   E. Right heart failure

5. The following are complications of chronic gastro-oesophageal reflux disease.
   A. Bronchospasm
   B. Headache
   C. Barrett's oesophagus

   D. Achalasia
   E. Oesophageal stricture

6. The following increase the risk of oesophageal carcinoma:
   A. Omeprazole
   B. Barrett's oesophagus
   C. Gastro-oesophageal reflux disease
   D. Smoking
   E. *H. pylori*

7. The following are features of Barrett's oesophagus:
   A. The presence of goblet cells
   B. Transitional cell metaplasia of the oesophageal mucosa
   C. Increased risk of oesophageal squamous cell carcinoma
   D. The presence of small bowel-type mucosa in the distal oesophagus
   E. Mucosal dysplasia

8. The following are associated with oesophageal varices:
   A. Splenomegaly
   B. Acute viral hepatitis
   C. Nodular regeneration and fibrosis of the liver
   D. Portal hypertension
   E. Reduced risk of bleeding with propranolol

9. The following reduce lower oesophageal sphincter tone:
   A. Alcohol
   B. Nifedipine
   C. Achalasia
   D. Isosorbide mononitrate
   E. Botulinum toxin

10. The following are recognized causes of gastric ulcers:
    A. Indometacin
    B. Proton pump inhibitors
    C. Gastric lymphoma
    D. *H. pylori*
    E. Alendronate

11. The following are causes of gastritis:
    A. *H. pylori*
    B. Indometacin
    C. Pantoprazole
    D. Renal failure
    E. Thyrotoxicosis

12. Gastric MALT lymphoma:
    A. Is a tumour arising from basophils in the gastric mucosa
    B. May be effectively treated by omeprazole, clarithromycin and amoxicillin
    C. Rarely metastasizes
    D. Can arise anywhere in the gastrointestinal tract
    E. Is a non-Hodgkin's lymphoma

13. The following are associated with a decreased risk of gastric adenocarcinoma:
    A. High dietary ascorbic acid
    B. Active *H. pylori* infection
    C. Gastric intestinal metaplasia
    D. Smoking
    E. Coeliac disease

14. The following are useful in the management of peptic duodenal ulcers:
    A. Omeprazole
    B. Aspirin
    C. Metronidazole
    D. Bismuth
    E. Mesalazine

15. The following are associated with coeliac disease:
    A. Primary biliary cirrhosis
    B. Hypothyroidism
    C. Hypersplenism
    D. Dermatitis herpetiformis
    E. Vitamin B_{12} deficiency

16. The following are histological features of coeliac disease:
    A. Crypt shortening
    B. Decreased lamina propria lymphocytes
    C. Villus shortening
    D. Crypt abscesses
    E. Jejunal ulceration

17. The following are true of carcinoid syndrome:
    A. Lung metastases result in right-sided cardiac valve lesions
    B. Flushing and diarrhoea may occur
    C. Octreotide is of little therapeutic use
    D. The primary tumour is commonly in the small bowel
    E. Serum 5-HIAA is a useful diagnostic test

18. The following would favour the diagnosis of ulcerative colitis rather than Crohn's disease:
    A. Non-caseating granulomata
    B. Crypt abscesses
    C. Enterovesical fistula formation
    D. Oral ulceration
    E. Failure to respond to oral prednisolone

19. The following are recognized manifestations of Crohn's disease:
    A. Uveitis
    B. Erythema multiforme
    C. Gallstones

D. Subacute small bowel obstruction
E. Ankylosing spondylitis

20. The following are risk factors for the development of colorectal cancer:
    A. NSAID consumption
    B. Familial polyposis coli
    C. Smoking
    D. Ulcerative colitis
    E. Diverticulosis

21. A 78-year-old man presents with increased stool frequency and rectal mucus. The following are likely diagnoses:
    A. Diverticular disease
    B. Colonic angiodysplasia
    C. Tubulovillous adenoma of the rectum
    D. Colorectal cancer
    E. Thyrotoxicosis

22. The following are more likely to indicate a diagnosis of irritable bowel syndrome than colorectal carcinoma:
    A. Rectal bleeding
    B. Weight loss
    C. Alternating diarrhoea and constipation
    D. Sensation of incomplete evacuation of stool
    E. Bloating

23. The following are sometimes useful in the management of the irritable bowel syndrome:
    A. Mebeverine
    B. Ibuprofen
    C. Peppermint
    D. Prednisolone
    E. Mesalazine

24. The following are causes of diarrhoea:
    A. Senna
    B. *Staph. aureus*
    C. Vasoactive intestinal peptide (VIP)
    D. Loperamide
    E. Hypothyroidism

25. The following are causes of an increased stool frequency:
    A. Vagotomy
    B. Diabetes mellitus
    C. Alcohol
    D. Hypocalcaemia
    E. Hyperparathyroidism

26. The following organisms cause diarrhoea mainly via the mechanism given:
    A. Cholera – mucosal inflammation
    B. *E. coli* – enterotoxin production
    C. *Campylobacter* – mucosal inflammation
    D. *Bacillus cereus* – colonic ulceration
    E. Giardia – malabsorption of water

27. The following are true of pseudomembranous colitis:
    A. Diagnosis is based on the presence of *Clostridium difficile* in stool
    B. It is best treated with intravenous vancomycin
    C. Risk of the disease is increased by intravenous cephalosporins
    D. It may result in bloody diarrhoea
    E. The causal bacterium is a normal commensal gut organism

28. The following are recognized causes of acute pancreatitis:
    A. Gallstones
    B. Prednisolone
    C. Thyroxine
    D. Coxsackie virus infection
    E. Hyperlipidaemia

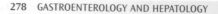

29. The following are indicators of poor prognosis in acute pancreatitis:
   A. Glucose < 6 mmol/L
   B. Hypocalcaemia
   C. Hypoxia
   D. Albumin > 30 g/L
   E. P_aco_2 < 5 kPa

30. The following favour a diagnosis of pancreatic carcinoma over acute viral hepatitis in painless jaundice:
   A. Weight loss
   B. Dilated bile ducts on ultrasound scanning
   C. Elevated alkaline phosphatase
   D. Unconjugated hyperbilirubinaemia
   E. Bilirubin > 300 μmol/L

31. The following are associated with an elevated serum gastrin:
   A. Omeprazole therapy
   B. Zollinger–Ellison syndrome
   C. Hyperchlorhydria
   D. Vagotomy
   E. Hypoglycaemia

32. The following are causes of a conjugated hyperbilirubinaemia:
   A. Gilbert's syndrome
   B. Carcinoma of the head of the pancreas
   C. Cholangiocarcinoma
   D. Viral hepatitis
   E. Haemolytic anaemia

33. The following are associated with acute hepatitis A infection:
   A. Elevated alanine transaminase
   B. Nausea and vomiting
   C. Bilirubin level always greater than 100 μmol/L
   D. Progression to chronic hepatitis
   E. Food-related outbreaks

34. The following statements are correct in the interpretation of hepatitis B serology:
   A. HBs (surface) antibody positive – previous exposure to infection
   B. HBe antigen positive – high infectivity risk
   C. HBc (core) antibody positive – seroconversion
   D. HBs antigen positive – successful immunization
   E. HBe antibody positive – seroconversion after acute infection

35. The following are associated with hepatitis C infection:
   A. Cryoglobulinaemia
   B. Hepatocellular carcinoma
   C. Primary sclerosing cholangitis
   D. Hepatic cirrhosis
   E. Ascites

36. The following are causes of viral hepatitis:
   A. Epstein–Barr virus
   B. Isolated hepatitis D virus
   C. Cytomegalovirus in immunosuppressed patients
   D. Coxsackie virus
   E. Adenovirus

37. The following are causes of fulminant hepatic failure:
   A. Paracetamol
   B. Hepatitis A
   C. Aspirin in childhood
   D. Halothane
   E. Haemochromatosis

38. The following are clinical features of cirrhosis of the liver except:
   A. Palmar erythema
   B. Caput medusae
   C. Macrocytosis

D. Portal hypotension

E. Bruising

39. The following are causes of transudative ascites:

A. Right heart failure

B. Peritoneal tuberculosis

C. Ovarian malignancy

D. Nephrotic syndrome

E. Liver cirrhosis

40. The following drugs may be associated with abnormalities of liver function except:

A. Ursodeoxycholic acid

B. Flucloxacillin

C. Ibuprofen

D. Verapamil

E. Thyroxine

Extended matching questions

Question 1 *Theme: diarrhoea*

A. E. coli

B. Thyrotoxicosis

C. Hypercalcaemia

D. Autonomic neuropathy

E. Laxative abuse

F. Osmotic diarrhoea

G. Ulcerative colitis

H. Tubulovillous adenoma

I. Diverticular disease

J. Coeliac disease

K. Giardiasis

L. Pseudomembranous colitis

For each of the following questions, select the best answer from the list above:

I. A 65-year-old man with known diabetes mellitus is reviewed as he has worsening diarrhoea. Upper gastrointestinal endoscopy, duodenal biopsy and barium enema were all normal. Stool culture carried out on three occasions did not reveal any abnormality. Blood testing revealed normal urea and electrolytes, calcium and liver function. What is the most likely cause for his diarrhoea?

II. A 38-year-old man is admitted with profuse mucus per rectum and generalized weakness. His potassium is noted to be 2.9 mmol/L. What is the most likely diagnosis?

III. A 27-year-old woman is admitted with abdominal discomfort, profuse bloody diarrhoea and a low-grade fever. Investigations reveal an iron deficiency anaemia. What is the most likely reason for her diarrhoea?

Question 2 *Theme: abdominal pain*

A. Sigmoid volvulus

B. Acute appendicitis

C. Cholecystitis

D. Duodenal ulceration

E. Bowel ischaemia

F. Diverticulosis

G. Crohn's disease

H. Irritable bowel syndrome

I. Acute pancreatitis

J. Colorectal carcinoma

K. Carcinoid syndrome

L. Ovarian cysts

M. Ectopic pregnancy

For each of the following questions, select the best answer from the list above:

I. A 76-year-old man complains of pain in the abdomen after eating. This is associated with mild diarrhoea. In the past he has had a myocardial infarction and several episodes of angina. He has type II diabetes mellitus. He smokes 20 cigarettes a day and drinks 10 units of alcohol a week. Suggest a likely cause for his pain.

II. A 32-year-old woman is referred by her GP with abdominal pain, nausea, weight loss and diarrhoea. She is also complaining of a bruise-like rash on her lower legs and mild joint pains. On examination she has multiple oral aphthous ulcers and tender bruise-like lesions over her shins.
What is the cause of her abdominal pain?

III. A 47-year-old woman is referred with left iliac fossa pain, bloating and alternating diarrhoea and constipation. Her weight is gradually increasing. The discomfort comes and goes but is not relieved by defaecation.
What is the most likely diagnosis?

Question 3 *Theme: malabsorption*

A. Pernicious anaemia
B. Coeliac disease
C. Whipple's disease
D. Primary biliary cirrhosis
E. Chronic pancreatitis
F. Cystic fibrosis
G. Bacterial overgrowth
H. Surgery for ileal Crohn's disease
I. Partial gastrectomy
J. Chronic alcohol-related liver disease
K. Carcinoma of the head of the pancreas

For each of the following questions, select the best answer from the list above:

I. A 15-year-old man is referred with a 6-year history of abdominal pain, bloating and weight loss. He is 1.78 m (5 feet 2 inches) tall and weighs 47 kg (7 stones 6 pounds). He has diarrhoea 2–3 times a day.
What is the most likely diagnosis?

II. A 56-year-old woman is noted to be vitamin B_{12}-deficient and anaemic. She has known autoimmune hypothyroidism but is otherwise well.

What is causing her B_{12} deficiency?

III. A 49-year-old man with a long history of alcohol abuse is reviewed due to worsening diarrhoea and abdominal pain. The stools are reported as foul-smelling and difficult to flush. His liver function tests are mildly deranged. What is the cause of his symptoms?

Short answer questions

1. Write short notes on the following:
   A. Post-hepatic jaundice
   B. Spider naevi
   C. Dupuytren's contracture
   D. Causes of hepatomegaly

2. Write short notes on the following:
   A. Causes of gastric ulcers
   B. *H. pylori*
   C. Hiatus hernias
   D. Reflux oesophagitis

3. Outline the role of the following in peptic ulcer disease:
   A. NSAIDs
   B. Proton pump inhibitors
   c. *H. pylori*

4. Write short notes on the following:
   A. Investigation of ulcerative colitis
   B. Histological features of Crohn's disease
   C. Management of toxic megacolon

5. Outline the role of the following in colorectal carcinoma:
   A. Genetic abnormalities
   B. Adenomatous polyps
   C. NSAIDs

6. Write short notes on the following:
   A. Management of acute pancreatitis
   B. Causes of chronic pancreatitis
   C. Investigation of painless jaundice

7. Write short notes on the following:
   A. Management of chronic hepatitis C infection
   B. Hepatocellular carcinoma
   C. Hepatitis D infection

8. Outline the disease states and the metabolic abnormalities associated with:
   A. Unconjugated hyperbilirubinaemias
   B. Elevated alanine transaminase
   C. Prolonged prothrombin time

Essay questions

1. Discuss the role of endoscopy in the diagnosis and treatment of gastrointestinal disease.

2. Outline the investigations you would consider in a 67-year-old man with a 1-month history of diarrhoea and rectal bleeding.

3. A 38-year-old man presents with epigastric pain and tenderness. Outline the investigations and possible causes of his symptoms. For each cause, list the appropriate treatments available.

4. Outline the management of a 48-year-old man with a history of alcohol abuse admitted with haematemesis and melaena.

5. Summarize the following:
   A. Drugs used in inflammatory bowel disease
   B. Extra-gastrointestinal manifestations of Crohn's disease
   C. Risk of malignancy in ulcerative colitis

6. A 26-year-old woman presents with mouth ulcers, abdominal pain and diarrhoea. On routine testing she is noted to be anaemic, haemoglobin 9.5 g/dL, MCV 72. Discuss the possible diagnoses, the appropriate investigations and the management of the most likely diagnosis. Outline the key points in the history and examination that you would elicit.

7. A 19-year-old man is referred as his mother has been diagnosed as having coeliac disease. Discuss the investigations you would carry out to determine whether he also has the disease and outline how you would explain coeliac disease and its implications to your patient.

8. A 65-year-old man presents with a 6-month history of diarrhoea, weight loss and rectal blood loss. Outline your management of the patient and give a differential diagnosis for his symptoms.

9. A 34-year-old woman returns from a trekking holiday in Indonesia. She has intermittent abdominal pain and diarrhoea. With reference to the likely causes, outline the investigations you would arrange and the treatments you would consider appropriate.

10. Discuss the key mechanisms of diarrhoea in humans, illustrating your answer with examples of the causes of each group and the management of the symptoms.

11. A 47-year-old man is referred due to increasing jaundice. He is noted to have been a heavy alcohol drinker for 20 years and smells of alcohol when he is reviewed. He has also been noted to be confused and at times drowsy. Outline your initial management of this patient and the long-term care he should receive.

12. What are the viral causes of hepatitis? In your answer outline the natural history and management of the important viruses you discuss.

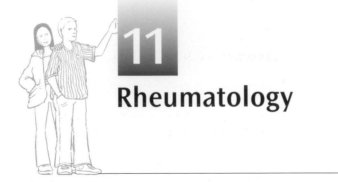

Rheumatology

If you need more detailed explanation refer to Kumar & Clark, Clinical Medicine, Chapter 10.

Examining the musculoskeletal system

Examination should include all of the following and be done in roughly this order:

EXAMINATION OF INDIVIDUAL JOINTS (K&C, p. 514)

❚ Ask the patient if the joint is painful; proceed with care if it is

Look for ❚ Swelling
❚ Erythema/rash
❚ Deformity
❚ Muscle-wasting

Feel for ❚ Tenderness
❚ Warmth
❚ Swelling
   — Hard swelling = bony
   — Fluctuant swelling = fluid/effusion
   — Boggy swelling = synovial swelling

Move the joint ❚ Passively first
❚ Assess for crepitus

EXAMINATION OF THE HANDS

▌ Expose both arms to the shoulders
▌ Ask if they are painful
▌ Describe particular features of osteoarthritis or rheumatoid arthritis if present (Table 11.1 and Fig. 11.1)
▌ Then proceed as for individual joints above
▌ Also examine the nails and feel for nodules on the forearms

EXAMINATION OF THE GAIT

▌ Ask the patient to walk a short distance away from you, turn, walk towards you and stand still

Arthritis

Osteoarthritis (OA) *(K&C, p. 333)*

▌ Pain and disability associated with joint space narrowing, altered cartilage structure and osteophyte formation

Epidemiology

▌ Most common type of arthritis
▌ Prevalence increases with age
▌ Most people > 60 years have some X-ray evidence of OA

Table 11.1 Some common particular features of osteoarthritis and rheumatoid arthritis in the hands

	Hand joints usually affected	Particular features
Osteoarthritis	DIP joints (Heberden's nodes) PIP joints (Bouchard's nodes) Carpometacarpal joint	Square hand
Rheumatoid arthritis	PIP joints MCP joints	Ulnar deviation Palmar subluxation of MCP joints Fixed flexion of PIP joints (Boutonnière deformity) Fixed hyperextension of PIP joints (swan neck deformity)

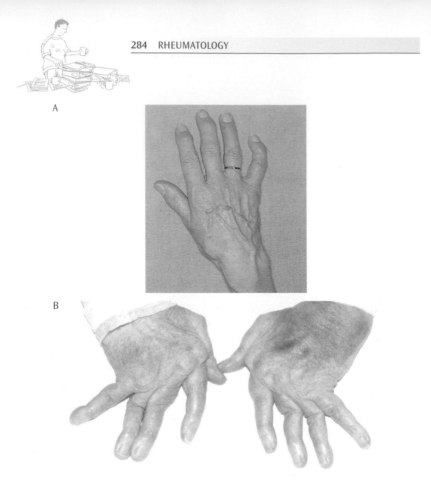

Fig. 11.1 The hands in arthritis. A. Nodal osteoarthritis. Heberden's and Bouchard's nodes and squaring of the thumb bases are seen. B. Rheumatoid arthritis.

Aetiology *Primary*
❙ Idiopathic

Secondary
❙ Trauma, e.g. previous fracture
❙ Chondrocalcinosis
❙ Haemochromatosis
❙ Acromegaly
❙ Haemophilia
❙ Avascular necrosis, e.g. steroids
❙ Sickle cell disease

Clinical features ❙ Joint pain
❙ Morning stiffness
❙ Joint swelling/instability

I Loss of function
I Crepitus
I Limitation of movement
I Joint instability
I Joint effusion
I Bony swelling
I Muscle wasting

Clinical subsets *Nodal OA*
I Familial
I ♀ ≫ ♂
I Develops in late middle age
I Polyarticular involvement of the hand (particularly distal interphalangeal (DIP) joints – Heberden's nodes)
I Generally good long-term functional outcome
I Predisposes to OA of the knee, hip and spine
I X-ray – marginal osteophyte and joint space loss

Erosive OA
I Rare
I DIP and proximal interphalangeal (PIP) joints equally affected
I Poor functional outcome
I X-ray – marked subchondral cysts
I May develop into rheumatoid arthritis

Generalized OA
I May occur in combination with nodal OA
I Hands, knees, first metatarsophalangeal (MTP) joints and hips
I Familial
I ♀ > ♂
I May be autoimmune

Large joint OA
I Knees and hips

Crystal-associated OA (chondrocalcinosis)
I Calcium pyrophosphate crystal deposition
I Knees and wrists commonly affected
I X-ray – may show calcification in the cartilage

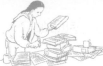

Investigations
I Inflammatory markers not elevated
I No autoantibodies
I X-rays abnormal if damage severe
I MRI can show early cartilage changes
I Arthroscopy may show early fissuring and surface erosion of cartilage

Management
I Treat symptoms and disability, not X-rays
I Explain diagnosis and reassure
I Weight loss and exercise
I Hydrotherapy (particularly lower limb joints)
I Heat/massage
I Analgesia
I Patients often use complementary medicine
I Joint replacements/other surgery

Rheumatoid arthritis (*K&C*, p. 537)

I A systemic disease with a chronic inflammatory symmetrical polyarthritis with synovitis and non-articular features

Epidemiology
I 1–3% of the population
I Can present at any age; commonly presents between 30 and 50 years
I ♀ > ♂ before menopause
I Familial or sporadic
I HLA-DR4 in 50–70%

Aetiology
I Unexplained
I Associated with T cell activation and presence of rheumatoid factors

Clinical features
I Slow onset
I Progressive symmetrical peripheral polyarthritis
I Joint pain and morning stiffness
I Eased by gentle activity
I Lethargy, malaise
I Joints warm and tender
I Limitation of movement
I Joint effusion
I Muscle-wasting
I Deformity
I Non-articular features (Fig. 11.2)

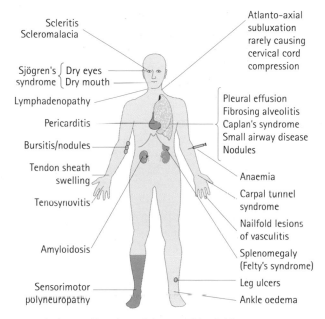

Scleritis
Scleromalacia

Atlanto–axial
subluxation
rarely causing
cervical cord
compression

Sjögren's { Dry eyes
syndrome { Dry mouth

Lymphadenopathy

Pericarditis

Bursitis/nodules

Pleural effusion
Fibrosing alveolitis
Caplan's syndrome
Small airway disease
Nodules

Tendon sheath
swelling

Tenosynovitis

Anaemia

Carpal tunnel
syndrome

Nailfold lesions
of vasculitis

Amyloidosis

Splenomegaly
(Felty's syndrome)

Sensorimotor
polyneuropathy

Leg ulcers

Ankle oedema

Fig. 11.2   Non-articular manifestations of rheumatoid arthritis.

Clinical subsets

Palindromic
❚ Monoarticular
❚ Progresses to other types

Transient
❚ Self-limiting
❚ Usually Rh factor-negative

Remitting
❚ Active for years then remits

Chronic persistent
❚ Most typical form
❚ Relapsing and remitting

Rapidly progressive
❚ Remorseless
❚ Progressive
❚ Rh factor-positive
❚ Associated with non-articular features

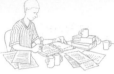

Joints affected	▌ Hands and wrists (see above) ▌ Shoulders ▌ Feet, knees and hips ▌ Cervical spine ▌ Or any other synovial joint
Investigations	▌ Anaemia, ↑ inflammatory markers ▌ Rheumatoid factors (in 70%) ▌ X-rays – erosions

Management
(*K&C*, p. 543)
	▌ Explain diagnosis and reassure
	▌ Multidisciplinary team approach
	▌ NSAIDs
	▌ Disease-modifying antirheumatic drugs (DMARDs)
	    — Sulfasalazine
	    — Methotrexate
	    — Gold
	    — Penicillamine
	▌ Corticosteroids (see Table 11.2 for side-effects)
	▌ Azathioprine and other immunosuppressants
	▌ Anticytokine therapies, e.g. anti-TNFα
	▌ Surgery

Septic arthritis (*K&C*, p. 554)

Aetiology	▌ Direct injury
	▌ Blood-borne infection
	▌ ↑ Susceptibility in
	    — Chronically inflamed joints
	    — Immunosuppressed patients
	    — Artificial joints

Table 11.2 Side-effects of steroids

General Weight gain Fluid retention	**Cardiovascular** Hypertension
Skin Acne Thin skin with easy bruising	**Eyes** Cataracts
Endocrine Diabetes Cushing's syndrome	**Bones** Osteoporosis

Organisms	▮ *Staphylococcus aureus* ▮ *Streptococcus* and other *staphylococci* ▮ *Neisseria gonorrhoeae* ▮ *Haemophilus influenzae* ▮ Gram-negative organisms
Clinical features	▮ Joint pain (may be severe) ▮ Muscle spasm ▮ Joint hot, red and swollen ▮ Signs of the source of infection
Investigations	▮ Urgent aspirate the joint — Microscopy and culture/gram stain — Elevated white cell count — Blood cultures
Management	▮ Two i.v. antibiotics for 2 weeks (start antibiotics immediately diagnosis suspected) ▮ Followed by 6 weeks of oral antibiotics ▮ Initial immobilization of the joint ▮ Early physiotherapy ▮ Consider surgical drainage and washout

SERONEGATIVE SPONDARTHROPATHIES (*K&C*, pp. 547–554)

▮ Conditions affecting the spine and peripheral joints which cluster in families and are associated with HLA-B27

Ankylosing spondylitis	▮ Episodic inflammation of spine and sacroiliac joints ▮ Asymmetrical large joint arthritis ▮ HLA-B27 in > 90% ▮ Associated with uveitis and costochondritis ▮ Inflammatory markers elevated ▮ X-rays — Erosions and sclerosis of affected joints — Syndesmophytes — Bamboo spine ▮ Treated with preventative exercises and NSAIDs

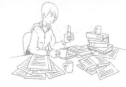

Psoriatic arthritis

Clinical features
- Arthritis in association with psoriasis
- May predate skin lesions
- DIP most common joints affected
- Dactylitis
- Erosions on X-rays (centre of joint unlike juxta-articular erosions in RA)
- 5% have arthritis mutilans
- Nail dystrophy in 85% of cases
- HLA-B27 in 50%

Management
- Treated with
  — NSAIDs
  — Steroid injections to joints
  — Sulfasalazine
  — Methotrexate/ciclosporin

Reactive arthritis

- Sterile synovitis following dysentery or a sexually acquired infection

Aetiology
- Trigger organism
  — *Salmonella*
  — *Shigella*
  — *Yersinia*
  — *Chlamydia*
  — *Ureasplasma*

Clinical features
- Acute asymmetrical lower limb arthritis
- ♂ > ♀
- Often also an enthesitis, e.g. plantar fasciitis
- Non-articular features
  — Acute anterior uveitis (see above)
  — Circinate balanitis
  — Keratoderma blenorrhagica
  — Nail dystrophy
  — Conjunctivitis

- Reiter's disease = urethritis, arthritis and conjunctivitis

Management
- Treatment usually symptomatic with NSAIDs

Inflammatory bowel disease (IBD)-associated arthritis
I 10–15% of patients with IBD
I Lower limb joints
I In ulcerative colitis treatment of bowel disease may improve arthritis
I In Crohn's disease arthritis persists even when bowel is disease inactive
I 5% have sacroiliitis (independent of activity of IBD)
I Treatment with intra-articular steroids and sulfasalazine

Gout
I Inflammatory arthritis associated with hyperuricaemia and urate crystal deposition

Epidemiology
I 5% of population have hyperuricaemia
I 0.2% of population have gout
I ♂ > ♀
I Commonly presents between 30 and 50 years
I Rare in women before the menopause
I Familial or sporadic
I HLA-DR4 positive in 50–70%

Aetiology
I Causes of hyperuricaemia (Table 11.3)

Clinical features
I Acute onset
I Acute painful, red, swollen joint
I Often affects first MTP joint
I Precipitated by
— Alcohol
— Excess food
— Dehydration
— Diuretics

Investigations
I Joint fluid microscopy – needle shape crystals
I Serum urate
I Urea and electrolytes

Management
I NSAIDs
I Colchicine (particularly if NSAIDs cannot be used)
I If attacks are frequent give allopurinol to reduce urate 4–6 weeks after acute attack
I Lifestyle advice, e.g. reduce alcohol intake

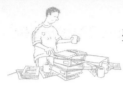

Table 11.3   Causes of hyperuricaemia

Impaired excretion of uric acid
Chronic renal disease (clinical gout unusual)
Drug therapy, e.g. thiazide diuretics, low-dose aspirin
Hypertension
Lead toxicity
Primary hyperparathyroidism
Hypothyroidism
Increased lactic acid production from alcohol, exercise, starvation
Glucose-6-phosphatase deficiency (interferes with renal excretion)

Increased production of uric acid
Increased purine synthesis de novo due to
    Hypoxanthine–guanine–phosphoribosyl transferase (HGPRT) reduction (an X-linked inborn error causing the Lesch–Nyhan syndrome)
Phosphoribosyl–pyrophosphate synthetase overactivity
    Glucose-6-phosphatase deficiency with glycogen storage disease type 1 (patients who survive develop hyperuricaemia due to increased production as well as decreased excretion)
Increased turnover of purines due to
    Myeloproliferative disorders, e.g. polycythaemia vera
    Lymphoproliferative disorders, e.g. leukaemia
    Others, e.g. carcinoma, severe psoriasis

Chronic tophaceous gout
I Very high serum urate
I White urate deposits (tophi) in skin particularly ear lobes and around joints
I Associated with renal failure or use of diuretics

Connective tissue disease

Systemic lupus erythematosus (SLE) (*K&C*, p. 557)
I Inflammatory multisystem disorder with arthralgia and rashes as common symptoms, and cerebral and renal disease as serious problems

Epidemiology
I ♀ > ♂
I Black > Caucasian
I Peak age of onset 20–40 years

Aetiology ❚ Familial
❚ ↑ HLA-B8 and DR3 in Caucasians
❚ Inherited deficiency of complement (C2 and 4)
❚ ?Related to female sex hormones
❚ Loss of immunological tolerance
❚ Environmental triggers
— Drugs – hydralazine, isoniazid, methyldopa, oral contraceptive pill/HRT
— Ultraviolet light

Clinical features ❚ Are the result of vasculitis (Fig. 11.3)

Investigations *Blood tests*
❚ Normochromic normocytic anaemia
❚ Leucopenia
❚ Thrombocytopenia
❚ +/− Autoimmune haemolytic anaemia

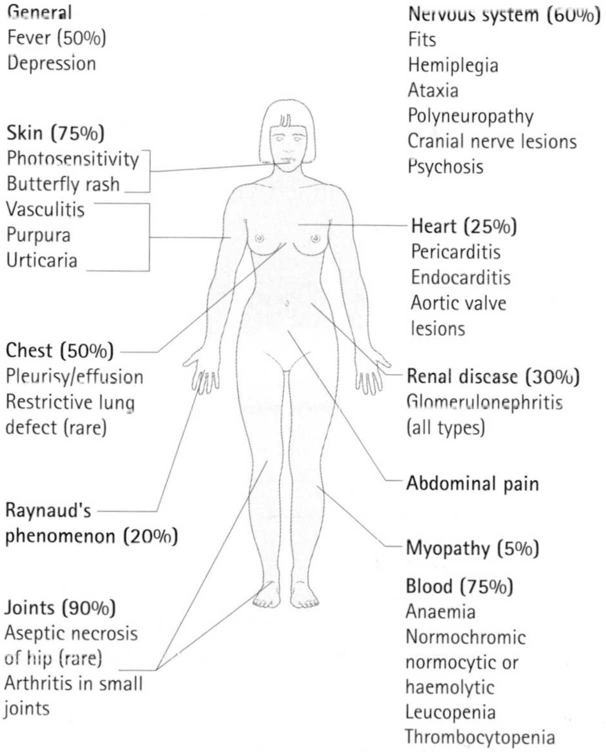

General
Fever (50%)
Depression

Skin (75%)
Photosensitivity
Butterfly rash
Vasculitis
Purpura
Urticaria

Chest (50%)
Pleurisy/effusion
Restrictive lung
defect (rare)

Raynaud's
phenomenon (20%)

Joints (90%)
Aseptic necrosis
of hip (rare)
Arthritis in small
joints

Nervous system (60%)
Fits
Hemiplegia
Ataxia
Polyneuropathy
Cranial nerve lesions
Psychosis

Heart (25%)
Pericarditis
Endocarditis
Aortic valve
lesions

Renal disease (30%)
Glomerulonephritis
(all types)

Abdominal pain

Myopathy (5%)

Blood (75%)
Anaemia
Normochromic
normocytic or
haemolytic
Leucopenia
Thrombocytopenia

Fig. 11.3   Clinical features of systemic lupus erythematosus.

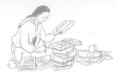

I ↑ ESR
I Normal CRP
I Antinuclear antibody (ANA) positive
I Double-stranded DNA positive in 50%, SLE-specific
I Low complement during attacks
I Rh factor-positive in 30–50%
I False positive syphilis serology
I Raised IgG and M

Histology
I e.g. Renal biopsy
I Characteristic histology and immunofluorescence

CT/MRI
I e.g. Brain, may show infarcts/haemorrhage

Management
I Explain diagnosis
I Avoid UV light if photosensitive
I NSAIDs for arthralgia
I Antimalarials (e.g. chloroquine) for skin and joint disease
I Steroids
I Immunosuppressants,
 — azathioprine/cyclophosphamide if severe

Course and prognosis
I Episodic
I Periods of complete remission
I 10-year survival 90%

Antiphospholipid syndrome (*K&C*, p. 560)
I A syndrome associated with the presence of antibodies to phospholipids

Clinical features
I Arterial and venous thromboses
I Recurrent miscarriage
I Thrombocytopenia
I Chorea, migraine and epilepsy
I Valvular heart disease
I Skin disease, e.g. livedo reticularis
I A few patients will have SLE

Investigation   ❚ Anticardiolipin antibodies
❚ Lupus anticoagulant antibodies
❚ ESR and ANA usually normal
❚ Prolonged APTT

Management   ❚ Anticoagulation
— Aspirin
— Heparin/warfarin

Systemic sclerosis (K&C, p. 561)

❚ A multisystem disease with widespread
obliterative damage to small blood vessels
associated with fibrosis of the skin and internal
organs

Clinical features   *Raynaud's phenomenon*
❚ 97% of cases
❚ Arterial spasm of hands and feet
❚ Three phases
— Pallor
— Cyanosis
— Erythema
❚ Numbness and pain

Skin
❚ Hands, face, feet, forearms
❚ Tight, waxy and tethered
❚ 'Beaking' of nose
❚ Microstomia
❚ Digital ulcers
❚ Telangiectasia
❚ Nail fold capillary loops

GI Tract
❚ Oesophagus
— Reflux
— Poor motility
— Dilatation
❚ Small bowel
— Bacterial overgrowth
— Malabsorption

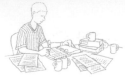
Renal
▌ Renal failure
▌ Malignant hypertension

Cardiorespiratory system
▌ Pulmonary fibrosis (common cause of death)
▌ Primary or secondary pulmonary hypertension
▌ Arrhythmias
▌ Conduction defects
▌ Pericarditis

Crest syndrome
▌ **C**alcinosis (calcium deposits in skin and elsewhere)
▌ **R**aynaud's phenomenon
▌ o**E**esophageal involvement
▌ **S**clerodactyly
▌ **T**elangiectasia

Investigations
▌ Normocytic normochromic anaemia
▌ Urea and electrolytes and urinalysis including creatinine clearance
▌ Autoantibodies
  — Speckled/nucleolar/anticentromere – 70–80%
  — Rheumatoid factor – 30%
▌ Chest X-ray – reticulonodular shadowing
▌ Other tests according to organ involved

Management
▌ Education, counselling and family support
▌ Hand-warmers and vasodilators for Raynaud's
▌ Proton pump inhibitors and motility agents
▌ Antibiotics and nutritional supplements
▌ Antihypertensives
▌ I.v. prostacyclin

Vasculitus (K&C, p. 564)

▌ Inflammation of the vessel wall (Table 11.4)

Table 11.4 Vasculitides

Name	Type of vessel	Clinical features	Diagnosis	Treatment
Giant cell arteritis (GCA) and polymyalgia rheumatica (PMR)	Large vessel (e.g. temporal artery)	> 50 years GCA Headache Scalp tenderness Jaw claudication Malaise tiredness Fever Sudden painless vision loss PMR Pain and stiffness in shoulders, neck, hips and spine Malaise Tiredness Fever Weight loss Depression Worse in mornings	Clinical features Raised ESR Temporal artery biopsy (shows a giant cell arteritis)	Steroids

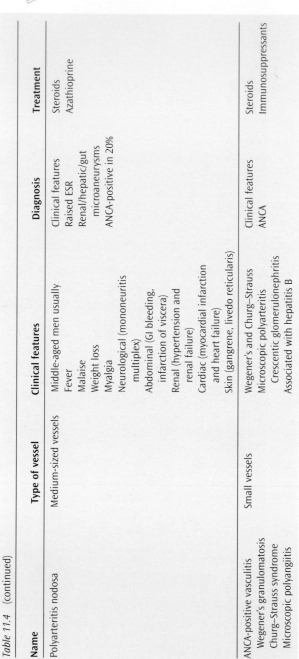

Table 11.4 (continued)

Name	Type of vessel	Clinical features	Diagnosis	Treatment
Polyarteritis nodosa	Medium-sized vessels	Middle-aged men usually Fever Malaise Weight loss Myalgia Neurological (mononeuritis multiplex) Abdominal (GI bleeding, infarction of viscera) Renal (hypertension and renal failure) Cardiac (myocardial infarction and heart failure) Skin (gangrene, livedo reticularis)	Clinical features Raised ESR Renal/hepatic/gut microaneurysms ANCA-positive in 20%	Steroids Azathioprine
ANCA-positive vasculitis Wegener's granulomatosis Churg–Strauss syndrome Microscopic polyangiitis	Small vessels	Wegener's and Churg–Strauss Microscopic polyarteritis Crescentic glomerulonephritis Associated with hepatitis B	Clinical features ANCA	Steroids Immunosuppressants

Table 11.4 (continued)

Non-ANCA vasculitis	Small vessels	Henoch–Schönlein purpura	Clinical features	Steroids if severe
Henoch–Schönlein purpura		Children mostly, after upper	Most self-limiting	
Cryoglobulinaemic vasculitis		respiratory tract infection		
		Purpura		
		Polyarthritis		
		Abdominal pain		
		Glomerulonephritis		
		Cryoglobulinaemic		
		Purpura		
		Glomerulonephritis		
		Arthralgia hepatitis C		
Behçet's syndrome	Small and large vessels	Japan and countries bordering the Mediterranean	Clinical features	Steroids
		Recurrent oral and genital ulceration		Ciclosporin
		Uveitis		Colchicine
		Erythema nodosum		
		Papulopustular and pseudofolliculitis skin lesions		
		Arthritis		
		GI symptoms		
		Neurological symptoms		

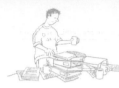

Bone disease (Table 11.5) *(K&C, p. 574)*

Osteoporosis *(K&C, p. 578)*

I Low bone mass and micro-architectural deterioration of bone leading to bone fragility and increased fracture risk
I In osteoporosis the bone is mineralized normally but deficient in quantity and quality including structural integrity

Epidemiology
I Common problem
I Lifetime risk of hip fracture in
— ♀ aged 60 years – 15%
— ♂ aged 60 years – 5%

Risk factors
I See Table 11.6

Clinical features
Vertebral crush fractures
I Back pain
I Weight loss
I Kyphosis

Fractures associated with falls
I Colles' fracture
I Fractured neck of femur

Investigations
I Ca^{++}, PO_4 and alkaline phosphatase normal
I X-rays identify fractures
I DXA scanning
— Measurement of bone density in lumbar spine and neck of femur

Table 11.5   Biochemical abnormalities in common bone disorders

Disease	Ca^{++}	PO_4	Alkaline phosphatase
Osteoporosis	→	→	→
Osteomalacia	↓	↓	↑
Paget's disease	→	→	↑
Bony secondary deposits	↑	↑ or →	↑

Table 11.6 Osteoporosis risk factors, associated disease and drug therapies

Risk factors	Cytotoxic therapy
Female sex	
Increasing age	**Disease**
Early menopause (including ovariectomy)	Endocrine
	Cushing's syndrome
White race	Hyperparathyroidism
Slender habitus	Hypogonadism (including orchidectomy)
Lack of exercise/immobility	
Smoking	Acromegaly
Family history	Type I diabetes mellitus
Excess alcohol	Joints
Nutrition (very low calcium diet, high protein intake for a long time)	Rheumatoid arthritis
	Other
	Chronic renal failure
	Chronic liver disease
Drug therapy	Mastocytosis
Corticosteroids	Anorexia nervosa
Heparin	Irritable bowel disease
Ciclosporin	

— Osteoporosis is defined as bone density < 2.5 SDs below the mean value of age-, sex- and race-matched controls

❙ Bone scan differentiates from bony metastases

Management ❙ Prevention
❙ Identification and monitoring of patients at risk

Non-drug therapies
❙ Diet rich in calcium and vitamin D
❙ Exercise
❙ Stopping smoking
❙ Reducing the risk of falls

Drugs
❙ HRT in post-menopausal women
❙ Androgens in hypogonadal men
❙ Bisphosphonates

Osteomalacia (*K&C*, p. 584)

❙ Defective bone mineralization associated with low levels of vitamin D
❙ In children the effects on the growth plates lead to rickets

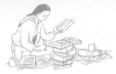
Aetiology ❙ See Table 11.7

Clinical features *Adults*
❙ Bone/muscle pain and tenderness
❙ Subclinical fractures
❙ Proximal myopathy
❙ Tetany (low calcium)

Children
❙ Bowed legs
❙ 'Rickety rosary' costochondritis
❙ Myopathy

Investigations ❙ $\downarrow Ca^{++}$, $\downarrow PO_4$, $\uparrow$ alkaline phosphatase
$\downarrow$ 25-hydroxy vitamin D
❙ X-ray – defective mineralization
❙ 'Looser's zones' on X-ray

Management ❙ Correction of cause
❙ Replacement of vitamin D

Table 11.7   Causes of rickets and osteomalacia

Vitamin D deficiency
Inadequate synthesis in skin
Low dietary intake
Malabsorption
  Coeliac disease
  Intestinal resection
  Chronic cholestasis, e.g. primary biliary cirrhosis

Renal disease
Chronic renal failure
Renal osteodystrophy
Bone disease due to dialysis
Tubular disorders, e.g. renal tubular acidosis, Fanconi's
  syndrome

Miscellaneous
Multiple myeloma
Vitamin D-dependent rickets types I and II
X-linked hypophosphataemia (vitamin D-resistant rickets)
Mesenchymal tumours

Paget's disease *(K&C,* p. 582)

I Disorder of bone remodelling associated with excessive bone resorption and excess structurally abnormal new bone formation

Epidemiology   I Europe (especially northern England) >> USA/Africa
I Patients > 40 years
I Asymptomatic X-ray evidence very common
I Patients less commonly have symptoms

Aetiology   I Genetic component
I Geographical/ethnic clusters
I Viral aetiology has been suggested

Clinical features   I Bone pain (spine/pelvis)
I Joint pain (near to involved bone)
I Deformities (tibia and skull)

Complications   *Nerve compression*
I VIII cranial nerve leads to deafness
I Also II, V and VII cranial nerves

Increased bone blood flow
I → High-output cardiac failure

Pathological fractures
I < 1% osteogenic sarcoma

Investigations   I Normal Ca^{++} and PO_4, ↑ alkaline phosphatase
I X-rays – excess abnormal bone

Management   I Simple analgesics for pain
I Bisphosphonates
I Surgery, e.g. joint replacement/osteotomy

Disorders of calcium metabolism

Hypercalcaemia *(K&C,* p. 1060)
Aetiology   I See Table 11.8

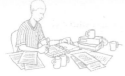

Table 11.8 Causes of hypercalcaemia

Excessive parathormone (PTH) secretion
Primary hyperparathyroidism (commonest by far), adenoma, hyperplasia or carcinoma
Tertiary hyperparathyroidism
Ectopic PTH secretion (very rare indeed)

Excess action of vitamin D
Iatrogenic or self-administered excess
Granulomatous diseases, e.g. sarcoidosis, TB
Lymphoma

Excessive calcium intake
'Milk-alkali' syndrome

Malignant disease (second commonest cause)
Secondary deposits in bone

Production of osteoclastic factors by tumours
PTH-related protein secretion
Myeloma

Other endocrine disease (mild hypercalcaemia only)
Thyrotoxicosis
Addison's disease

Drugs
Thiazide diuretics
Vitamin D analogues
Lithium administration (chronic)
Vitamin A

Miscellaneous
Long-term immobility
Familial hypocalciuric hypercalcaemia

Clinical features
❚ Tiredness
❚ Malaise
❚ Depression
❚ Renal stones
❚ Polyuria
❚ Bone pains
❚ Abdominal pain
❚ Peptic ulcer disease
❚ Ectopic calcification, e.g. corneal

Investigations
❚ Ca^{++}, PO_4, alkaline phosphatase
❚ Urea and electrolytes
❚ Chest X-ray
❚ Parathormone (PTH)
❚ Thyroid-stimulating hormone (TSH)
❚ Serum electrophoresis

Management
❚ Rectify cause
❚ i.v. Saline rehydration
❚ Bisphosphonates

Hypocalcaemia (K&C, p. 1062)

Aetiology	▌ See Table 11.9
Clinical features	▌ Paraesthesiae ▌ Circumoral numbness ▌ Cramps ▌ Anxiety ▌ Tetany ▌ Fits ▌ Dystonia ▌ Psychosis ▌ Chvostek's sign – tapping over the facial nerve produces twitching of facial muscles ▌ Trousseau's sign – compression of the upper arm (e.g. with blood pressure cuff) produces tetany spasms of the hands
Investigations	▌ Ca^{++}, PO_4, alkaline phosphatase ▌ Urea and electrolytes ▌ X-rays ▌ Parathyroid hormone ▌ Vitamin D
Management	▌ Rectify cause ▌ Calcium/vitamin D

Table 11.9   Causes of hypocalcaemia

Increased phosphate levels Chronic renal failure (common) Phosphate therapy	**Vitamin D deficiency** Osteomalacia Vitamin D resistance
Hypoparathyroidism Surgical – after neck exploration (thyroidectomy parathyroidectomy – common) Congenital deficiency (DiGeorge syndrome) Idiopathic hypoparathyroidism (rare) Severe hypomagnesaemia	**Resistance to PTH** Pseudohypoparathyroidism **Drugs** Calcitonin Bisphosphonates **Miscellaneous** Acute pancreatitis (quite common) Citrated blood in massive transfusion (not uncommon)

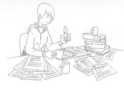

Disorders of collagen (K&C, p. 585)

I Collagen is part of the extracellular matrix
I It consists of three polypeptide chains wound
round one another in a triple helical conformation

Ehlers–Danlos syndrome (K&C, p. 585)

I Ten different types, mainly autosomal dominant
I Varying degrees of
— Skin fragility
— Skin hyperextensibility
— Joint hypermobility

Clinical features
I Easy bruising
I Extensible velvety skin
I Hypermobile joints

Pseudoxanthoma elasticum (K&C, p. 1311)

I Abnormal collagen and elastin

Clinical features
Skin
I Loose, lax, wrinkled ('plucked chicken skin')
I Particularly in the flexures

Other
I GI bleeding
I Angioid streaks in the eye
I Early myocardial infarction
I Claudication

Marfan's syndrome (K&C, p. 803)

I Autosomal dominant
I Mutation of the collagen fibrillin
I Chromosome 15

Clinical features
I Tall stature
I Arachnodactyly (long thin digits)
I Long arm span
I High arched palate
I Recurrent joint dislocations
I Inguinal/femoral herniae
I Spontaneous pneumothorax
I Emphysema

▌ Aortic/mitral incompetence
▌ Aortic aneurysm
▌ Dislocation of the lens

Self-assessment questions

Multiple choice questions

1. The following are features of osteoarthritis:
   A. Joint swelling
   B. Treatment with methotrexate
   C. Surgery may be indicated for hip disease
   D. Raised inflammatory markers
   E. Subchondral cysts on X-ray

2. In rheumatoid arthritis the following may be found:
   A. Rheumatoid factors in 90% of cases
   B. Treatment with methotrexate
   C. Pulmonary fibrosis
   D. Atlanto axial subluxation
   E. HLA-DR3 in 50% of patients

3. In septic arthritis:
   A. Treatment should wait for results of antibiotic sensitivities
   B. Disease usually resolves without treatment
   C. The joint is red
   D. Disease is associated with a high serum urate
   E. Surgery is contraindicated

4. Regarding autoantibodies:
   A. ANA occurs in 90% of cases of antiphospholipid syndrome
   B. Rheumatoid factor occurs in 50% of cases of systemic lupus erythematosus (SLE)
   C. Rheumatoid factor occurs in 60% of cases of systemic sclerosis
   D. Double-stranded DNA is specific for SLE
   E. Anticentromere antibodies occur in systemic sclerosis

5. In SLE the following may be found:
   A. Butterfly skin rash
   B. Pleural effusion
   C. Thrombocytopenia
   D. Hemiplegia
   E. 'Beaking' of the nose

6. In systemic sclerosis:
   A. Steroids are used
   B. Malabsorption is caused by villous atrophy
   C. Pulmonary fibrosis is a common cause of death
   D. Raynaud's phenomenon occurs in few cases
   E. Hands are rarely affected

7. In osteoporosis:
   A. Plasma calcium is low
   B. Diagnosis is made when bone density rises 2.5 SDs above the mean for sex- and race-matched controls
   C. Fracture risk can be reduced by bisphosphonates
   D. Men and women are equally affected
   E. Calcaneal fractures are common

8. In polymyalgia rheumatica:

A. The ESR is usually low

B. There can be an association with giant cell arteritis

C. Disease is unresponsive to steroids

D. Presentation can be with depression

E. Symptoms are worse at night

9. Osteomalacia:

A. Is treated with steroids

B. Is associated with normal bone biochemistry

C. In children causes ricketts

D. Can be caused by inadequate exposure to sunlight

E. Occurs in primary biliary cirrhosis

10. Causes of hypercalcaemia include:

A. Secondary deposits in bone

B. Addison's disease

C. Hypoparathyroidism

D. Thiazide diuretics

E. Massive blood transfusion

11. In hypocalcaemia:

A. Tapping on the facial nerve may induce twitching of the facial muscles

B. Tetany may occur

C. Treatment with bisphosphonates can be useful

D. It is mandatory to check parathormone levels

E. i.v. calcium is contraindicated

12. In relation to serum bone biochemistry:

A. Calcium is normal and alkaline phosphatase elevated in Paget's disease

B. Phosphate is high in hypocalcaemia associated with chronic renal failure

C. Calcium is low and alkaline phosphatase elevated in osteomalacia

D. Calcium is low in hypoparathyroidism

E. Calcium is high and phosphate low in hyperparathyroidism

Extended matching questions

Question 1 *Theme: back pain*

A. Osteoporosis
B. Osteoarthritis
C. Rheumatoid arthritis
D. Ankylosing spondylitis
E. Gout
F. Reactive arthritis
G. Systemic lupus erythematosus
H. Osteomalacia
I. Paget's disease

For each of the following questions, select the best answers from the list above:

I. A 28-year-old male who has intermittent episodes of back pain has a raised ESR and is HLA-B27-positive. X-rays show syndesmophytes. What is the most likely diagnosis?

II. A 60-year-old male smoker presents with progressive increasing episodes of back pain. His symptoms are worse in the mornings when he has stiffness. X-rays show no erosions. The ESR and alkaline phosphatase are normal. What is the most likely diagnosis?

III. A 72-year-old female presents with an episode of severe back pain. She fractured her wrist recently during a

fall and has a long history of asthma. She has normal alkaline phosphatase and calcium.
What is the most likely diagnosis?

Question 2 *Theme: painful hands*

A. Systemic sclerosis
B. Osteoarthritis
C. Rheumatoid arthritis
D. Gout
E. Reactive arthritis
F. Systemic lupus erythematosus
G. Septic arthritis
H. Psoriatic arthritis

For each of the following questions, select the best answers from the list above:

I. A 56-year-old businessman has acute episodes of pain in the joints of his hands and feet. The episodes occur particularly in the distal and interphalangeal joints of the hands and first metatarsophalangeal joint of the great toe. His body mass index is 30 and the serum urate is elevated. What is the most likely diagnosis?

II. A 35-year-old female presents with episodes of pain in the metacarpophalangeal joints of the hands. She has a fever and a rash on the face and the following blood results: rheumatoid factor positive, Antinuclear antibody positive, ESR 15, CRP 145.
What is the most likely diagnosis?

III. A 72-year-old female presents with pains in the joints of her hands and her neck. On examination she has bony expansion of the distal interphalangeal joints of both hands. ESR is 35.
What is the most likely diagnosis?

Short answer questions

1. Write short notes on the following:
   A. Side-effects of steroids
   B. Reactive arthritis
   C. Gout
   D. Antibiotics in septic arthritis

2. Write short notes on the following:
   A. CREST syndrome
   B. Antiphospholipid syndrome
   C. Skin changes associated with systemic sclerosis
   D. Raynaud's phenomenon

3. Write short notes on the following:
   A. Henoch–Schönlein purpura
   B. Behçet's disease
   C. Paget's disease
   D. DXA scanning

4. Write short notes on the following:
   A. Causes of hypocalcaemia
   B. Emergency management of hyper- and hypocalcaemia
   C. Hyperparathyroidism
   D. Marfan's syndrome

Essay questions

1. Outline the important features of the history, examination and investigation of a 50-year-old woman with pains in the joints of the hands.

2. Discuss the non-articular features of rheumatoid arthritis.

3. Describe the clinical features of SLE.

4. Describe how you would tell a 30-year-old woman that she has SLE.

5. Outline the approach to prevention and treatment of osteoporosis.

6. Discuss the investigation of a 40-year-old male patient with low back pain.

7. Outline the investigations you would carry out in a patient found to have an elevated serum calcium.

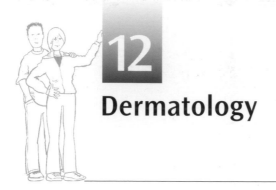

12 Dermatology

If you need more detailed explanation refer to Kumar & Clark, Clinical Medicine, Chapter 22.

Examining the skin

Examination of a rash (K&C, p. 1273)

Look at the rash   **I** For useful terms see Table 12.1

Table 12.1   *Useful terms to describe skin lesions*

Term	Meaning
Atrophy	Thinning of skin
Bulla	Large fluid-filled blister
Crusting	Dried exudate
Ecchymosis	Large 'bruise'
Erosion	Small denuded area of skin
Excoriation	Scratch mark
Fissure	Deep linear crack
Lichenification	Thickened skin with normal markings
Macule	Flat, circumscribed non-palpable lesion
Nodule	Large papule (> 0.5 cm)
Papule	Small palpable circumscribed lesion
Petechia	Pinpoint-sized macule of blood in the skin
Plaque	Large flat-topped palpable lesion
Purpura	Larger macule of blood in the skin which does not blanch on pressure
Pustule	Pus-filled lesion (white/yellow)
Scaly	Visible flakes/shedding of skin surface
Telangiectasia	Abnormal visible dilatation of blood vessels
Ulcer	Larger denuded area of skin
Vesicle	Small fluid-filled blister
Weal	Raised erythematous swelling (dermal swelling)

Note its distribution   *Useful terminology*
I Flexural/extensor (remember psoriasis is usually extensor and eczema is usually flexural)
I Localized/widespread
I Symmetrical/unilateral
I Facial
I Centripetal (trunk > limbs)
I Acral (hands and feet)
I Linear/annular
I Reticulate (lacy network)

Feel the rash   I Use gloves if necessary

PROCEED TO EXAMINE

I Nails
I Hair
I Mouth

Cutaneous infection

BACTERIAL INFECTIONS (*K&C*, pp. 1274–1276)

Impetigo   I Weeping exudative areas with honey-coloured crust
I Highly infectious
I 90% due to *Staphylococcus aureus*

Management   I Topical/oral antibiotics

Cellulitis   I Hot tender area of confluent erythema
I Often on lower legs
I Can affect face (erysipelas)
I Caused by streptococci

Risk factors   I Diabetes mellitus

Management   I Oral / i.v. antibiotics

VIRAL INFECTIONS (*K&C*, pp. 1276–1277)

Herpes simplex   I Vesicular lesions
I May be recurrent, e.g. cold sores

Management   I Topical/oral aciclovir

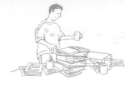

Herpes zoster (shingles)

I Reactivation of infection
I There may be a prodrome of tingling pain
I Unilateral blistering eruption
— Single dermatomal distribution usually
— Otoscopy demonstrates vesicles in the external auditory meatus

Management
I Analgesia
I Oral aciclovir

Complications
I Post-herpetic neuralgia (pain)
I Ocular involvement (trigeminal nerve)

FUNGAL INFECTIONS (MYCOSES) (*K&C*, pp. 1278–1280)

Dermatophyte infections

Tinea corporis
I Body ringworm
I Slightly itchy asymmetrical scaly patch with central clearing and raised edge

Tinea cruris
I Groin ringworm

Tinea pedis
I Athlete's foot

Tinea capitis
I Scalp ringworm

Management
I Antifungal cream
I Oral agents for feet/severe infections

Candida albicans
I Flexural areas
I Red areas with ragged edges
I Satellite lesions

Risk factors
I Immunosuppression including steroids
I Diabetes mellitus

Management
I Topical/oral antifungal agents

INFESTATIONS (*K&C*, pp. 1281–1282)

Scabies
I *Sacoptes scabiei*
I Itchy red papules in web spaces
I Skin burrows visible
I Diagnosis by skin scrapings

Treatment
- Malathion or permethrin
- Treat all skin below neck
- Treat all close contacts

Eczema (dermatitis) (*K&C*, p. 1282)

- Acute – inflamed weeping skin with vesicles
- Subacute – erythema, dry/flaky skin, crusted
- Chronic – lichenified skin

Epidemiology
- 40% of population have an episode associated with atopy
- Atopic individuals have a tendency to
  — Asthma
  — Eczema
  — Hay fever
  — Allergic rhinitis

Aetiology
- Genetic – polygenic
- Environmental triggers
  — Detergents/chemicals
  — Infection
  — Stress/anxiety
  — Animal fur
  — Foods (dairy products in the very young)

Clinical features
- Itchy erythematous scaly patches
- Often flexural
- May be associated with nail pitting

Investigations
- May have raised IgE or eosinophils
- Skin-patch testing

Management
- Avoid irritants
- Topical steroids
- Emollients
- Antibiotics for secondary infection
- Antihistamines
- Second-line agents
  — Ultraviolet (UV) light
  — Oral steroids
  — Ciclosporin/azathioprine

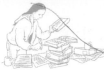

Complications ▌ Infection (staphylococcal/streptococcal)
▌ Conjunctivitis

Psoriasis (K&C, p. 1287)

▌ Common disorder characterized by red scaly
plaques

Epidemiology ▌ 2% of the population
▌ ♂ = ♀

Aetiology ▌ T lymphocyte-driven
▌ Genetic – polygenic
▌ Environmental triggers
— Infection
— Drugs, e.g. lithium
— UV light
— Alcohol
— Stress/anxiety

Clinical features *Chronic plaque psoriasis*
▌ Purplish/red scaly plaques, particularly on extensor
surfaces
▌ Scalp frequently involved
▌ Can occur in areas of skin trauma (Köbner
phenomenon)
▌ 50% associated with nail changes
— Nail pitting
— Distal separation of nail plate (onycholysis)
— Yellow/brown discoloration
— Subungual hyperkeratosis
— If severe, loss of nail plate

Flexoral psoriasis
▌ Occurs in older patients
▌ Patches in
— Groin
— Natal cleft
— Submammary areas

Guttate psoriasis
▌ Raindrop-like lesions on trunk

ERYTHRODERMA

Suggested by
Widespread inflammation of the skin

Common causes
Atopic eczema
Psoriasis
Drugs, e.g. sulphonamides, gold
Seborrhoeic dermatitis

Management
Bed rest
Liberal i.v. fluids
Keep warm
Emollients
Beware of sepsis
Treat/remove the cause

Complications (can be life-threatening)
High-output cardiac failure
Hypothermia
Dehydration
Hypoalbuminaemia
Increased basal metabolic rate
Capillary leak syndrome

I Occurs in children/young adults 2 weeks after a streptococcal sore throat

Arthritis associated with psoriasis
I See page 290

Management I Avoid irritants
I Topical steroids
I Calcipotriol (vitamin D_3 analogue)
I Coal tar
I Phototherapy, e.g. PUVA (psoralen + UVA)
I Methotrexate if severe

Complications I Erythroderma (*K&C*, p. 1296)

Skin cancer (*K&C*, p. 1304)

I There are three common types (Table 12.2)
I All are related to exposure to sunlight

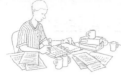

Table 12.2   Features of the three common skin cancers

Type	Clinical features	Spread	Management
Basal cell carcinoma (rodent ulcer)	Occur in later life Slow-growing nodule May ulcerate Pearly edge Telangiectasia Can erode local structures	No metastases	Surgical excision Radiotherapy
Squamous cell carcinoma	Rapidly growing nodule which ulcerates More common in immunosuppressed patients, e.g. renal transplant patients Also occurs in areas of chronic Inflammation	Metastases occur	Surgical excision
Malignant melanoma	Can occur in young patients Transformation of 'moles' Consider in all bleeding pigmented lesions or 'changing moles'	Early metastases	Wide excision Radiotherapy Immunotherapy Chemotherapy for metastases

Cutaneous features of systemic disease *(K&C*, pp. 1296–1300)

Erythema nodosum
- Painful dusky/blue nodules
- Commonly on the shins
- Associations – see Table 12.3

Table 12.3   Aetiology of erythema nodosum and erythema multiforme

Erythema nodosum	Erythema multiforme
Streptococcal infection	Herpes/Epstein–Barr virus infection
Drugs (e.g. antibiotics, oral contraceptive pill)	Drugs (e.g. antibiotics, barbiturates)
Tuberculosis	Mycoplasma infections
Inflammatory bowel disease	Connective tissue disease, e.g. SLE
Sarcoid	HIV
Leprosy	Carcinoma/lymphoma
Idiopathic	

Erythema multiforme	❚ Erythematous lesion with central pallor (target lesions) ❚ Symmetrical, particularly on limbs ❚ May blister ❚ Mucosal involvement = Stevens–Johnson syndrome ❚ Associations – see Table 12.3
Pyoderma gangrenosum	❚ Erythematous nodules with ulceration ❚ Large areas of ulceration ❚ Bluish/black edge ❚ Purulent surface ❚ Associations — Inflammatory bowel disease — Rheumatoid arthritis — Myeloma/leukaemia/lymphoma — Liver disease — Idiopathic
Management	❚ Topical/oral steroids ❚ Treatment of underlying condition ❚ Ciclosporin
Acanthosis nigricans	❚ Thickened hyperpigmented skin in the flexures, e.g. axilla ❚ Associations — Insulin resistance — Malignancy (particularly GI tract)
Chronic discoid lupus	❚ Red scaly atrophic plaques +/– telangiectasia ❚ Face/exposed areas of skin ❚ May be associated with alopecia ❚ Triggered/exacerbated by UV light ❚ 30% antinuclear factor-positive ❚ 5% develop systemic lupus erythematosus (SLE)
Management	❚ Topical steroids ❚ Hydroxychloroquine ❚ Oral steroids/azathioprine/ciclosporin

Systemic lupus erythematosus (skin manifestations)

❚ Macular erythema on cheeks/nose/forehead (butterfly rash)

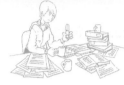

Pruritus

Medical conditions associated with itching
- Iron deficiency
- Malignancy, e.g. lymphoma
- Diabetes mellitus
- Chronic renal failure
- Cholestasis
- Chronic liver disease
- Thyroid disease
- HIV
- Polycythaemia rubra vera

Leg ulcers (*K&C*, pp. 1308–1309)

Aetiology
- Venous hypertension
- Arterial insufficiency
- Neuropathic (e.g. diabetes mellitus)
- Neoplastic (e.g. squamous cell carcinoma)
- Vasculitis
- Infection, e.g. syphilis
- Blood disorders, e.g. sickle cell disease
- Trauma

Venous ulcers
- Most common cause
- Associated with varicose veins or previous thrombosis
- Often recurrent and chronic
- Painless
- Medial aspect of leg
- Exclude arterial insufficiency with Doppler

Management
- Topical therapy to ulcer
- Compression bandaging and elevation of legs
- Antibiotics for overt infection
- Diuretics for oedema
- Analgesia if painful
- Skin grafting if resistant to therapy

Arterial ulcers
- Punched out
- Painful
- Leg cold and pale
- Absent pulses

I History of hypertension, claudication, smoking, angina
I Investigate with Doppler studies/angiogram

Management I Analgesia
I Topical treatment of ulcer
I Vascular reconstruction

Neuropathic ulcer I Over pressure areas, e.g. metatarsal heads
I Result of trauma
I Polyneuropathy, e.g. diabetes mellitus
I Painless

Management I Keep clean
I Avoid trauma

Self-assessment questions

Multiple choice questions

1. The following are risk factors for skin infections:
   A. Sunlight exposure
   B. Diabetes mellitus
   C. Steroids
   D. Phenytoin
   E. HIV infection

2. In dermatology the following are true:
   A. A bulla is fluid-filled
   B. Acral lesions affect the scalp
   C. An ecchymosis is a large bruise
   D. Purpura blanches on pressure
   E. Ringworm is a fungal infection

3. In eczema:
   A. The rash is rarely itchy
   B. The rash is often on the extensor surfaces
   C. Stress can be a trigger factor
   D. Ciclosporin is the usual treatment
   E. There can be an association with asthma

4. Psoriasis:
   A. Is more common in males
   B. Can be triggered by stress
   C. Most commonly affects extensor surfaces
   D. Rarely involves the scalp
   E. Is usually treated with topical steroids

5. Basal cell carcinoma:
   A. Is associated with early metastases
   B. May have telangiectasia
   C. Never ulcerates
   D. Is treated with chemotherapy
   E. Is most common in young adults

6. Malignant melanoma:
   A. Is associated with early metastases
   B. Often arises in a mole
   C. Is associated with UV exposure
   D. Is treated by wide excision and adjuvant therapy
   E. Only occurs in the skin

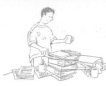

7. Erythema nodosum:
  A. Often occurs on the legs
  B. Is associated with Crohn's disease
  C. Is associated with use of oral contraceptives
  D. Occurs in tuberculosis
  E. Is most commonly associated with a streptococcal infection

8. In erythema multiforme:
  A. Uniform red patches occur
  B. Lesions in the mouth occur in Stevens–Johnson syndrome
  C. Disease can be caused by barbiturates
  D. Disease may occur in immunosuppressed patients
  E. Rash is often asymmetrical

9. Leg ulcers:
  A. Are most commonly caused by arterial insufficiency
  B. Are always painful if venous
  C. Associated with neuropathy occur over metatarsal heads
  D. May need treatment with antibiotics
  E. Are rarely recurrent

Extended matching questions

Question 1 *Theme: erythematous rash*

  A. Eczema
  B. Psoriasis
  C. Meningococcal septicaemia
  D. Squamous cell carcinoma
  E. Systemic lupus erythematosus
  F. Impetigo
  G. Erysipelas
  H. Erythema multiforme
  I. Erythema nodosum
  J. Typhoid fever

For each of the following questions, select the best answer from the list below:

I. A 39-year-old female presents with an erythematous rash on her legs. She has just returned from holiday in north Africa. The lesions are purplish, painful and warm to the touch. She has a medical history of Crohn's disease and at present has a flare-up of her symptoms with diarrhoea.
What is the most likely diagnosis?

II. A 12-year-old female presents with an erythematous rash on her arms. She has a history of asthma. She also says that she is having difficulty sleeping because of itching. The rash is flexural in distribution and she has nail pitting.
What is the most likely diagnosis?

III. A 28-year-old male presents with a rash on his hands. It is weeping fluid and in parts has yellow crusting areas. His girlfriend has a similar rash. It responds to treatment with antibiotics.
What is the most likely diagnosis?

Question 2 *Theme: skin ulcers*

  A. Venous ulcers
  B. Squamous cell carcinoma
  C. Malignant melanoma
  D. Erythema multiforme
  E. Erythema nodosum
  F. Pyoderma gangrenosum
  G. Impetigo
  H. Erythrasma
  I. Leprosy

For each of the following questions, select the best answer from the list below:

I. A 39 year old female presents with a painless ulcer on her right shin. She

recently injured this area whilst on holiday in Africa. She has a medical history of Crohn's disease. She is worried that the ulcer is rapidly increasing in size.
What is the most likely diagnosis?

II. An 82-year-old female presents with an ulcer just above the medial malleolus. She has been treated with dressings by the community nurses for 6 weeks without improvement. She has previously had surgery for varicose veins and is on aspirin for angina. The skin around the ulcer is pigmented and brownish.
What is the most likely diagnosis?

III. A 48-year-old male presents with an ulcer on his ear. He is a keen gardener. He has had an area of crusting skin there for some time. There is an enlarged hard post-auricular lymph node.
What is the most likely diagnosis?

Short answer questions

1. Write short notes on the following:
   A. Herpes zoster infection
   B. Impetigo
   C. Ringworm
   D. Cellulitis

2. Write short notes on the following:
   A. Squamous cell carcinoma
   B. Guttate psoriasis
   C. Nail changes associated with psoriasis

3. Write short notes on the following:
   A. Pyoderma gangrenosum
   B. Acanthosis nigricans
   C. Chronic discoid lupus

Essay questions

1. Outline the differential diagnosis of a red rash in the groin of an 85-year-old woman.

2. Discuss how you would explain the diagnosis of eczema to an 18-year-old man.

3. Describe the causes, treatment and complications of erythroderma.

4. Outline the investigation of a patient presenting with pruritus.

5. Discuss the treatment of venous leg ulcers.

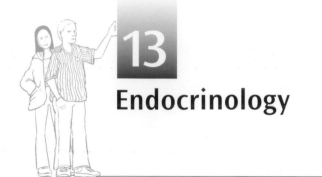

13

Endocrinology

For a more detailed explanation see Kumar and Clark's *Clinical Medicine*, Chapter 18.

Hormones
- Transmit information between cells or organs
- Allow adjustment to internal and external environment

Endocrine organs
- Synthesize and release hormones
- Maintain homeostatic mechanisms

Endocrine disorders
- Caused by abnormalities in hormone
  — Synthesis
  — Secretion
  — Control
  — Function
- Common disorders are shown in Table 13.1
- Much rarer conditions, however, provide classical cases for both written and clinical examinations and will be included in this chapter

Common pathologies
- Affect endocrine glands or their target organs
- Organ-specific autoimmune disorders
- Endocrine tumours

Table 13.1   Some common endocrine disorders

Diabetes mellitus	Osteoporosis
Thyroid disease	Primary hyperparathyroidism
Subfertility	Short stature
Menstrual disorders	Delayed puberty
Excess hair growth	

Clinical history in endocrine disease

I See Table 13.2

Examining the endocrine system

I Overall appearance (i.e. spot diagnosis), e.g. acromegaly, Graves' disease, should be assessed
I All clinical 'systems' may be involved in endocrine disorders
I Full examination of all systems is expected
I Certain parts of the examination may be discriminatory in diagnosis

Laboratory tests in endocrinology

(*K&C*, p. 1002)

I Hormones may be measured in blood/plasma or urine
I Markers of function
— Glucose in diabetes
— Calcium in hyperparathyroidism

Table 13.2   *Points to note in taking an endocrine history*

Past medical history	Social history
Diabetes mellitus	Alcohol or drug abuse
Hypertension	Diet, e.g. salt/iodine intake
Previous pregnancies/fertility	**Drug history**
Previous surgery – thyroid/ parathyroid, ovarian, testicular	Details of *all* drugs taken at present and previous regular medications
Childhood milestones and development	Corticosteroids
Puberty	Sex hormones, e.g. HRT, oral contraceptive pill
Previous radiation exposure – neck (thyroid), gonads	
Family history	
Autoimmune disorders	
Endocrine disorders	
Diabetes mellitus	

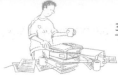

> ## CLINICAL EXAMINATION IN ENDOCRINOLOGY
> Overall appearance
> Height, weight and nutritional status
> Blood pressure (including postural measurements)
> Neck – look for goitre
> Thyroid status (see box, p. 327)
> Eyes – look for exophthalmos, Graves' eye disease
> Visual fields – pituitary tumours
> Secondary sexual characteristics and testicular examination
> Skin and hair – pigmentation, bruising, telangiectasia, acne
> Urine – check for glucose, protein, β-human chorionic
>   gonadotrophin

BASAL LEVELS

Blood or plasma levels

- Useful measurements for hormones with a long half-life, e.g. thyroxine (T_4 and T_3)
- Also applied to certain conditions in which normal values are known, e.g.
  — Time of day – cortisol and adrenocorticotrophic hormone (ACTH)
  — Period of menstrual cycle – follicle stimulating hormone (FSH), oestrogen, progesterone
  — Posture – aldosterone

24-hour urine collections

- Provide an average of a whole day's secretion of a hormone
- Require normal renal function and accurately timed and complete urine collection

DYNAMIC TESTS

- Test ability of a gland to respond appropriately to stimulation or suppression
- Failure of normal negative feedback causing uncontrolled hormone secretion
  — From within the gland
  — From an ectopic source
- Failure of a normal positive response to stimulation of a gland

I Examples are given below but the principles may be utilized in many hormonal axes and specific tests are listed in the relevant sections of this chapter

Stimulation test – Synacthen test

I Normal adrenal response to a dose of synthetic **ACTH** is an increase in plasma cortisol levels

I In primary adrenal failure, maximal stimulation produces a diminished or absent response

I If adrenal failure is secondary to lack of pituitary secretion of ACTH then a normal or enhanced cortisol response is seen

Suppression test – dexamethasone suppression test

I Normal response to a dose of synthetic steroid is a reduction in pituitary release of ACTH and a subsequent fall in adrenal cortisol release and plasma levels

I Uncontrolled endogenous production of ACTH from a pituitary tumour or ectopic source leads to inadequate suppression of plasma cortisol level

Thyroid disorders (K&C, p. 1035)

Control of thyroxine secretion

I See Figure 13.1 and Table 13.3

Examination of thyroid gland and status

I See information box on page 327

Goitre

Aetiology in a euthyroid patient

I Simple non-toxic goitre
— Iodine deficiency
— Treated Graves' disease
— Puberty

I Solitary nodule
— Thyroid adenoma
— Thyroid cyst
— Thyroid carcinoma

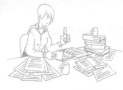

Fig. 13.1
The hypothalamic-pituitary-thyroid axis.
TRH: Thyrotrophin releasing hormone
TSH: Thyroid stimulating hormone

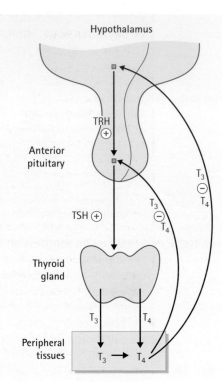

Aetiology in a hypothyroid patient

❙ Hashimoto's thyroiditis
❙ After radioiodine-treated Graves' disease

Aetiology in a hyperthyroid patient

❙ Graves' disease

Table 13.3 Biochemistry of thyroid disorders

	Hormone levels		Dynamic and other tests
	T4	**TSH**	
Hyperthyroidism	↑	↓	Autoantibodies
Primary hypothyroidism	↓	↑	Autoantibodies
Secondary hypothyroidism	↓	↓ or normal	

EXAMINATION OF THYROID GLAND AND STATUS

General inspection
Look for signs of thyroid disease

Examine the neck
Look for a goitre

Ask the patient to take a sip of water and hold it in the mouth, then ask him or her to swallow while watching the neck – look for movement of goitre with swallowing

Stand behind the patient and feel the thyroid with both hands, starting in the centre below the thyroid cartilage over the trachea, and moving laterally to the two lobes which extend behind the sternomastoid muscle. Ask the patient to swallow while palpating. Assess the goitre for size, nodularity or diffuse enlargement, discrete nodules and firmness

Palpate for lymph nodes

Auscultate – listen over the thyroid for a bruit

Assess thyroid status
Pulse – count the rate and note the presence or absence of atrial fibrillation

Palms – warm and sweaty

Tremor of outstretched arms

Examine the eyes
Exophthalmos
Lid retraction
Lid lag

Examine the reflexes
Slow relaxation in hypothyroidism

Hypothyroidism (K&C, p. 1037)

Aetiology
- Hashimoto's thyroiditis
- After radioiodine-treated hyperthyroidism
- Thyroidectomy

Clinical features
- Weight gain
- Lethargy
- Patient feels the cold
- Constipation
- Poor appetite
- Menstrual disturbances
- Myxoedema facies; thickened skin
- Brittle hair

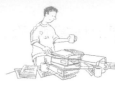

I Periorbital puffiness
I Bradycardia
I Slow relaxing reflexes

Investigations I Biochemistry (Table 13.3)
I Haematology
— Macrocytosis
— Anaemia
I Anti-thyroid antibodies

Management I Thyroxine replacement
I Caution in cardiac disease
I Monitor TSH

Graves' disease (*K&C*, p. 1040)

Clinical features I Heat intolerance
I Weight loss
I Increased appetite
I Diarrhoea
I Irritability
I Sleeplessness, tiredness
I Exertional breathlessness
I Goitre
I Tachycardia/atrial fibrillation
I Tremor
I Hyperkinesia
I Proximal muscle wasting
I Cardiac failure
I Pretibial myxoedema

Eye signs (Graves' disease)
I Exophthalmos
I Lid lag
I Lid retraction
I Ophthalmoplegia

Management *Medical treatment*
I Carbimazole
I Radioiodine

Surgical treatment for
I Malignancy
I Pressure symptoms
I Failure of medical treatment

Pituitary disorders

Functions of the anterior pituitary
▌ See Figure 13.2 and Table 13.4

Control of growth hormone secretion
▌ See Figure 13.3

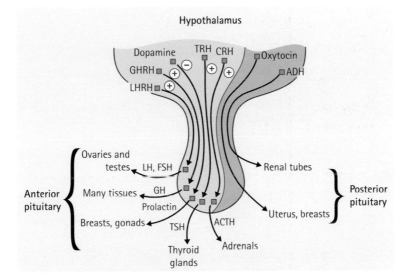

Fig. 13.2   The hypothalamic-pituitary axis.
LHRH: Luteinizing hormone releasing hormone
FSH: Follicle stimulating hormone
GHRH: Growth hormone releasing hormone
TRH: Thyrotrophin releasing hormone

TSH: Thyroid stimulating hormone
CRH: Corticotrophin releasing hormone
ACTH: Adrenocorticotrophic hormone
ADH: Antidiuretic hormone

Table 13.4   Biochemistry of the hypothalamic-anterior pituitary axis

	Hormone levels	Dynamic and other tests
Acromegaly	Growth hormone ↑	Oral glucose load (growth hormone (GH) fails to suppress)
Prolactinoma	Prolactin ↑	
Panhypopituitarism	Luteinizing hormone (LH)/ follicle stimulating hormone (FSH) ↓ GH ↓ TSH ↓ ACTH ↓	Luteinizing hormone releasing hormone (LHRH) test Insulin stress test TRH test Synacthen test

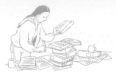

Acromegaly (*K&C*, p. 1033)

Clinical features
- Often insidious non-specific onset
- Headaches
- Polyuria
- Impotence
- Visual field defects, e.g. bitemporal hemianopia
- Nerve compression, e.g. carpal tunnel syndrome

Aetiology
- Pituitary tumour
- Typical facies, e.g.
  — Thick greasy skin
  — Protrusion of lower jaw
  — Gaps between teeth
- Large 'spade-like' hands
- Cardiac failure
- Diabetes mellitus
- Hypertension

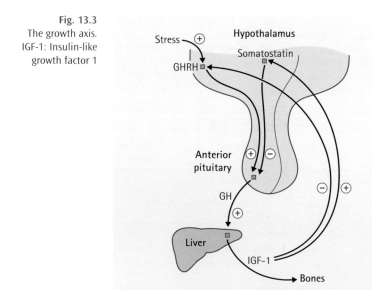

Fig. 13.3
The growth axis.
IGF-1: Insulin-like
growth factor 1

Management ❚ Bromocriptine
❚ Surgical hypophysectomy

Hypopituitarism (*K&C*, p. 1011)

Aetiology *Congenital*
❚ Kallmann's syndrome

Infective
❚ Basal meningitis
❚ Encephalitis
❚ Syphilis

Vascular
❚ Sheehan's syndrome

Tumours
❚ Pituitary
❚ Hypothalamic
❚ Craniopharyngiomas
❚ Meningiomas
❚ Gliomas
❚ Metastases (especially breast)
❚ Lymphoma

Infiltrates
❚ Sarcoidosis
❚ Langerhan's histiocytosis
❚ Haemochromatosis

Others
❚ Radiation
❚ Anorexia nervosa
❚ Trauma or previous surgery

Clinincal features ❚ Due to progressive loss of anterior pituitary
hormones (listed in order of frequency)

Growth hormone
❚ Growth failure
❚ Short stature

Prolactin
❚ Failure of lactation

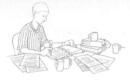

Gonadotrophins
❚ Delayed puberty
❚ Infertility
❚ Amenorrhoea
❚ Loss of body hair

TSH
❚ Hypothyroidism

ACTH
❚ Adrenal failure (without pigmentation)

Investigations   ❚ Determine hormone deficiencies
❚ Pituitary imaging, e.g. CT scan, MRI scan

Management   ❚ Treat cause
❚ Hormone replacement

Adrenal hormone abnormalities

Control of cortisol secretion
❚ See Figure 13.4

Cushing's syndrome (*K&C*, p. 1052)
❚ Overproduction of corticosteroids or excess corticosteroid treatment

Aetiology   *ACTH-dependent*
❚ Pituitary adenoma
❚ Ectopic ACTH-secreting tumours

Non-ACTH-dependent
❚ Adrenal adenoma
❚ Adrenal carcinoma
❚ Steroid treatment

Others
❚ Alcohol-induced pseudo-Cushing's syndrome

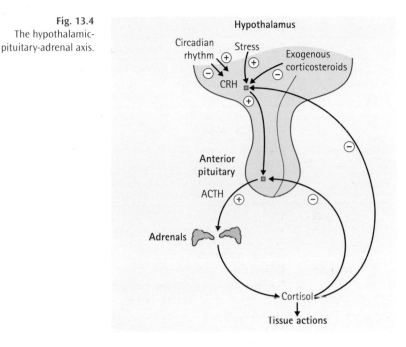

Fig. 13.4
The hypothalamic-pituitary-adrenal axis.

Clinical features
I Weight gain
I Thin skin
I Bruising
I Menstrual disturbances
I Psychosis
I Red face
I Central obesity
I Buffalo hump
I Hirsutism
I Proximal myopathy
I Hypertension
I Diabetes mellitus

Investigations
I See Table 13.5
I Serum electrolytes
  — Sodium ↓
  — Potassium ↑

Management
Pituitary-dependent
I Trans-sphenoidal resection of tumour

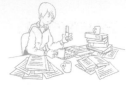

Table 13.5 Biochemistry of the pituitary-adrenal axis

	Hormone levels	Dynamic and other tests
ACTH-secreting pituitary adenoma (Cushing's disease)	24-hour urine cortisol ↑ Midnight cortisol ↑	Dexamethasone suppression test
Ectopic ACTH secretion	24-hour urine cortisol ↑ Midnight cortisol ↑	Dexamethasone suppression test
Adrenal adenoma	24-hour urine cortisol ↑ Midnight cortisol ↑	Dexamethasone suppression test
Pituitary failure	9 am cortisol ↓	Synacthen test (normal response)
Primary adrenal failure	9 am cortisol ↓	Synacthen test (diminished response)

Adrenal adenomas
❚ Medical treatment with metyrapone, to induce remission before adrenalectomy

Ectopic ACTH
❚ Remove tumour if possible
❚ Control Cushing's with metyrapone

Primary hypoadrenalism – Addison's disease *(K&C, p. 1050)*
❚ Destruction of adrenal cortex causing reduced production of glucocorticoid, mineralocorticoid and sex steroids

Aetiology ❚ See Table 13.6

Clinical features ❚ Tiredness
❚ Debility
❚ Nausea, vomiting

Table 13.6 Causes of primary hypoadrenalism

Common	Uncommon
Autoimmune disease (approx 90%) Tuberculosis (< 10% in UK) Surgical removal	Haemorrhage/infarction Meningococcal septicaemia Venography Malignant destruction Amyloid

- Anorexia, weight loss
- Abdominal pain
- Diarrhoea
- Depression
- Menstrual disturbance
- Pigmentation – mouth, palmar creases
- Postural hypotension
- Dehydration
- Loss of body hair

Investigations
- See Table 13.5

Management
- Replacement of glucocorticoids and mineralocorticoids with oral hydrocortisone and fludrocortisone

Parathyroids

Hyperparathyroidism (*K&C*, p. 1060)

Aetiology *Primary*
- Adenoma (80% solitary)
- Hyperplasia
- Carcinoma

Secondary
- Hyperplasia in hypocalcaemia
- Chronic renal failure
- Osteomalacia

Tertiary
- Autonomous secretion after prolonged hypocalcaemia

Clinical features
- Anorexia ⎤
- Abdominal pain ⎥ Due to
- Constipation ⎥ hypercalcaemia
- Polydipsia and polyuria ⎥
- Renal calculi ⎦
- Pain
- Pathological fractures

Investigations
- See Table 13.7

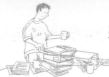

Table 13.7 Biochemistry of disorders of calcium homeostasis

	Hormone levels	Dynamic and other tests
Osteoporosis	PTH normal	
Primary hyperparathyroidism	PTH ↑	Serum calcium ↑ Serum phosphate ↓
Tertiary hyperparathyroidism	PTH ↑	Serum calcium ↑ Serum phosphate ↓
Primary hypoparathyroidism	PTH undetectable	Serum calcium ↓
Pseudohypoparathyroidism	PTH normal	Serum calcium ↓

Management
- Treat underlying cause
- Parathyroidectomy if Ca^{++} > 3 or symptoms
- Treat hypercalcaemia (page 303)

Hypoparathyroidism (K&C, p. 1062)

Aetiology
- Post-surgical
- Post-radiotherapy
- Autoimmune

Clinical features
- Tetany
- Paraesthesiae
- Cramps
- Fits

  Due to hypocalcaemia

- Cataracts

Investigations
- See Table 13.7

Osteoporosis
- Reduction in bone density below normal for age and sex (page 300)

Sex hormone and reproductive disorders

Amenorrhoea – primary or secondary (K&C, p. 1021)

Aetiology *Pituitary causes*
- Hyperprolactinaemia
- Hypopituitarism

Table 13.8   Biochemistry of ovarian disorders

	Hormone levels	Dynamic and other tests
Polycystic ovary syndrome	Androgens ↓	

Primary ovarian failure	FSH ↑
	LH ↑
	Oestrogen ↓
		LHRH test
		Clomiphene
		  stimulation
		  test

I Thyrotoxicosis
I Anorexia nervosa

Ovarian causes (Table 13.8)
I Surgery
I Primary ovarian failure
I Polycystic ovary syndrome
I Congenital adrenal hyperplasia
I Chromosomal abnormalities
I Turner's syndrome

Salt and water balance disorders

Control of salt and water homeostasis
　　　　I See Figure 13.5

Diabetes insipidus (K&C, p. 1057)
　　　　I Deficiency of antidiuretic hormone (ADH) or
　　　　　insensitivity to its action

Aetiology　I Cranial causes
　　　　　— Idiopathic
　　　　　— Familial (DIDMOAD – diabetes insipidus,
　　　　　　diabetes mellitus, optic atrophy, deafness)
　　　　　— Tumours, e.g. craniopharyngioma, glioma,
　　　　　　metastases (breast)
　　　　　— Infiltration, e.g. sarcoidosis, histiocytosis
　　　　　— Sheehan's syndrome (pituitary infarction
　　　　　　following post- or antepartum haemorrhage)

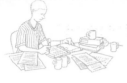

Fig. 13.5
The thirst axis.

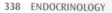

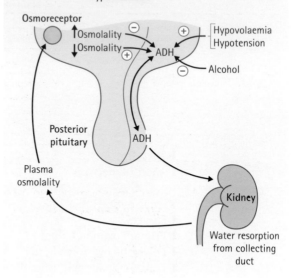

Hypothalamus

Osmoreceptor

↑Osmolality ⊖
↓Osmolality ⊕

ADH

⊕

Hypovolaemia
Hypotension

⊖ Alcohol

Posterior
pituitary

ADH

Plasma
osmolality

Kidney

Water resorption
from collecting
duct

▌ Nephrogenic causes
 — Idiopathic
 — Renal tubular acidosis
 — Hypokalaemia
 — Hypercalcaemia
 — Drugs, e.g lithium, demeclocycline,
   glibenclamide

Clinical features ▌ Polyuria
  ▌ Thirst
  ▌ Nocturia
  ▌ Polydipsia
  ▌ Dehydration
  ▌ High urine output (10–15 L/day)

Differential ▌ Primary polydipsia (excessive water
diagnosis   drinking/normal ADH secretion)

Investigations ▌ See Table 13.9

Table 13.9 Biochemistry of the hypothalamic-posterior pituitary axis

	Hormone levels	Dynamic and other tests
Cranial diabetes insipidus	ADH ↓ (not measured routinely)	Water deprivation test High plasma osmolality Low urine osmolality Normal response to DDAVP
Nephrogenic diabetes insipidus	ADH ↑ (not measured routinely)	Water deprivation test High plasma osmolality Low urine osmolality No response to DDAVP
Inappropriate ADH	ADH ↑ (not measured routinely)	Plasma osmolality low Urine osmolality high

WATER DEPRIVATION TEST

Free fluid overnight

08.00 hrs
No access to fluids
Record hourly
    Urine and plasma osmolality
    Urine volume
    Body weight
Stop and allow fluid if body weight loss > 3%

16.00 hrs
2 μg desmopressin injection i.m.
Continue fluid restriction according to urine output

04.00 hrs
Stop

Normal
Normal plasma osmolality maintained up to urine concentration > 800 mosm/kg

Cranial DI
Urine fails to concentrate
Plasma osmolality rises
Abnormality is corrected with desmopressin

Nephrogenic DI
As for cranial DI but not corrected by desmopressin

Management
❚ Treat underlying cause
❚ Synthetic vasopressin analogue
❚ DDAVP
❚ Carbamazepine
❚ Chlorpropamide

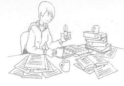
Syndrome of inappropriate ADH secretion (SIADH) *(K&C, p. 1059)*

I Inappropriate ADH secretion leads to retention of water and hyponatraemia

Aetiology   *Tumours*
I Squamous cell carcinoma of lung
I Prostate cancer
I Pancreatic cancer

Lungs
I Pneumonia
I TB

CNS
I Meningitis
I Tumours
I Head injury
I Chronic subdural haematoma
I SLE vasculitis

Drugs
I Chlorpropamide
I Carbamezepine
I Phenothiazines

Clinical features   I Confusion
I Nausea
I Fits
I Coma

Management   I Underlying cause
I Fluid restriction
I Dimethylchlortetracycline

Endocrine causes of hypertension *(K&C, pp. 1063–1067)*

Control of the renin-angiotensin-aldosterone system
I See Figure 13.6

Primary hyperaldosteronism (Table 13.10)
I Rare (< 1% of all hypertension)

Fig. 13.6
The renin-
angiotensin-
aldosterone system.
ACE: Angiotensin-
converting enzyme

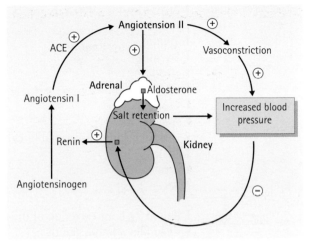

Aetiology   ▮ Conn's syndrome (adrenal adenoma 60%)
▮ Bilateral adrenal hyperplasia (40%)

Management   ▮ Surgery for tumours
▮ Aldosterone antagonists, e.g. spironolactone

Phaeochromocytoma

▮ Very rare
▮ Tumour of the sympathetic nervous system (90% adrenal)
▮ Secretion of norepinephrine and epinephrine leading to
— Peripheral vasoconstriction
— Inotropic effects
— Tachycardia
— High blood pressure

Table 13.10   Biochemistry of hyperaldosteronism

	Hormone levels	Dynamic and other tests
Primary hyperaldosteronism (Conn's syndrome)	Renin ↓ Aldosterone ↑	Serum K ↓ Serum Na ↑ Metabolic alkalosis
Secondary hyperaldosteronism	Renin ↑ Aldosterone ↑	Serum K ↓ Serum Na ↑ Metabolic alkalosis

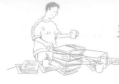
Clinical features
- Anxiety, panic attacks
- Palpitations
- Tremor
- Sweating
- Headache
- Flushing
- GI upset
- Weight loss
- Hypertension (paroxysmal or continuous)
- Tachycardia
- Arrhythmias
- Fever

Investigations
- Raised 24-hour excretion of urinary catecholamines
- CT or MRI adrenal glands
- MIBG scan ^{131}I metaiodobenzylguanidine is specifically taken up in sites of sympathetic activity
  — Positive in 90% of phaeochromocytomas

Management
- Remove tumour
- α- and β-blockade (α first with phenoxybenzamine, then β with propranolol) prior to surgery to prevent dangerous swings in blood pressure

Multiple endocrine neoplasia (MEN)
- Simultaneous or metachronous occurrence of tumours in a number of endocrine glands with autosomal dominant inheritance

Type 1
- Parathyroid – adenomas, hyperplasia
- Pituitary – adenomas
- Pancreas – islet cell tumours (e.g. insulinoma), gastrinoma
- Adrenal adenoma
- Thyroid adenoma

Type 2a
- Adrenal – phaeochromocytoma
- Thyroid – medullary carcinoma
- Parathyroid – adenomas, adenocarcinoma

Type 2b
- Type 2a plus Marfanoid phenotype plus visceral ganglioneuromas

Diabetes mellitus (K&C, p. 1069)

I Syndrome characterized by chronic hyperglycaemia due to relative insulin deficiency or resistance or both

WHO CLASSIFICATION OF DIABETES

Type 1
(K&C, p. 1071)

I β cell destruction usually leading to absolute insulin deficiency
I Autoimmune or idiopathic

Type 2
(K&C, p. 1074)

I Variable combination of insulin resistance and defects in insulin secretion

Other specific types

Genetic defects

I Defects of β cell function or insulin function

Endocrinopathies

I Cushing's syndrome
I Acromegaly
I Phaeochromocytoma
I Hyperthyroidism

Diseases of the endocrine pancreas

I Trauma
I Pancreatectomy
I Chronic pancreatitis
I Fibrocalculous pancreatic diabetes
I Cystic fibrosis
I Haemochromatosis
I Cancer

Drug-induced

I Corticosteroids
I Thiazides

WHO CRITERIA FOR DIAGNOSIS OF DIABETES (K&C, p. 1077)

I See Table 13.11 and Figure 13.7

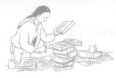

Table 13.11   WHO criteria for the diagnosis of diabetes (glucose mmol/L)

	Whole blood	Plasma
Diabetes mellitus		
Fasting	≥ 6.1	≥ 7.0
2 hrs after oral glucose load	≥ 10.0	≥ 11.1
Impaired glucose tolerance		
Fasting	< 6.1	< 7.0
2 hrs after oral glucose load	≥ 6.7 – < 10.0	≥ 7.8 – < 11.1
Impaired fasting glucose		
Fasting	≥ 5.6 – < 6.1	≥ 6.1 – < 7.0
2 hrs after oral glucose load	< 6.7	< 7.8

PRESENTING CLINICAL FEATURES (*K&C*, p. 1067)

Due to hyperglycaemia
- Thirst
- Polyuria
- Weight loss
- Ketoacidosis
- Lack of energy
- Visual blurring
- *Candida* infections
- Asymptomatic, picked up on blood/urine testing

Due to complications
- Skin infections
- Retinopathy
- Polyneuropathy
- Impotence
- Arterial disease
- Renal disease

Clinical features of complications (*K&C*, pp. 1092–1100)

Macrovascular and microvascular disease
- Atheroma
- Strokes
- Myocardial ischaemia
- Renal disease
- Peripheral vascular disease
- Retinopathy

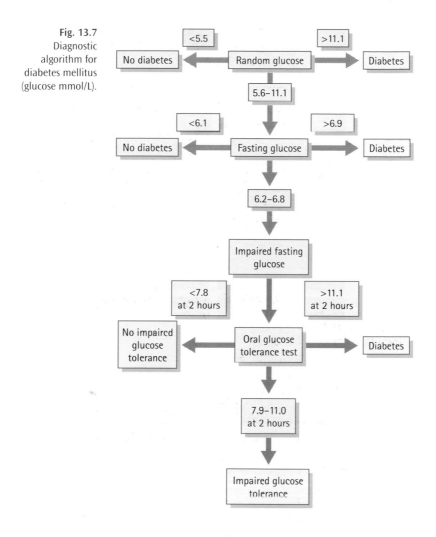

Fig. 13.7 Diagnostic algorithm for diabetes mellitus (glucose mmol/L).

<5.5		>11.1
No diabetes ←	Random glucose	→ Diabetes

5.6–11.1

<6.1		>6.9
No diabetes ←	Fasting glucose	→ Diabetes

6.2–6.8

Impaired fasting glucose

<7.8 at 2 hours		>11.1 at 2 hours
No impaired glucose tolerance ←	Oral glucose tolerance test	→ Diabetes

7.9–11.0 at 2 hours

Impaired glucose tolerance

Eyes ▌ See Figure 13.8

Kidney ▌ Glomerulosclerosis
▌ Microalbuminuria
▌ Persistent proteinuria
▌ End-stage renal failure (associated with anaemia, raised ESR and hypertension)
▌ Ischaemia
▌ Ascending infection

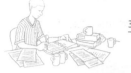

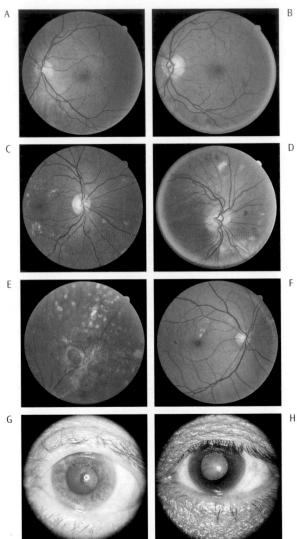

Fig. 13.8   Features of diabetic eye disease. A. The normal macula (centre) and optic disc.
B. Dot and blot haemorrhages (early background retinopathy). C. Hard exudates are present
in addition in background retinopathy. D. Multiple cotton-wool spots indicate pre-
proliferative retinopathy requiring routine ophthalmic referral. E. Multiple frond-like new
vessels, the hallmark of proliferative retinopathy. White fibrous tissue is forming near the
new vessels, a feature of advanced retinopathy. (This eye also illustrates multiple xenon arc
laser burns superiorly.) F. Exudates appearing within a disc width of the macula are a feature
of an exudative maculopathy. G and H. Central and cortical cataracts can be seen against the
red reflex with the ophthalmoscope. (Reproduced with permission from Kumar and Clark
(2002). *Clinical Medicine*: Saunders, Edinburgh.)

Neuropathy
- Peripheral polyneuropathy (loss of ankle jerks and malleolar vibration sense)
- Glove and stocking sensory neuropathy
- Mononeuritis multiplex
- Peripheral and cranial nerve
- Autonomic neuropathy:
  — Diarrhoea
  — Postural hypotension
  — Impotence
  — Gastroparesis
- Diabetic amyotrophy – painful asymmetrical wasting of quadriceps
- Charcot's joints

Diabetic foot
(Table 13.12)
- Ischaemic and/or neuropathic ulcers

Infections
- Only increased in poor glycaemic control
- Skin sepsis, e.g. staphylococcal or candida
- Urinary tract infection
- Pneumonia
- TB

MANAGEMENT OF DIABETES MELLITUS (*K&C*, p. 1078)

- Based on self-monitoring and management by the patient, helped and advised by specialists
- Requires good education and understanding of disease by the patient, including
  — Monitoring blood sugar

Table 13.12 The diabetic foot

	Ischaemic	Neuropathic
Symptoms	Claudication Rest pain	Usually painless
Signs	Trophic changes Cold Pulseless Painful ulcers Ulcers on heels and toes	High arch, clawed toes Warm Bounding pulse Painless ulcers Ulcers on sole and where shoes rub

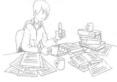

— Self-injection of insulin
— Managing hypoglycaemic events
— How to recognize complications
— When to contact specialists for help

Glycaemic control (K&C, p. 1078)

Diet ❙ All patients need education regarding a diabetic diet

Insulin ❙ See Table 13.13

Drugs *Sulphonylureas, e.g. gliclazide*
❙ May cause hypoglycaemia and weight gain

Biguanides, e.g. metformin
❙ Do not cause hypoglycaemia
❙ May aid weight loss

α-glucosidase inhibitors, e.g. acarbose
❙ Do not cause hypoglycaemia

Insulin sensitizers, e.g. rosiglitazone
❙ Might cause hepatotoxicity

Insulin formulations (K&C, p. 1080)

❙ Synthetic human insulins are almost exclusively used
❙ Insulin is given regularly by subcutaneous injection
❙ Insulin regimes are developed to suit individual patients and may be tailored according to specific needs for certain situations, e.g. missing meals, heavy exercise

Soluble insulin ❙ Fast-acting and short-acting
❙ Good for fine control
❙ Needs frequent administration

Table 13.13   Indications for insulin treatment

Anyone who has been in ketoacidosis
Patients presenting under 40 years old
Failure of oral therapy

Prolonged acting   **❙** Mixed in varying degrees with soluble insulin to
insulin   give a prolonged duration of action but with less
accuracy and slower onset of action

Complications of insulin treatment (K&C, p. 1083)
❙ Lipoatrophy and lipohypertrophy at injection site
❙ Weight gain
❙ Hypoglycaemia

Monitoring diabetic control (K&C, p. 1085)
Home monitoring   **❙** Urine reagent strips – simple but not very accurate
❙ Blood glucose reagent strips – more immediately
accurate

Hospital blood tests   **❙** HbA$_{1c}$ (glycosylated haemoglobin)
❙ Fructosamine (glycosylated plasma protein)
❙ Both give an index of average blood glucose
concentration over the past 6 weeks

Diabetes clinic   **❙** Every visit
checkup visits   — Review self-monitoring
— Review current treatment (including diet)
— Ongoing patient education

HYPOGLYCAEMIA

Clinical features
Sweating
Tremor
Pounding heart
Pallor
Drowsiness
Confusion
Coma
Fits

Management
Mild
    Oral rapidly absorbed carbohydrate, e.g glucose drink, tea
    with sugar or sweets
Severe
    i.v. 50% glucose injection 20–50 ml (after taking blood to
    confirm hypoglycaemia but before waiting for result)
    1 mg i.m. glucagon injection

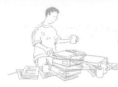

I Annual review
— Weight
— Blood pressure
— Biochemical assessment of control
— Visual acuity and retinal examination
— Check feet for condition, pulses, sensation and ankle jerks
— Urinalysis for proteinuria
— Blood lipids
— Renal function

DIABETIC EMERGENCIES

Diabetic ketoacidosis (*K&C*, p. 1088)
I Uncontrolled diabetes with acidosis and ketosis due to insulin deficiency (p. 351)

Non-ketotic hyperosmolar state (*K&C*, p. 1091)
I Severe hyperglycaemia without ketosis usually in type II diabetes

Clinical features
I Severe dehydration
I Stupor
I Coma
I Underlying illness (e.g. pneumonia)

Investigations
I High plasma osmolarity
I High serum sodium
I Very high plasma glucose
I High urea
I Normal arterial pH

Management
I Treat underlying cause
I Intravenous insulin to correct hyperglycaemia
I Normal saline to correct fluid depletion – beware rapid changes of osmolality due to reducing plasma sodium or glucose levels too fast
I Subcutaneous prophylactic heparin
I Mortality is up to 25%

DIABETIC KETOACIDOSIS

Clinical features
Prostration
Hyperventilation (Kussmaul's breathing)
Nausea and vomiting
Abdominal pain
Confusion
Coma
Dehydration
Ketones on breath
Hyperglycaemia
Ketonuria or ketonaemia
Acidosis

Principles of management
Replace fluid loss
Replace electrolyte loss
Restore acid–base balance (usually achieved by correcting
    circulating volume and stopping ketone production with
    insulin)
Replace deficient insulin
Continuous i.v. infusion of soluble insulin
Monitor blood glucose
I.v. glucose in i.v. fluids to prevent hypoglycaemia
(Do not stop insulin)
Seek underlying cause and treat appropriately

Emergency treatment
Insulin
    Intravenous insulin 6 units stat then
    6 units/hour by continuous infusion with blood glucose
        monitoring
Fluid
    Normal saline
    1 L in 30 minutes then
    1 L in 1 hour then
    1 L in 2 hours then
    1 L in 4 hours then
    1 L every 6 hours for 24 hours
    i.e. at least 4 L in first 24 hours
Check serum potassium hourly initially and add
    20 mmol/L of i.v. fluid when < 4 mmol
Monitor central venous pressure if shocked at presentation
Insert urinary catheter if anuric for > 2 hours
Antibiotics if septic
Subcutaneous heparin to prevent thrombosis

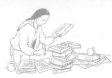

Self-assessment questions

Multiple choice questions

1. The following statements about TSH are correct:
   A. It is produced by the parathyroid glands
   B. It is reduced in primary hypothyroidism
   C. It is a sensitive marker of under-treatment during thyroxine replacement
   D. In a normal TRH stimulation test TSH secretion should be inhibited
   E. Levels are low in Graves' disease

2. The following are common features of Graves' disease:
   A. Atrial fibrillation
   B. Goitre
   C. Oedema
   D. Anorexia
   E. Weight loss

3. The following are common features of hypothyroidism:
   A. Heat intolerance
   B. Pretibial myxoedema
   C. Hoarse voice
   D. Weight gain
   E. Depression

4. The following statements about pituitary function are correct:
   A. Suspected diabetes insipidus is investigated with a water deprivation test
   B. Prolactin production, unlike that of other pituitary hormones, is principally controlled by an inhibitory factor
   C. ACTH and cortisol production display a circadian rythym
   D. Sheehan's syndome is commoner in men than women
   E. TSH is secreted from the posterior pituitary

5. In patients with untreated active acromegaly:
   A. About 25% of patients have impaired glucose tolerance
   B. Arthritis is a common feature
   C. An oral glucose tolerance test is used to confirm the diagnosis
   D. Serum IGF-1 levels are low
   E. The incidence of carcinoma of the colon is increased

6. The following are common features of panhypopituitarism:
   A. Diabetes mellitus
   B. Failure of lactation
   C. Infertility
   D. Pigmentation
   E. Increased urinary catecholamines

7. The following biochemical findings are often seen in an acutely unwell patient presenting with an Addisonian crisis:
   A. Hypernatraemia
   B. Hyperkalaemia
   C. A low ACTH
   D. Hypercalcaemia
   E. A raised TSH

8. The following statements about Cushing's syndrome are correct:
   A. The commonest cause is an ACTH-secreting tumour of the pituitary
   B. There is impaired glucose tolerance in 75% of cases

C. Severe hypokalaemia may be indicative of ectopic ACTH production

D. Proximal myopathy is a common feature

E. Alcohol excess may mimic the biochemical findings of Cushing's disease

9. The following are true of ectopic ACTH secretion:

A. There is failure of suppression of cortisol secretion during a high-dose dexamethasone suppression test

B. It may be caused by a bronchial carcinoma

C. It may cause increased skin pigmentation

D. It is associated with small atrophic adrenal glands

E. Diagnosis may require inferior petrosal venous sinus blood sampling

10. The following are features of cranial diabetes insipidus:

A. It may be associated with optic atrophy

B. It may be associated with postpartum haemorrhage

C. It is caused by treatment with lithium

D. It responds to treatment with DDAVP

E. It is treated with fluid restriction

11. The following are causes of nephrogenic diabetes insipidus:

A. Sheehan's syndrome

B. Pancreatic islet cell antibodies

C. Excessive water drinking

D. Hypercalcaemia

E. Hypokalaemia

12. The following are features of SIADH:

A. Hypernatraemia

B. Low urine osmolality

C. Diagnosis requires serum ADH measurement

D. It may present with fits

E. Treatment includes fluid restriction

13. The following are true of phaeochromocytoma:

A. It is the cause of 10% of all hypertension

B. It is caused by a tumour of adrenal cortex in 90% of cases

C. alpha- and β-adrenergic blockers are used prior to surgery to prevent swings in blood pressure

D. It is seen in MEN type 2

E. It is associated with coarctation of the aorta

14. The following are seen in MEN type 2a:

A. Marfanoid phenotype

B. Phaeochromocytoma

C. Pancreatic islet cell tumours

D. Pituitary tumours

E. Medullary carcinoma of the thyroid

15. The following statements about diabetes mellitus are correct:

A. The diagnosis is made on the basis of a fasting glucose > 7.8 mmol/L

B. When it presents in pregnancy (gestational diabetes) it usually resolves after delivery

C. In patients with proliferative diabetic retinopathy thrombolysis is contraindicated in the event of a myocardial infarction

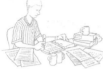

D. The glycated haemoglobin (HbA_{1c}) level is used to assess diabetic control

E. The mortality following anterior myocardial infarction is twice as high in diabetic as in non-diabetic patients

16. Regarding type II diabetes:
   A. Treatment with metformin works by increasing pancreatic insulin production
   B. Retinopathy is much rarer than in type I diabetes
   C. The thiazolidinediones are a new class of drug for treatment
   D. It only affects adults over the age of 40
   E. The incidence in the UK is falling

17. In type I diabetes:
   A. Patients control their blood glucose by regular self-injection of i.m. insulin
   B. There is a strong genetic association with HLA-DR3/DR4
   C. The average life expectancy is less than in type II diabetes
   D. There is an association with coeliac disease

E. Patients on insulin are unable to hold a UK driving licence

18. The following statements about diabetic ketoacidosis are correct:
   A. It cannot occur in patients with type II diabetes
   B. The plasma potassium is usually raised at presentation
   C. When treatment is started the plasma potassium often falls
   D. The plasma anion gap is normal
   E. It can result in a low plasma phosphate level

19. In diabetic ketoacidosis
   A. Patients should be treated immediately with subcutaneous insulin
   B. Acidosis usually corrects with insulin and fluid replacement
   C. Patients should eat normally as soon as possible
   D. A fast respiratory rate indicates concurrent pneumonia
   E. Insulin therapy is no longer needed when the blood glucose returns to normal

Extended matching questions

Question 1 *Theme: polyuria*

A. Diabetes mellitus
B. Diabetes insipidus
C. Chronic renal failure
D. Primary hyperparathyroidism
E. Chronic hypokalaemia
F. Urinary tract infection
G. Diuretic therapy
H. Compulsive water drinking
I. Supraventricular tachycardia

For each of the following questions, select the best answer from the list above:

I. A 48-year-old female with a previous Whipple's operation (pancreatoduodenectomy) for Zollinger–Ellison syndrome presents with a 3-month history of polyuria and constipation.
   What is the most likely diagnosis?

II. A 27-year-old female presents with polyuria 2 months after home delivery of a healthy 3.2 kg son. She needed urgent hospital admission after the birth for blood transfusion for postpartum haemorrhage.
What is the most likely diagnosis?

III. A 16-year-old male presents with a 4-week history of thirst, polyuria, malaise and loss of appetite. Serum urea and electrolytes are normal apart from $HCO_3 = 19$ mmol/L.
What is the most likely diagnosis?

Question 2 *Theme: weight loss*

A. Thyrotoxicosis
B. Coeliac disease
C. Carcinoma of the stomach
D. Diabetes mellitus
E. Addison's disease
F. Anorexia nervosa
G. Breast cancer
H. Crohn's disease
I. Amphetamine abuse

For each of the following questions, select the best answer from the list above:

I. A 57-year-old female on B_{12} injections for pernicious anaemia presents with anxiety, palpitations, intermittent diarrhoea and weight loss of 6 kg over 3 months.
What is the most likely diagnosis?

II. A 29-year-old male presents with night sweats, fever, abdominal pain and weight loss of 10 kg since he returned from Bangladesh 3 months ago. Examination shows increased pigmentation in the palmar creases and postural hypotension.
What is the most likely diagnosis?

III. A 36-year-old female from Galway presents with a 6-month history of weight loss and abdominal cramps. Blood tests show iron deficiency and folate deficiency.
What is the most likely diagnosis?

Short answer questions

1. Describe the clinical features of the following
   A. Hyperthyroidism
   B. Acromegaly
   C. Primary hypoadrenalism

2. Write short notes on the following
   A. Multiple endocrine neoplasia
   B. Phaeochromocytoma
   C. Goitre

3. Briefly discuss the causes of the following
   A. Cushing's syndrome
   B. Adrenal failure
   C. Diabetes insipidus

4. Write short notes on the following
   A. Thyroid related eye abnormalities
   B. SIADH
   C. Causes of polyuria

5. List the following
   A. The hormones secreted by the anterior pituitary and their functions
   B. The causes of hypopituitarism
   C. The biochemical changes seen in primary hyperaldosteronism

Essay questions

1. Discuss the use of thyroid function tests in thyroid disorders.

2. Describe the clinical features, diagnosis and treatment of Graves' disease.

3. Describe the functions of the anterior pituitary.

4. Discuss the use of dynamic tests in pituitary disease.

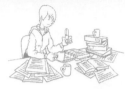

5. Describe how you would investigate a patient with a suspected diagnosis of Cushing's syndrome.

6. Describe the functions of the posterior pituitary.

7. How would you investigate a patient to exclude an endocrine cause of hypertension?

8. Discuss the important points in managing a young patient with a new diagnosis of type I diabetes requiring insulin treatment.

9. Describe the important points to be addressed in a yearly diabetes checkup.

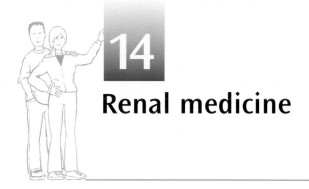

Renal medicine

For more detail see Kumar and Clark's
Clinical Medicine, Chapter 11.

Functions of the kidney *(K&C, p. 588)*

Excretory ▌ Waste products

Regulatory ▌ Control of body fluid volume and composition

Endocrine ▌ Erythropoietin
▌ Renin-angiotensin
▌ Prostaglandins

Metabolic ▌ Vitamin D

Examining the renal system

▌ All systems need to be examined but pay special attention to the following

Kidneys ▌ Position
▌ Size
▌ Shape
▌ Scars from previous surgery

Urine *(K&C, p. 593)*
Urinalysis ▌ Chemical (Stix) testing
▌ Blood

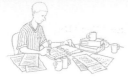

> **PALPATION OF THE KIDNEYS**
> Place one hand posteriorly on the flank with the other hand anteriorly
> Gently push up from below aiming to 'ballot' the kidney
> Differences between kidney and spleen
> ❙ Kidneys are ballotable
> ❙ Spleen has a notch
> ❙ You cannot get above the spleen
> ❙ Spleen is dull to percussion

❙ Protein
❙ Glucose
❙ Bacterial nitrites

Microscopy
❙ White cells
❙ Red cells
❙ Bacteria
❙ Casts

Volume
❙ Oliguria
❙ Polyuria
❙ Specific gravity and osmolality
❙ Urinary pH

Investigations in nephrology

IMAGING (*K&C*, p. 596)

Plain X-rays
❙ Renal calcification
❙ Renal calculi

Excretory urography
❙ Intravenous urogram
❙ Anatomy of renal tract
❙ Excretion of contrast

Ultrasound
❙ Renal masses
❙ Renal cysts
❙ Dilatation of renal tract – obstruction
❙ Renal size
❙ Bladder emptying

CT and MRI	▌ Retroperitoneal masses
Arteriography	▌ Extrarenal arterial imaging
Dynamic scintigraphy	▌ DPTA – shows perfusion ▌ Shows glomerular filtration ▌ Demonstrates obstruction
Static scintigraphy	▌ DMSA – renal function ▌ Visualization of kidney

RENAL BIOPSY (K&C, p. 600)

▌ Transcutaneous under ultrasound control

| Indications | ▌ Nephrotic syndrome
▌ Unexplained renal failure
▌ Diagnosis of systemic disease |
| Contraindications | ▌ Single kidney
▌ Small kidneys
▌ Haemorrhagic disorders
▌ Uncontrolled hypertension |

BIOCHEMICAL RENAL FUNCTION TESTS (K&C, p. 590)

Serum urea and creatinine	▌ Rise due to failure of excretion when glomerular filtration rate (GFR) is reduced by 50–60% (i.e. may be normal in the presence of significant decrease in renal function)
Creatinine clearance	▌ Estimates GFR ▌ $= \dfrac{V \text{ (urine volume)} \times U \text{ (urine creatinine concentration)}}{P \text{ (plasma creatinine concentration)}} \times 100$
Arterial blood gases	▌ Metabolic acidosis in renal failure due to failure to excrete fixed acid and renal bicarbonate loss

Glomerulonephritis (K&C, p. 601)

▌ A group of disorders
  — With immunologically mediated injury to glomerulus

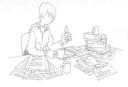
— Which involves both kidneys
— With secondary injury after initial immune insult
— Which may be part of generalized disease
— Classified by histology

Pathogenesis ❙ Deposition of immune complexes
❙ Deposition of anti-glomerular basement
membrane (anti-GBM) antibody

Aetiology *Immune complex nephritis*
❙ Unknown antigen
❙ Viruses
— Mumps
— Measles
— Hepatitis B and C
— Epstein–Barr virus (EBV)
— Coxsackie
— Varicella
— HIV
❙ Bacteria
— Group A β-haemolytic streptococci
— *Streptococcus viridans*
— Staphylococci
— *Treponema pallidum*
— Gonococci
— Salmonellae
❙ Parasites
— *Plasmodium malariae*
— *Schistosoma*
— Filiariasis
❙ Host antigens
— DNA (systemic lupus erythematosus – SLE)
— Cryoglobulins
— Malignant tumours
❙ Drugs
— Penicillamine

Anti-GBM antibody
❙ Antibodies to type IV collagen

Secondary mechanisms
❙ Complement activation

I Fibrin deposition
I Platelet aggregation
I Neutrophil-driven inflammation
I Kinin activation

Clinical features   I GN presents in one of four ways
— Asymptomatic proteinuria +/– microscopic haematuria
— Acute nephritic syndrome (Fig. 14.1)
— Nephrotic syndrome (Fig. 14.2)
— Chronic renal failure

Investigations   I 24-hour urinary protein (twice)
I Urine microscopy
I Assessment of renal function
I Excretory urography

SPECIFIC TYPES OF GN (Table 4.1) (*K&C*, pp. 604–607)

IgA nephropathy
Pathology   I Focal proliferative GN
I Mesangial deposits of IgA

Clinical features   I Microscopic haematuria
I Children and young adults

Prognosis   I Usually good
I 20% eventually develop renal failure

Henoch–Schönlein purpura
Pathology   I Focal segmental GN

Clinical features   I Purpuric rash
I Abdominal colic
I Joint pain
I ♂ > ♀ (2:1)
I Often after recent respiratory infection

Prognosis   I Usually good

Goodpasture's syndrome
Pathology   I Severe proliferative crescentic GN

Table 14.1 Types of glomerulonephritis

Histology	Example of causes	Clinical presentation
Proliferative glomerulonephritis		
Diffuse	Post-streptococcal	Acute nephritic syndrome
Focal segmental	SLE	Haematuria
	Henoch–Schönlein purpura	Proteinuria
Crescentic	Wegener's granulomatosis	Progressive renal failure
	Goodpasture's syndrome	
Mesangiocapillary		
Type1	Hepatitis B and C	Haematuria
		Proteinuria
Type 2	Measles	Nephrotic syndrome
Membranous	Unknown	Nephrotic syndrome
	Malaria	
Minimal change	Unknown	Nephrotic syndrome (especially in children)
IgA nephropathy	Henoch–Schönlein purpura	Asymptomatic haematuria
Focal glomerulosclerosis	Diabetes mellitus	Proteinuria
		Nephrotic syndrome

Clinical features ▌ Haemoptysis
▌ Progressive renal failure

Prognosis ▌ Usually progresses to renal failure

ACUTE NEPHRITIC SYNDROME (*K&C*, p. 606)

▌ Classically occurs 3 weeks after streptococcal throat infection or otitis media
▌ See Figure 14.1

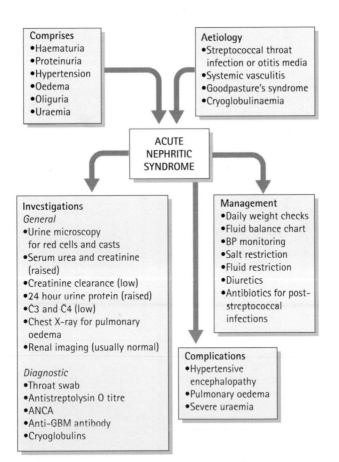

Comprises
- Haematuria
- Proteinuria
- Hypertension
- Oedema
- Oliguria
- Uraemia

Aetiology
- Streptococcal throat infection or otitis media
- Systemic vasculitis
- Goodpasture's syndrome
- Cryoglobulinaemia

ACUTE NEPHRITIC SYNDROME

Investigations
General
- Urine microscopy for red cells and casts
- Serum urea and creatinine (raised)
- Creatinine clearance (low)
- 24 hour urine protein (raised)
- C3 and C4 (low)
- Chest X-ray for pulmonary oedema
- Renal imaging (usually normal)

Diagnostic
- Throat swab
- Antistreptolysin O titre
- ANCA
- Anti-GBM antibody
- Cryoglobulins

Management
- Daily weight checks
- Fluid balance chart
- BP monitoring
- Salt restriction
- Fluid restriction
- Diuretics
- Antibiotics for post-streptococcal infections

Complications
- Hypertensive encephalopathy
- Pulmonary oedema
- Severe uraemia

Fig. 14.1   Acute nephritic syndrome.

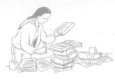

NEPHROTIC SYNDROME (*K&C*, p. 611)

❙ See Figure 14.2

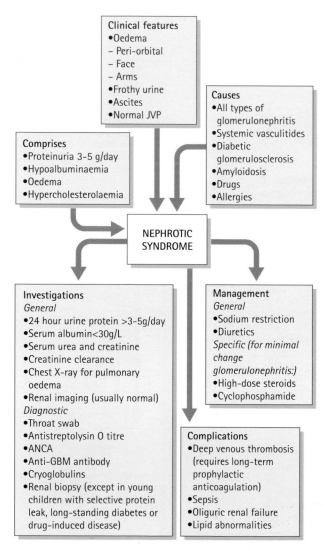

Clinical features
- Oedema
  - Peri-orbital
  - Face
  - Arms
- Frothy urine
- Ascites
- Normal JVP

Causes
- All types of glomerulonephritis
- Systemic vasculitides
- Diabetic glomerulosclerosis
- Amyloidosis
- Drugs
- Allergies

Comprises
- Proteinuria 3–5 g/day
- Hypoalbuminaemia
- Oedema
- Hypercholesterolaemia

NEPHROTIC SYNDROME

Investigations
General
- 24 hour urine protein >3–5g/day
- Serum albumin<30g/L
- Serum urea and creatinine
- Creatinine clearance
- Chest X-ray for pulmonary oedema
- Renal imaging (usually normal)
Diagnostic
- Throat swab
- Antistreptolysin O titre
- ANCA
- Anti-GBM antibody
- Cryoglobulins
- Renal biopsy (except in young children with selective protein leak, long-standing diabetes or drug-induced disease)

Management
General
- Sodium restriction
- Diuretics
Specific (for minimal change glomerulonephritis:)
- High-dose steroids
- Cyclophosphamide

Complications
- Deep venous thrombosis (requires long-term prophylactic anticoagulation)
- Sepsis
- Oliguric renal failure
- Lipid abnormalities

Fig. 14.2 Nephrotic syndrome.

GLOMERULAR DISORDERS IN SYSTEMIC DISEASE

Systemic vasculitis (K&C, p. 608)
- SLE – all types of glomerulonephritis
- Polyarteritis nodosa (PAN) – renal failure
- Microscopic polyarteritis – crescentic glomerulonephritis
- Wegener's granulomatosis – glomerulonephritis

Cryoglobulinaemia (K&C, p. 609)
- Monoclonal or polyclonal expansion of abnormal immunoglobulins which precipitate reversibly in the cold (cryoglobulins)

Aetiology
- Viral infections, e.g. hepatitis B and C, cytomegalovirus (CMV), EBV
- Fungal infections
- Malaria
- Infective endocarditis
- Autoimmune diseases

Clinical features
- Glomerulonephritis
- Purpura
- Raynaud's phenomenon
- Systemic vasculitis
- Polyneuropathy
- Hepatic involvement

Diabetes mellitus
- See Chapter 13, page 345

Amyloidosis (K&C, p. 610)
- A disorder of protein metabolism with extracellular deposition of insoluble fibrillar proteins in organs and tissues

Types
- AL amyloidosis
- Familial amyloidosis
- Secondary amyloidosis

AL amyloidosis (K&C, p. 118)
Pathology
- Plasma cell production of amyloidogenic immunoglobulin light chains (AL)
- AL chains are excreted in urine (Bence Jones proteins)

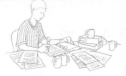

I Associated with myeloma and Waldenström's macroglobulinaemia

Clinical features
I Nephrotic syndrome
I Cardiomyopathy
I Autonomic neuropathy
I Sensory neuropathy
I Carpal tunnel syndrome
I Hepatomegaly
I Splenomegaly
I Bruising
I Macroglossia

Familial amyloidosis (K&C, p. 1118)

Pathology
I Autosomal dominant inherited mutant protein formation
I Mutant protein forms amyloid fibrils

Mutant proteins
I Transthyretin (commonest)
I Apolipoprotein A-1
I Fibrinogen
I Lysosyme

Clinical features
I Peripheral sensorimotor neuropathy
I Autonomic neuropathy
I Conduction defects in heart

Secondary amyloidosis

Pathology
I Amyloid is formed from acute phase protein serum amyloid A (SAA)

Aetiology
I Rheumatoid arthritis
I Inflammatory bowel disease
I Familial Mediterranean fever
I Tuberculosis
I Bronchiectasis
I Osteomyelitis

Clinical features
I Renal disease
I Hepatosplenomegaly

Diagnosis of amyloidosis
I Rectal or gum biopsy
I Amyloid stains red with Congo red and has green birefringence in polarized light

Management of amyloidosis
- Treat associated disorder
- Treat nephrotic syndrome or cardiac failure
- Chemotherapy for AL
- Liver transplant for transthyretin-associated amyloidosis

Haemolytic uraemic syndrome (HUS) (K&C, p. 610)
- Follows gastroenteritis or respiratory tract infection, *E. coli* 0157
- Comprises
  — Intravascular haemolysis
  — Thrombocytopenia
  — Acute renal failure

Thrombotic thrombocytopenic purpura (K&C, p. 611)
- Microangiopathic haemolysis
- Renal failure
- Neurological disturbance

Multiple myeloma
- Monoclonal expansion of B cells which secrete light chains (immunoglobulin fragments)
- Acute renal failure
- Myeloma kidney
- Renal amyloid deposits

Contrast nephropathy
- Caused by iodinated radiological contrast media
- Dose-dependent effect
- Risk increased with
  — Pre-existing renal impairment
  — Hypovolaemia
  — Low cardiac output
  — Diabetes mellitus
  — Hyperviscosity
- Risk reduced by
  — *n*-Acetyl cysteine
  — Pre-hydration with saline

Urinary tract infection (K&C, p. 615)

- Common in women; 90% of attacks are isolated
- Uncommon in men

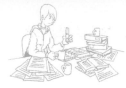

BACTERIAL INFECTIONS

Causative organisms

- *E. coli* – 70%
- *Proteus mirabilis* – 10%
- *Staphylococcus saprophyticus* or *epidermidis* – 10%
- *Klebsiella aerogenes* – 5%
- *Enterococcus faecalis* – 5%

Associated diseases

- Diabetes mellitus
- Sickle cell disease or trait
- Analgesic abuse
- Stones
- Obstruction
- Polycystic kidneys
- Vesico-ureteric reflux

Clinical features

- Cystitis
  — Frequency of micturition
  — Dysuria
  — Suprapubic pain/tenderness
  — Haematuria
  — Smelly urine
- Pyelonephritis
  — Loin pain/tenderness
  — Fever
  — Systemic upset

Investigations

- Symptomatic women
  — Dipstix + for nitrites and leucocytes
  — > 10^2 coliforms/mL + pyuria *or* }
  — > 10^5 any pathogenic organism/mL *or* } MSU
  — Any growth from suprapubic bladder aspiration
- Symptomatic men
  — > 10^3 pathogenic organisms/mL
- Asymptomatic patients
  — > 10^5 pathogenic organisms/mL (× 2)
- Causes of sterile pyuria
  — *Chlamydia*
  — TB

Radiology ❙ Excretory urography
— Women with ≥ 3 attacks
— All men
— All children
❙ Abdominal X-ray and ultrasound
— Acute pyelonephritis

Management ❙ Oral antibiotics
— Amoxicillin
— Nitrofurantoin
— Trimethoprim
— Oral cephalosporin
❙ Intravenous antibiotics
— For acute pyelonephritis with high fever, vomiting or systemic upset
— Cefuroxime
— Gentamicin
— Ciprofloxacin

Tuberculosis of the renal tract (*K&C*, p. 620)

❙ Affects the renal cortex spreading to the papillae and into the urine, ureters and bladder
❙ May cause ureteric obstruction and hydronephrosis

Investigations ❙ Culture of acid-fast bacillae from early morning urine (EMU) samples

Renal calculi (*K&C*, p. 625)

Prevalence ❙ 2% of UK population

Types of urinary stone ❙ See Table 14.2

Aetiology ❙ Dehydration
❙ Hypercalcaemia
❙ Hypercalciuria
❙ Hyperoxaluria
❙ Hyperuricaemia

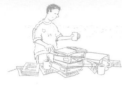

Table 14.2 Types of urinary stone

Type	Frequency
Calcium oxalate	65%
Calcium phosphate	15%
Magnesium ammonium phosphate	10–15%
Uric acid	3–5%
Cystine	1–2%

▌ Infection
▌ Cystinuria
▌ Renal tubular acidosis
▌ Primary renal disease

Clinical features ▌ Asymptomatic
▌ Renal colic
▌ Haematuria
▌ Urinary tract infection
▌ Obstruction

Investigations ▌ Midstream urine (MSU) and culture
▌ Serum urea and electrolytes, creatinine
▌ Serum calcium
▌ Serum urate
▌ Plain abdominal X-ray
▌ Excretion urography
▌ Urinary calcium, oxalate and uric acid
▌ Sieve urine to trap stones for analysis

Management ▌ Analgesia (opiates, NSAIDs)
▌ High fluid intake
▌ Stones < 0.5 cm pass spontaneously
▌ Stones > 1 cm require intervention
▌ Obstruction or infection requires intervention

Intervention *Percutaneous nephrolithotomy*
▌ Endoscopic extraction of renal pelvis stones
  through a percutaneous tract

Extracorporeal shock-wave lithotripsy (ESWL)
I Fragmentation of stones with shock waves focused in from an external source

Urinary tract obstruction (K&C, p. 631)

I See Table 14.3

Hydronephrosis   I Dilatation of renal pelvis above obstruction

Clinical features   I Loin pain/tenderness
I Anuria – bilateral obstruction
I Polyuria
I Bladder outflow obstruction (hesitancy, poor stream, terminal dribbling)
I Palpable enlarged kidney(s)

Investigations   I Urea and electrolytes
I Ultrasound
I Excretion urography
I Cystoscopy

Management   I Relieve obstruction by temporary drainage via nephrostomy or urethral or suprapubic catheter
I Treat underlying cause
I Prevent and/or treat infection

Table 14.3   Causes of urinary tract obstruction

Within lumen	Neuropathic bladder
Calculus	Urethral stricture
Blood clot	Calculus
Sloughed papilla	Gonococcal infection
Tumour	**Outside pressure**
Within wall	Tumours
Ureteric stricture	Aortic aneurysm
TB	Prostatic obstruction
Calculus	Retroperitoneal fibrosis
Post-surgical	Accidental ligation of ureter
Schistosomiasis	Phimosis

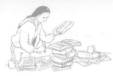

Surgical drainage
▌ Urinary diversion
▌ Ureteric stents

Acute renal failure (*K&C*, pp. 637–642)

▌ Abrupt deterioration in renal function which is usually reversible

Pre-renal uraemia   ▌ Impaired perfusion of kidneys

Aetiology   ▌ Hypovolaemia (acute blood loss, dehydration, sepsis)
▌ Hypotension
▌ Cardiac failure
▌ Renal artery stenosis

Management   ▌ Correct hypovolaemia or hypotension
▌ Monitor central venous pressure to maintain adequate vascular volume

Acute uraemia due to renal causes
Aetiology   ▌ Acute tubular necrosis (Fig. 14.3)
▌ Vasculitis
▌ Pre-eclampsia
▌ Haemolytic uraemic syndrome
▌ Rhabdomyolysis

Post-renal uraemia
▌ Urinary tract obstruction

Investigations in acute renal failure
Determine whether pre-renal, renal or post-renal   ▌ Exclude bladder outflow obstruction – insert urinary catheter
▌ Ultrasound – to exclude upper urinary tract obstruction
▌ Fluid challenge – to differentiate pre-renal from renal

Urinalysis   ▌ Dipstick for protein and blood
▌ Myoglobin

Serum biochemistry   ▌ Urea and electrolytes
— ↑ Urea

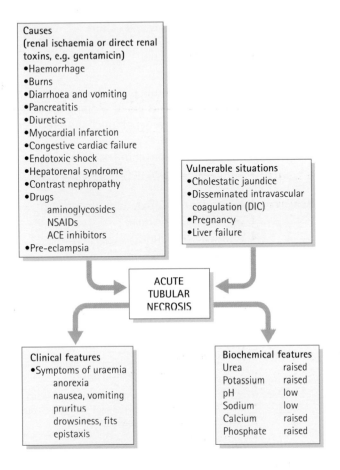

Causes
(renal ischaemia or direct renal toxins, e.g. gentamicin)
- Haemorrhage
- Burns
- Diarrhoea and vomiting
- Pancreatitis
- Diuretics
- Myocardial infarction
- Congestive cardiac failure
- Endotoxic shock
- Hepatorenal syndrome
- Contrast nephropathy
- Drugs
    aminoglycosides
    NSAIDs
    ACE inhibitors
- Pre-eclampsia

Vulnerable situations
- Cholestatic jaundice
- Disseminated intravascular coagulation (DIC)
- Pregnancy
- Liver failure

ACUTE TUBULAR NECROSIS

Clinical features
- Symptoms of uraemia
    anorexia
    nausea, vomiting
    pruritus
    drowsiness, fits
    epistaxis

Biochemical features

Urea	raised
Potassium	raised
pH	low
Sodium	low
Calcium	raised
Phosphate	raised

Fig. 14.3 Acute tubular necrosis.

- Creatinine
    — ↑ K^+
- Calcium and phosphate
- Albumin
- Alkaline phosphatase
- Urate
- Drug levels

Haematology
- Full blood count and blood film
    — Relatively normal Hb
- ESR
- Coagulation studies

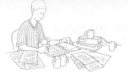

Microbiology ❙ Urine microscopy and culture
❙ Blood cultures

Management of acute uraemia

General management ❙ Admit to renal unit or ITU for support of all systems, with the aim of keeping the patient alive while waiting for renal function to recover

Diet ❙ Sodium and potassium restriction
❙ Protein restriction only if trying to avoid dialysis

Fluid balance ❙ Assessment of input–output chart
❙ Signs of fluid overload
❙ Serum electrolytes
❙ Daily weight check

Treat sepsis ❙ Avoid nephrotoxic drugs and alter dose for renally excreted drugs

HYPERKALAEMIA

Check result is compatible with patient's clinical condition (if not repeat sample)

Do ECG to look for changes of hyperkalaemia (peaked T waves, widened QRS complexes – Fig. 14.4) and put patient on cardiac monitor

For $K^+ > 6.0$ or with symptoms or ECG changes, give:
i.v. calcium gluconate 10 mL 10%
i.v. 100 mL 50% dextrose plus 10 units soluble rapid-acting insulin over 30 minutes, monitoring blood glucose for hypoglycaemia
Oral calcium resonium 15–30 g 2–3 times daily *or*
Rectal calcium resonium retention enema 50 g daily
Nebulized salbutamol 10 mg

Dialysis or haemofiltration if no correction

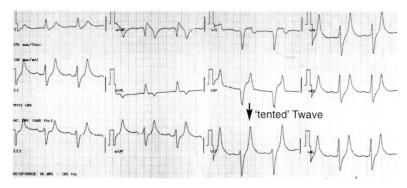

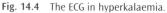

Fig. 14.4   The ECG in hyperkalaemia.

Dialysis and haemofiltration in acute renal failure

Indications   **I** Symptomatic uraemia
I Complications of uraemia, e.g. pericarditis
I Severe biochemical derangement
I Uncontrolled hyperkalaemia
I Pulmonary oedema
I Acidosis
I Removal of toxic drugs, e.g aspirin overdose, gentamicin

Options   **I** Peritoneal dialysis
I Continuous haemofiltration

Prognosis   **I** 50% mortality

Chronic renal failure (K&C, p. 643)

I Long-standing progressive impairment of renal function

Prevalence   **I** 600/million/year in UK
I End-stage renal failure – 200/million/year in UK

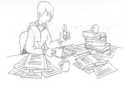

Aetiology ❚ See Table 14.4

Clinical features | *History*
❚ Duration of symptoms
❚ Drug ingestion, especially NSAIDs, analgesics and herbal therapies
❚ Past surgery
❚ Previous chemotherapy
❚ Family history of renal disease

Symptoms
❚ Asymptomatic
❚ Malaise, loss of energy
❚ Insomnia
❚ Nocturia, polyuria
❚ Itching
❚ Nausea, vomiting, diarrhoea
❚ Paraesthesiae
❚ 'Restless legs' syndrome
❚ Bone pain
❚ Peripheral or pulmonary oedema
❚ Anaemia
❚ Amenorrhoea and impotence

Signs
❚ Short stature
❚ Anaemia

Table 14.4   *Causes of chronic renal failure*

Congenital	**Tubulo-interstitial disease**
Polycystic kidney disease	Nephritis
Alport's syndrome	Idiopathic
Glomerular disease	Drugs
Primary glomerulonephritis	Reflux nephropathy
Secondary glomerulonephritis	TB
(SLE, diabetes, amyloidosis)	Schistosomiasis
Vascular disease	**Obstruction**
Atherosclerosis	Stones
Vasculitis	Prostate disease
SLE	Pelvic tumours
	Retroperitoneal fibrosis

❚ Pigmentation on sun-exposed areas
❚ Brown nails
❚ Fluid overload
❚ Signs of underlying disease

Investigations   *Urine*
❚ Urinalysis
❚ Microscopy
❚ Culture
❚ 24-hour creatinine clearance

Biochemistry
❚ Urea and electrolytes
— ↑ Urea
— ↑ normal K^+
❚ Creatinine ↑
❚ Calcium and phosphate
— ↓ Calcium

Haematology
❚ Full blood count
— Anaemia

Radiology
❚ Renal tract ultrasound
❚ Plain abdominal X-ray
❚ CT scan of abdomen and pelvis

Immunology
❚ Urinary Bence Jones proteins
❚ Serum electrophoresis and immunoglobulins
❚ Autoantibodies
❚ Complement levels

Microbiology
❚ Antistreptolysin O titre — post Strep. infection
❚ Malaria film
❚ Hepatitis B and C serology

Histology
❚ Renal biopsy

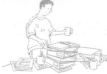
Complicaltions
- Anaemia (erythropoietin)
- Renal osteodystrophy (osteomalacia, rickets, hyperparathyroidism, osteoporosis, osteosclerosis)
- Pruritus
- Delayed gastric emptying
- Peptic ulceration (↑ gastrin)
- Pancreatitis
- Constipation
- Gout
- Hyperlipidaemia
- Hyperprolactinaemia
- Impotence and male infertility
- Amenorrhoea and female infertility
- Short stature
- Cardiovascular disease
- Cardiac failure
- Sudden death
- Stroke

Management

General
- Treat underlying disease if possible
- Control hypertension
- Early referral to nephrologist when serum creatinine > 350 μmol/L *or* in diabetics > 250 μmol/L

Diet
- Calcium supplements
- Low phosphate diet
- Sodium and potassium restriction
- Protein restriction
- Fluid restriction

Anaemia
- Erythropoietin
- Iron therapy

Renal replacement therapy

HAEMODIALYSIS *(K&C, p. 650)*

- Blood from the patient is pumped through semipermeable membranes against a dialysate fluid allowing diffusion of molecules along concentration gradients

I Requires rapid blood flow through a large-bore double-lumen central venous catheter or arteriovenous fistula

Frequency   I Usually 4–5 hours 3 times per week

Complications   I Hypotension whilst on dialysis

HAEMOFILTRATION

I Removal of plasma water and dissolved electrolytes (potassium, sodium, urea and phosphate) by flow across a semipermeable membrane and replacement with a solution of desired biochemical composition

I Mostly used in acute renal failure

Frequency   I Usually continuous

PERITONEAL DIALYSIS (*K&C*, p. 653)

I Uses peritoneum as semipermeable membrane

I Dialysis fluid is run into peritoneal cavity through a tube in the anterior abdominal wall

I Urea, creatinine and phosphate pass into the dialysate from the blood in peritoneal capillaries along a diffusion gradient

I Water and electrolytes go in through osmosis

Frequency   I Dialysis fluid is exchanged usually 3–5 times per day

I Fluid exchange takes about 40 minutes

RENAL TRANSPLANTATION (*K&C*, p. 656)

I A kidney, explanted from either a cadaveric or living related donor, is anastomosed to the iliac vessels of the recipient

I The ureter is placed into the bladder

I Immunosuppression is required for the rest of the patient's life

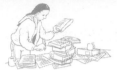

Prognosis ▌ 80% of grafts survive 5–10 years
▌ 60% of grafts survive for 10–30 years

Cystic renal diseases

▌ Solitary or multiple simple renal cysts are common, affecting
▌ 50% of the population > 50 years old
▌ Usually asymptomatic

Autosomal dominant polycystic kidney disease *(K&C, p. 658)*

▌ Inherited disorder
▌ Presents in adulthood
▌ Multiple bilateral renal cysts
▌ Associated with hepatic cysts

Prevalence ▌ 1:400–1000

Responsible genes ▌ PKD 1 on chromosome 16
▌ PKD 2 on chromosome 4

Clinical features ▌ Acute loin pain +/– haematuria (due to haemorrhage, infection or stone formation)
▌ Loin discomfort (due to large kidneys)
▌ Subarachnoid haemorrhage (secondary to berry aneurysm rupture)
▌ Hypertension
▌ Liver cysts
▌ Chronic renal failure
▌ Large irregular palpable kidneys
▌ Hepatomegaly
▌ Ultrasound shows multiple renal cysts

Complications ▌ Progression to chronic renal failure
▌ Pain
▌ Cyst infection
▌ Renal stones
▌ Hypertension
▌ Liver cysts
▌ Berry aneurysms (8%)

Screening ❚ Children and siblings of patients should have renal ultrasound after age 20

Tumours of the urogenital tract and prostate

Renal cell carcinoma (K&C, p. 661)
❚ Average age at presentation 55 years
❚ ♂ > ♀ (2:1)

Clinical features ❚ Haematuria
❚ Loin pain
❚ Mass in flank
❚ Malaise
❚ Weight loss
❚ Polycythaemia (excess erythropoietin)

Investigations ❚ Excretion urography
❚ Ultrasound
❚ MRI (for tumour staging)
❚ Raised ESR

Management ❚ Nephrectomy
❚ α-interferon/interleukin-2

Prognosis ❚ 60–70% 5-year survival for localized tumour
❚ 15–35% 5-year survival for lymph node involvement
❚ 5% 5-year survival for distant metastases

Urothelial tumours (K&C, p. 662)
❚ Transitional cell carcinoma, most common in the bladder
❚ ♂ > ♀ (4:1)
❚ Present most commonly after 40 years

Risk factors ❚ Cigarette smoking
❚ Industrial carcinogen exposure (β-naphthylamine, benzidine)
❚ Drugs (phenacetin, cyclophosphamide)
❚ Chronic inflammation (schistosomiasis causes squamous cell carcinoma)

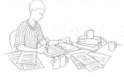
Clinical features ▮ Painless haematuria
▮ Clot retention

Investigations ▮ Urine cytology
▮ Excretion urography
▮ Cystoscopy

Management ▮ Local tumour ablation – endoscopic diathermy
▮ Local tumour resection – endoscopic transurethral bladder tumour resection (TURBT)
▮ Cystectomy
▮ Radiotherapy
▮ Local or systemic chemotherapy

Prognosis ▮ 80% 5-year survival (T1 N0 M0)
▮ 5% 5-year survival (distant metastases)

Prostate cancer (*K&C*, p. 664)

▮ Fourth commonest cause of cancer death in men
▮ Malignant change in prostate gland is very common in older men
▮ About 80% > 80 years
▮ Usually dormant or asymptomatic

Clinical features ▮ Bladder outflow obstruction
▮ Distant metastases to bone, lung or brain

Investigations ▮ Cystoscopy
▮ Transrectal ultrasound
▮ Prostatic biopsy
▮ Prostate-specific antigen (PSA)
▮ Bone scan

Management *Local disease*
▮ Radical prostatectomy
▮ Radiotherapy

Metastatic disease
▮ Orchidectomy
▮ LHRH analogues (buserelin, goserelin)

Prognosis ▮ Variable

Testicular tumours (*K&C*, p. 664)
- Commonest in young men aged 30–35
- Seminomas 30%
- Teratomas 70%
- Higher risk in undescended testes and history of orchidopexy

Clinical features
- Testicular swelling (painless or painful)
- Distant metastases

Investigations
- Testicular ultrasound
- Surgical exploration and biopsy via the groin

Staging
- Chest X-ray
- α-fetoprotein
- β-human chorionic gonadotrophin
- Abdominal CT scan

Management   *Seminomas*
- Radiotherapy

Teratomas
- Orchidectomy
- Chemotherapy

Diseases of the prostate

Benign prostatic enlargement (*K&C*, p. 663)
- Common over 60 years

Clinical features
- Bladder outflow obstruction
- Urinary tract infection
- Stones
- Acute urinary retention
- Chronic retention with overflow incontinence
- Bilateral hydronephrosis
- Smooth enlarged prostate on rectal exam

Investigations
- Urine culture
- Assessment of renal function

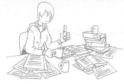

ACUTE URINARY RETENTION

Clinical features
Anuria
Pain
Urgency
Palpable bladder

Management
Urethral catheterization
Suprapubic catheterization
Look for a cause

▌ PSA
▌ Cystoscopy

Management   ▌ Observation

Medical
▌ α-receptor blockers
▌ Finasteride

Surgical
▌ Transurethral resection of prostate (TURP)
▌ Prostatic stents

Self-assessment questions

Multiple choice questions

1. IgA nephropathy:
   A. Is commoner in older patients
   B. Presents after streptococcal infections
   C. Presents with a purpuric rash
   D. Is caused by anti-GBM antibody
   E. Usually progresses to chronic renal failure

   B. Is caused by immune complex deposition
   C. Causes proliferative crescentic glomerulonephritis
   D. Usually progresses to chronic renal failure
   E. Is treated by nephrectomy

2. Goodpasture's syndrome:
   A. May present with haemoptysis

3. Acute nephritic syndrome:
   A. Occurs after streptococcal infections
   B. Comprises oedema and low albumin

C. May cause acute renal failure
D. Urine microscopy shows red cell casts
E. Is commonly complicated by hypercholesterolaemia

4. In nephrotic syndrome:
   A. Urine protein excretion is > 3 g/day
   B. The renal lesion is always proliferative glomerulonephritis
   C. The urine may be frothy
   D. The JVP is normal
   E. Renal biopsy is contraindicated

5. Urinary tract infection:
   A. Is commoner in females
   B. Is always symptomatic
   C. Usually indicates an abnormal renal tract in females
   D. May be treated with oral antibiotics
   E. Is most commonly caused by E. coli infection

6. Pyelonephritis
   A. May present with loin pain and fever
   B. May be secondary to urinary tract obstruction
   C. Is associated with diabetes mellitus
   D. Requires investigation of the renal tract
   E. May be complicated by septicaemia

7. Renal calculi:
   A. Are most commonly composed of uric acid
   B. May be asymptomatic
   C. May be caused by hyperkalaemia
   D. Are usually radiolucent
   E. Over > 2 cm pass spontaneously

8. Symptoms of bladder outflow obstruction include:
   A. Anuria
   B. Oliguria
   C. Polyuria
   D. Dysuria
   E. Incontinence

9. Pre-renal uraemia:
   A. Is caused by under-perfusion of the kidneys
   B. May be due to gastrointestinal bleeding
   C. May correct with fluid replacement
   D. Usually requires emergency dialysis
   E. Presents with pericarditis

10. Complications of acute renal failure include:
    A. Gastrointestinal bleeding
    B. Encephalopathy
    C. Hyperkalaemia
    D. Pericarditis
    E. Septicaemia

11. Acute tubular necrosis:
    A. May be caused by gentamicin toxicity
    B. May be part of multisystem failure
    C. May be caused by a reaction to intravenous radiological contrast
    D. Rarely requires dialysis
    F. Has a good overall prognosis

12. Causes of chronic renal failure include:
    A. Polycystic kidney disease
    B. Diabetes mellitus
    C. Cirrhosis of the liver
    D. Herbal therapies
    E. Gilbert's syndrome

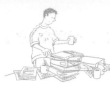

13. Clinical features of chronic renal failure commonly include:
   A. Lethargy
   B. Itching
   C. Alopecia
   D. Visual disturbance
   E. Nocturia

14. Complications of chronic renal failure commonly include:
   A. Anaemia
   B. Gout
   C. Paget's disease
   D. Hypertension
   E. Peptic ulcers

Extended matching questions

Question 1 *Theme: right-sided abdominal pain*

A. Pyelonephritis
B. Right ovarian cyst
C. Renal calculi
D. Appendicitis
E. Polycystic kidney disease
F. Crohn's disease
G. Gallstones
H. Right lower lobe pneumonia
I. Pancreatitis
J. Renal cell carcinoma
K. Hydronephrosis
L. Hepatitis
M. Irritable bowel syndrome

For each of the following questions, select the best answer from the list above:

I. A 39-year-old advertising executive, who suffers with gout, presents with sudden onset of excruciating colicky pain in the right loin. On examination he is distressed and tender in the right flank. He is apyrexial. Urinalysis shows blood^{+++} and no nitrite.
What is the most likely diagnosis?

II. A 49-year-old woman with chronic multiple sclerosis, confined to a wheelchair, presents with fever, confusion and vomiting. She is incontinent of urine with a permanent indwelling catheter. She is pyrexial with a temperature of 39°C. There is reduced air entry to the right lung base. Her Po_2 is 7.6 and urinalysis shows protein^{++}, blood$^+$, nitrite$^+$.
What is the most likely diagnosis?

III. A 39-year-old man presents with a 6-month history of a chronic dull ache in the right flank with a feeling of fullness on that side. Eighteen months ago he had emergency neurosurgical clipping of a berry aneurysm after suffering a subarachnoid haemorrhage. What is the most likely diagnosis?

Question 2 *Theme: acute renal failure*

A. Hepatorenal syndrome
B. Contrast nephropathy
C. Gentamicin toxicity
D. Acute GI haemorrhage
E. Hypertensive nephropathy
F. Haemolytic uraemic syndrome
G. Goodpasture's syndrome
H. Wegener's granulomatosis
I. Prostatic obstruction
J. Retroperitoneal fibrosis
K. Renal artery stenosis

For each of the following questions, select the best answer from the list above:

I. A 48-year-old alcoholic cirrhotic female was admitted 2 days ago with constipation and confusion. She has become pyrexial with low blood pressure and oliguria. Her blood tests show acute renal failure.
What is the most likely diagnosis?

II. A 90-year-old man is admitted in a dehydrated, febrile and confused state. He was seen by his GP for a 'stomach upset' 2 days ago. His full blood count shows anaemia and thrombocytopenia with red-cell fragments on the blood film. His biochemistry shows acute renal failure.
What is the most likely diagnosis?

III. A 74-year-old male is admitted with symptoms of a urinary tract infection. In the past 2 days he has developed increasing abdominal pain, fever and anuria. On examination he has a mass in the pelvis which is tender and dull to percussion. His blood tests show acute renal failure.
What is the most likely diagnosis?

Short answer questions

1. Write short notes on the following
   A. Cryoglobulinaemia
   B. Haemolytic uraemic syndrome (HUS)
   C. Secondary amyloidosis

2. Write short notes on the following
   A. The common causes of chronic renal failure
   B. Write short notes on peritoneal dialysis in chronic renal failure
   C. Anaemia in chronic renal failure

3. Write short notes on the following
   A. Management of acute hyperkalaemia in acute renal failure

   B. The biochemical abnormalities which occur in acute renal failure
   C. The indications for renal replacement therapy in acute renal failure

4. Write short notes on
   A. Sterile pyuria
   B. Associated risk factors for urinary tract infection
   C. The diagnostic criteria for urinary tract infection

Essay questions

1. Indicate how you would investigate a patient with nephrotic syndrome.

2. Outline the causes of urinary tract obstruction and how you would investigate a patient with bilateral hydronephrosis.

3. Describe how you would investigate a patient with acute renal failure.

4. Describe the commonly used renal replacement therapy options for acute renal failure.

5. How would you investigate a 40-year-old woman presenting with chronic renal impairment?

6. Describe the options for renal replacement therapy in chronic renal failure.

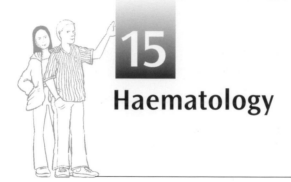

15

Haematology

Haematology comprises the study of the components of the blood and the bone marrow, along with disorders of the lymphoreticular system. Common disorders include the anaemias and haematological malignancy.

Basic science in haematology

COMPONENTS OF BLOOD

Cellular
- Erythrocytes (red cells)
- Reticulocytes (immature red cells)
- Leucocytes (white cells)
  - Lymphocytes
  - Monocytes
  - Eosinophils
  - Basophils
  - Neutrophils
- Platelets

Non-cellular

Plasma
- Liquid component of blood
- Includes
  - Fibrinogen
  - Clotting factors
  - Immunoglobulins
  - Albumin
  - Other plasma proteins
  - Electrolytes

Serum ▮ Fluid remaining after the formation of a fibrin clot (i.e. no fibrinogen)

HAEMOPOIESIS (Fig. 15.1) *(K&C, p. 405)*

Sites of haemopoiesis
▮ Embryonic yolk sac – week 3
▮ Liver and spleen – weeks 6–7
▮ Bone marrow – week 8
▮ All bones – at birth
▮ Central skeleton
▮ Proximal long bones } adulthood

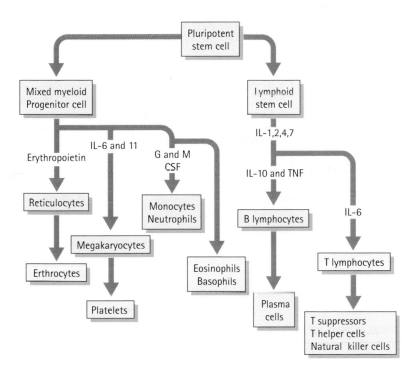

Fig. 15.1 Haemopoiesis. All blood cells derive from the pluripotent stem cell. Differentiation into cell lineages depends on a range of cytokines, hormones and growth factors.
IL: Interleukin
G-CSF: Granulocyte colony stimulating factor
M-CSF: Monocyte colony stimulating factor
TNF: Tumour necrosis factor

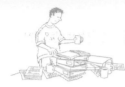

Stem cells
- Progenitor cells for blood cells
- Proliferation and differentiation
- → Mature blood cells
- Self-renewal, so source cells not depleted

Growth factors
- Glycoproteins, e.g. granulocyte colony-stimulating factor (G-CSF)
- Stimulate proliferation and differentiation
- Used to increase number of white cells, e.g. after chemotherapy

LABORATORY VALUES (Table 15.1)

Red cell indices
- Size, number and haemoglobin content of erythrocytes
- Important in the classification of anaemia

Erythocyte sedimentation rate (ESR)
- Rate of fall of red cells in a column of blood
- Measure of acute phase proteins and therefore of inflammation

Table 15.1 Blood cell indices

Measurement	Units	Male	Female
Haemoglobin (Hb) Hb concentration in blood	g dL^{-1}	13–18	11.5–15.5
Packed cell volume (PCV) Ratio of cell volume to plasma	L/L	0.42–0.53	0.35–0.45
Red cell count (RCC)	10^{12}/L	4.5–6.0	3.9–5.0
Mean corpuscular volume (MCV) Red cell size	fl	80–96	
Mean corpuscular Hb (MCH) Amount of Hb in each cell	pg	27–33	
Mean corpuscular Hb concentration (MCHC) Red cell Hb concentration	g dL^{-1}	32–35	
White cell count (WCC)	10^{9}/L	4.0–11.0	
Platelet count	10^{9}/L	150–400	
Reticulocyte count Proportion of immature red cell	%	0.5–2.0	

I Increases with age
I Higher in ♀ than ♂

Plasma viscosity I Measure of acute phase proteins
I No sex and little age variation

Reticulocyte I Immature red cells
count I Measure of erythropoiesis
I Normally < 2%
I Increased by high marrow activity, e.g.
— After bleeding
— Anaemia
— Haemolysis

HAEMOGLOBIN (K&C, p. 408)

Structure I Four globin (protein) chains
I Four haem (iron-containing) molecules
I Molecular weight 68 000

Function I Haem moiety can bind oxygen and CO_2
I Acts as transporter for these gases

Genetics I Adult Hb (Hb A) consists of two α and two β
globins
I Hb A_2 consists of two α and two δ globins (2% of
adult Hb)
I Fetal Hb consists of two α and two γ globins

Anaemia (K&C, p. 410)

I A haemoglobin level below the reference range

Classification I By erythrocyte volume (MCV)

Macrocytic – large red cells
I B_{12} deficiency
I Folate deficiency
I Alcohol
I Liver disease
I ↑ Reticulocytes
I Hypothyroidism

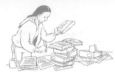

Microcytic – small red cells
❙ Iron deficiency
❙ Thalassaemia
❙ Sideroblastic anaemia
❙ Anaemia of chronic disease

Normocytic – normal red cells
❙ Acute blood loss
❙ Anaemia of chronic disease
❙ Haemolysis
❙ Infection
❙ Pregnancy
❙ Hypopituitarism
❙ Hypothyroidism (may be macrocytic)
❙ Renal failure

Clinical features

Symptoms
❙ Fatigue
❙ Headache   }   Common in general population
❙ Faintness
❙ Breathlessness
❙ Angina on effort
❙ Intermittent claudication
❙ Palpitations

Signs
❙ Pallor
❙ Tachycardia
❙ Systolic flow murmur
❙ Cardiac failure
❙ Koilonychia – spoon-shaped nails in iron deficiency
❙ Jaundice – haemolytic anaemia
❙ Bone deformity – thalassaemia major
❙ Leg ulcers – sickle cell disease

Investigations
❙ White cell count – if low may be dilutional or bone marrow failure
❙ Reticulocyte count – bone marrow activity
❙ Blood film for erythrocyte morphology – may show dimorphic picture (both large and small red cells); seen in combined iron and folate deficiency

Iron deficiency anaemia (K&C, p. 412)

Iron metabolism
- Iron requirements
  — ♂ 0.5–1 g/day
  — ♀ 1.2–1.7 g/day
- Dietary iron 15–20 g/day
- 10% absorbed
- Absorbed in duodenum and jejunum
- Transported in blood bound to transferrin
- Stored as ferritin and haemosiderin

Causes of iron deficiency
- Blood loss (commonly menstrual)
- Growth or pregnancy (↑ requirement)
- Decreased absorption (e.g. gastrectomy)
- Low dietary intake

Clinical features
- Koilonychia and brittle nails/hair
- Angular stomatitis
- Dysphagia   ⎤ Plummer–Vinson or
- Glossitis   ⎦ Paterson–Kelly syndrome

Investigations
- Blood count and film
- ↓ Serum ferritin
- ↓ Serum iron and ↑ iron-binding capacity

Management
- Treat cause
- Oral iron – ferrous sulphate or gluconate
- I.m. iron if unable to tolerate oral

Anaemia of chronic disease (K&C, p. 417)

Aetiology
- Reduced erythropoiesis
- Reduced red cell survival
- Chronic infection
  — Osteomyelitis
  — Infective endocarditis
  — TB
- Chronic inflammation
  — Rheumatoid arthritis
  — Systemic lupus erythematosus (SLE)
  — Polymyalgia rheumatica
- Malignancy

Investigations
- Low iron and iron-binding capacity
- Normal or high ferritin

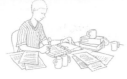
Sideroblastic anaemia (K&C, p. 416)

Aetiology   ▌ Abnormal haem metabolism
▌ Inherited (X-linked) or acquired
— Myelodysplastic syndrome
— Drugs, e.g. isoniazid
— Alcohol/lead

Megaloblastic anaemia (K&C, p. 417)

Aetiology   ▌ B_{12} deficiency (Fig. 15.2 and Table 15.2)
▌ Folate deficiency (Table 15.3)
▌ Myelodysplasia

Table 15.2   Causes of B_{12} deficiency anaemia

Low dietary intake
Vegan diet – B_{12} high in meat, fish, eggs and milk

Impaired absorption (stomach)
Pernicious anaemia
Gastrectomy   } Lack of intrinsic factor
Congenital lack of intrinsic factor

Impaired absorption (small bowel)
Pancreatic insufficiency – failure to cleave off R-binders
Terminal ileal disease – loss of absorption site
Bacterial overgrowth – bacterial utilization of B_{12}

Abnormal metabolism
Transcobalamin II deficiency – congenital lack of B_{12} transporter

---

Table 15.3   Causes of folate deficiency

Nutritional	Inhibited metabolism
Poor intake	Drugs
Old age	Anticonvulsants, e.g.
Poor diet	phenytoin
Starvation	Methotrexate
Alcohol abuse	Trimethoprim
Anorexia	Increased cell turnover,
Malignancy	e.g. malignancy
GI disease	Inflammatory disease
↑ **Utilization**	Metabolic disease, e.g.
Physiological	homocystinuria
Pregnancy	Haemodialysis
Lactation	
Pathological	
Increased red cell synthesis, e.g. haemolysis	

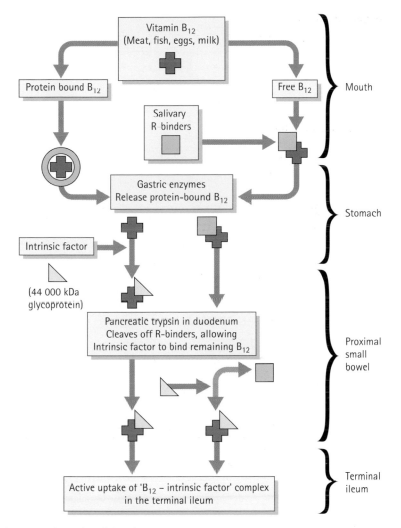

Fig. 15.2   Absorption of vitamin B_{12}.

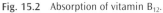

Investigations   ❙ ↑ MCV > 96 fl (macrocytosis)
❙ Blood film – hypersegmented neutrophils
❙ Serum B_{12}
❙ Serum folate
❙ Red cell folate – better measure of tissue folate
❙ Schilling test (Fig. 15.3)

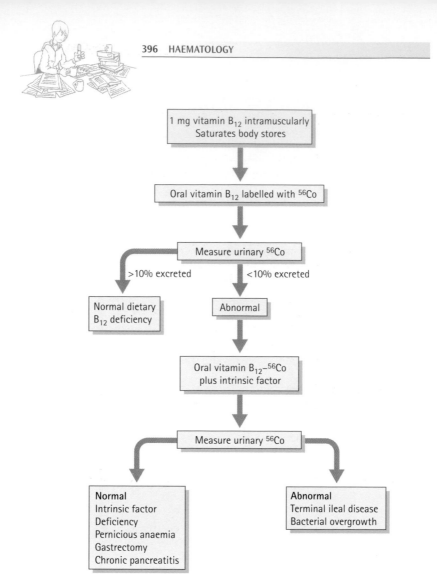

Fig. 15.3 Schilling tests. These are designed to diagnose the cause of vitamin B_{12} deficiency.

Pernicious anaemia (*K&C*, p. 418)

    ❙ → Megaloblastic anaemia

Aetiology ❙ Autoimmune disease
              ❙ Anti-intrinsic factor antibodies in 50%
              ❙ Anti-parietal cell antibodies in 90%
              ❙ → Intrinsic factor deficiency
              ❙ → B_{12} malabsorption

Disease associations
- Autoimmune thyroid disease
- Addison's disease
- Vitiligo
- Blond hair and blue eyes
- Higher risk of gastric cancer in males

Pathology
- Gastric mucosal atrophy
- Achlorhydria (loss of gastric acid synthesis)

Clinical features
- Pallor and mild jaundice
- Glossitis (sore red tongue)
- Angular stomatitis
- Progressive polyneuropathy
- Subacute combined degeneration of the cord
- → Paraesthesia, weakness and ataxia
- → Paraplegia
- Rarely, optic atropy or dementia

Management
- 1 mg vitamin B_{12} per day for 7 days i.m.
- Then 1 mg every 3 months for life

Folate deficiency (*K&C*, p. 420)
- → Megaloblastic anaemia (Table 15.3)

Folate absorption
- Found in spinach, broccoli, liver and kidney
- Cooking destroys folate
- Daily requirement 100 μg
- B_{12} required for folate metabolism

Clinical features
- Anaemia
- Glossitis
- No neuropathy

Management
- Oral folate 5 mg per day

Prophylaxis
- Advised prior to and during pregnancy
- Reduces risk of neural tube defects

Sickle cell disease (*K&C*, p. 430)
Aetiology
- Mutation → abnormal β globin (Hb S)
- → Sickle cell trait (heterozygote Hb AS)
- Or sickle cell disease (homozygote Hb SS)
- Hb S is insoluble when deoxygenated

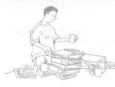

Table 15.4   Causes of macrocytosis without anaemia

Physiological
Pregnancy
Newborn babies

Pathological
Alcohol excess
Liver disease
Reticulocytosis
Hypothyroidism
Aplastic anaemia
Drugs, e.g. azathioprine

| → Hb forms crystals and deforms red cells
| → Sickle shape
| → Reduced red cell survival and microvascular obstruction

Epidemiology | 25% of Africans carry abnormal gene
| Also India, Middle East and southern Europe

Precipitation of crisis | Infection
— Notably chest → hypoxia

ACUTE SICKLE CRISIS

Give
High-flow oxygen
I.v. access and fluids

History
Previous crises
Chest or cardiac crises
Previous ITU admissions
Recent fever or evidence of infection
Recent travel

Check for
Chest sickling
Pleuritic pain, cough, crackles, pleural rub
Hypoxia on blood gases

Investigations
Full blood count – extent of anaemia and leucocytosis
Chest X-ray if there are chest signs
Urea and electrolytes for renal dysfunction

Analgesia
i.v. or i.m. pethidine, diamorphine or fentanyl

— Parvovirus → aplasia
— Haemolysis due to sepsis
▌ Sequestration of red cells in liver and spleen
▌ Dehydration → increased plasma viscosity

Clinical features ▌ Onset after 6 months (as Hb F level drops)
▌ Haemolytic anaemia
▌ Recurrent painful crises
▌ Bone pain
▌ Chest – pleuritic pain, common cause of death
▌ Cerebral – fits, neurological signs
▌ Kidneys – papillary necrosis, inability to concentrate urine
▌ Spleen – splenic infarcts → hyposplenism
▌ Liver – pain and abnormal liver function
▌ Penis – priapism

Long-term
▌ Hyposplenism → risk of infection
▌ Chronic leg ulcers
▌ Gallstones
▌ Necrosis of femoral heads
▌ Chronic renal disease

Investigations ▌ Full blood count
— Anaemia
— Infection (leucocytosis)
▌ Blood film
— Sickling
— Hyposplenism
▌ Hb electrophoresis demonstrates Hb S

Management *Acute*
▌ I.v. fluids
▌ Oxygen
▌ Antibiotics if evidence of infection
▌ Adequate analgesia
▌ Exchange transfusions if severe crisis

Long-term
▌ Pneumococcal vaccine
▌ *Haemophilus influenzae* vaccine

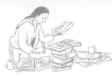

I Folic acid
I Transfusions if very anaemic
I Hydroxyurea increases Hb F production

Thalassaemia (*K&C*, p. 427)

Aetiology
I Inherited failure of synthesis of one globin type
I Accumulation of remaining globin type
I → Haemolysis and ineffective erythropoiesis

β-thalassaemia
Minor
I Carrier state (heterozygote)
I Symptomless
I Low MCV and MCH

Major
I Homozygote
I Severe anaemia requiring transfusions
I Onset 3–6 months old
I Anaemia and infections
I Extramedullary haemopoiesis
I → Skull expansion and bossing

Treatment
I Regular transfusions to suppress haemopoiesis and avoid deformity and anaemia
I Iron chelation to reduce overload
I Bone marrow transplantation

α-thalassaemia
I Deletion in one to four of the four α globin genes
I All four deleted → fetal death (hydrops fetalis)
I Three of four → moderate anaemia
I Two of four → carrier state, no anaemia

Haemolytic anaemia (*K&C*, p. 435)

I Anaemia due to the premature breakdown of erythrocytes, resulting in reduced red cell survival
I If haemolysis is acute, anaemia, jaundice and haemoglobinuria are seen

Aetiology
Inherited
I Sickle cell disease
I Thalassaemia
I Hereditary spherocytosis

I Hereditary elliptocytosis
I Glucose-6-phosphate dehydrogenase deficiency
  — X-linked recessive
  — → Haemolysis due to drugs, e.g. aspirin
  — Favism (fava beans → haemolysis)
  — Haemolysis due to infection
I Pyruvate kinase deficiency
  — Autosomal recessive
  — → Anaemia and splenomegaly

Acquired
I Autoimmune haemolytic anaemia (Table 15.5)
  — Autoantibodies against red cell membrane
  — Positive direct Coombs' test (Fig. 15.4)
I Drug-induced autoimmune haemolysis
  — Quinine
  — Penicillin
  — Methyldopa
I Haemolytic disease of the newborn
  — Maternal anti-red cell IgG crosses placenta
  — → Fetal red cell destruction (Rhesus disease)
I Paroxysmal nocturnal haemoglobinuria
  — Red cell destruction by complement
  — → Haemolysis due to infection or surgery
  — → Early morning haemoglobinuria
  — Increased risk of venous thrombosis

Table 15.5   Autoimmune haemolytic anaemia (AIHA)*

	Warm AIHA	Cold AIHA
Antibody type	IgG	IgM
Optimal antibody binding	37°C	< 37°C
Direct Coombs' test	Strong positive	Positive
Causes	Idiopathic (primary) SLE Lymphomas Chronic lymphatic leukaemia Malignancy Drugs, e.g. methyldopa	Idiopathic (primary) Lymphomas Infectious mononucleosis *Mycoplasma* infection

*These anaemias are classified based on the temperature at which the autoantibody best binds to the red cell membrane.

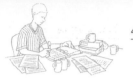

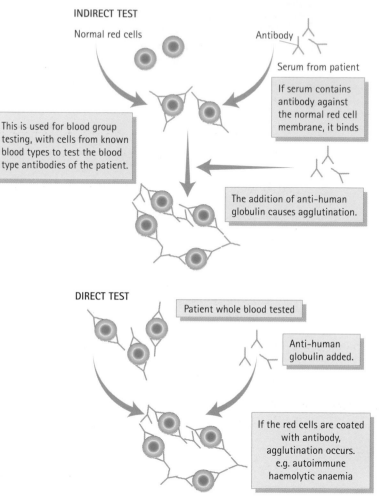

INDIRECT TEST

Normal red cells

Antibody

Serum from patient

This is used for blood group testing, with cells from known blood types to test the blood type antibodies of the patient.

If serum contains antibody against the normal red cell membrane, it binds

The addition of anti-human globulin causes agglutination.

DIRECT TEST

Patient whole blood tested

Anti-human globulin added.

If the red cells are coated with antibody, agglutination occurs. e.g. autoimmune haemolytic anaemia

Fig. 15.4 Coombs'/antiglobulin tests. A. Indirect tests are designed to establish whether there is an anti-red cell antibody in the patient's serum. They are used for blood group testing, using cells from known blood types to test the blood type antibodies of the patient. B. Direct tests establish whether there is an autoantibody already attached to the patient's red cells.

❚ Mechanical haemolysis
— Cardiac prosthetic valves
— Marching
— Microangiopathic haemolytic anaemia

▌ Others
— Extensive burns
— Renal and liver disease
— Malaria

Blood groups and blood transfusion (K&C, p. 445)

▌ The blood group of a particular patient is determined by red cell surface antigens
▌ The two common and most important groupings are ABO and Rhesus status
▌ The process of typing blood is based on a series of indirect Coombs' tests to analyse the blood for the presence of these antigens
▌ Cross-matching blood for transfusion is carried out by looking for agglutination when blood cells to be donated are mixed with the patient's serum (Fig. 15.4A)

ABO blood group
(Table 15.6)

▌ Presence of A or B antigens on red cells
▌ Presence of anti-A or anti-B in serum
▌ Mixing incompatible blood → haemolysis

Rh blood group

▌ Presence or absence of D antigen
▌ Antibodies form if a D-negative patient is given D-positive blood

Table 15.6   The ABO and Rhesus blood groups

Group	Genotype	Red cell antigens	Antibodies	Frequency	Notes
O	OO	None	Anti-A and anti-B	44%	Universal donor
A	AO or AA	A	Anti-B	45%	
B	BO or BB	B	Anti-B	8%	
AB	AB	A and B	None	3%	Universal recipient
D-positive	C or D or E	D	None		Three genes determine genotype: C, D and E
D-negative	CDE	None	Anti-D*		* After exposure

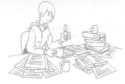

Fetal Rhesus D syndrome
- RhD-negative mother with a D-positive child will be sensitized at the first delivery
- Subsequent D-positive fetuses will be subjected to anti-D antibodies → hydrops fetalis
- Prophylaxis with anti-D antibodies given to the mother at each delivery suppresses the mother's own antibody production, protecting future fetuses

Blood products
- Whole blood ~ 500 mL
- Packed cells – 250 mL of plasma removed
- Red cell concentrate – all plasma removed
- Platelet concentrate
- Fresh frozen plasma – replacement of clotting factors
- Cryoprecipitate – factor VIII, fibrinogen and von Willebrand factor
- Human albumin
- Normal immunoglobulin

Procedure for blood transfusion (*K&C*, p. 446)
- Type patient's blood
- Cross-match donor blood with patient serum
- Donor blood is coded and labelled with the patient's name; a record sheet with the unit number of the donor blood and the patient's name and identification number is produced

When administering blood
- Two members of staff check the following

Between the patient and record sheet
- Name of the patient
- Date of birth of the patient
- Identification number of the patient

Between the blood and record sheet
- Blood unit number
- Blood group
- Name, age and date of birth of the patient

Complications of blood transfusion (*K&C*, p. 447)
- Incompatibility → poor red cell survival

Transfusion reactions

I Usually ABO incompatibility
I Haemolysis and haemoglobinuria
I Rigors
I Dyspnoea
I Hypotension
I Renal failure
I Disseminated intravascular coagulation

Febrile transfusion
reactions

I Mild fever and flushing
I Rarely due to haemolysis

Transmission
of infection

I Previously HCV + HIV
I All blood screened

Blood coagulation (Fig. 15.5) *(K&C, p. 453)*

Vessel wall injury leads to

I Vasoconstriction → reduced blood flow
I Platelet activation → serotonin and thromboxane
I Coagulation → fibrin clot formation

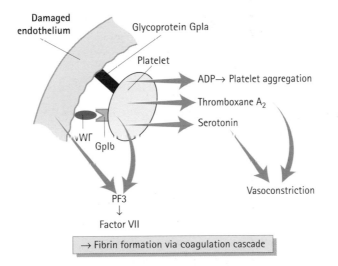

Fig. 15.5 Clot formation on a damaged vessel.
vWF: von Willebrand factor
Gpla: Glycoprotein Ia
Gplb: Glycoprotein Ib
PF-3: Platelet factor 3
ADP: Adenosine diphosphate

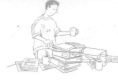

Platelet adhesion
- Adhesion to collagen exposed by vessel damage via glycoprotein Ia receptor on platelets and in combination with von Willebrand factor via glycoprotein Ib receptors
- Fibrinogen then binds to platelets, is converted to fibrin and forms cross-links, producing a platelet plug

Platelet prostaglandin
- Prostaglandin metabolism → thromboxane production
- → Vasoconstriction and platelet activation
- Process is inhibited by aspirin

Coagulation cascade (Fig. 15.6) *(K&C, p. 455)*
- Enzymatic reactions
- → Activation of coagulation proteins
- → Conversion of fibrinogen to fibrin

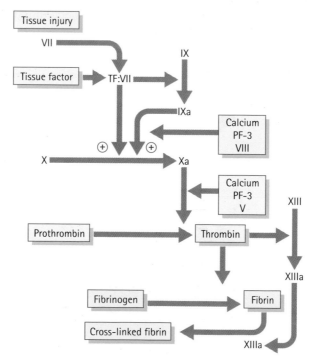

Fig. 15.6 The coagulation cascade *in vivo*.

I Old classification into extrinsic and intrinsic
I This is based on in vitro coagulation; in vivo cascade differs

Coagulation factors
I Synthesized in the liver
I Enzyme precursors (XII, XI, X, IX)
I Enzyme cofactors (V, VIII)

Coagulation inhibitors
I Anti-thrombin inactivates clotting factors
I Activated protein C destroys factors V and VIII and initiates fibrinolysis
I Protein S – cofactor for protein C

Fibrinolysis (Fig. 15.7)
I Plasminogen converted to plasmin by tissue plasminogen activator (t-PA)
I Converts fibrin to fibrin degradation products and D-dimer fragments

Measurements of coagulation

Prothrombin time (PT, normal 10–12 seconds)
I Lengthened by factor VII, X, V or II abnormality
I Also increased by warfarin

International normalized ratio (INR, normal = 1–1.2)
I Comparison of prothrombin time to a known standard
I Used to monitor warfarin

Fig. 15.7
The breakdown of fibrin.

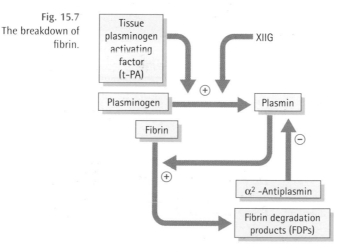

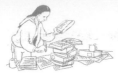
Activated partial thromboplastin time (APTT, normal 23–31 seconds)	▮ Abnormalities of factors XI, IX, VIII, X, V, II or I ▮ Increased by heparin
Thrombin time (TT, normal 12 seconds)	▮ Prolonged by fibrinogen deficiencies and heparin
Bleeding time	▮ Standard cut made and time taken for bleeding to stop is measured
Correction tests – addition of normal plasma	▮ If this corrects an abnormal test, then a factor deficiency is the cause of the coagulopathy ▮ If no correction occurs, it suggests the presence of an inhibitor in the patient's plasma
D-dimer assay	▮ Increased during fibrinolysis, e.g. after pulmonary embolus
Fibrin degradation products (FDPs)	▮ Increased by fibrinolysis, e.g. pulmonary embolus

INHERITED COAGULATION DEFECTS (K&C, p. 460)

Haemophilia A
▮ X-linked inheritance found in 1:5000 men
▮ Factor VIII:C deficiency

Factor VIII < 1% of normal
▮ Frequent spontaneous bleeding
▮ Joint bleeds → deformity

Factor VIII < 5% of normal
▮ Severe bleeding after injury

Factor VIII > 5% of normal
▮ Mild disease
▮ Prolonged bleeding after trauma

Investigations
▮ See Table 15.7

Table 15.7   Blood results in coagulopathy

	Prothrombin time (PT)	Activated partial thromboplastin time (APTT)	Bleeding time	Factor VIII:C level	Von Willebrand factor (vWF)
Platelet disorders	Normal	Normal	↑	Normal	Normal
Vitamin K Deficiency	↑	↑	Normal	Normal	Normal
Haemophilia A and B	Normal	↑	Normal	↓	Normal
Von Willebrand's disease	Normal	↑	↑	↓	↓

Management
- Factor VIII:C i.v.
- DDAPV (vasopressin) intranasal spray (increases factor VIII:C levels)
- Minor bleeding – aim for 30% of normal
- Major bleeding – aim for 50% of normal
- Surgery – aim for 100% preoperatively

Complications of treatment
- Antibodies against factor VIII:C
- Complications of blood transfusion

Haemophilia B (Christmas disease) (K&C, p. 462)
- X-linked inheritance found in 1:30 000 men
- Factor IX deficiency
- Clinically identical to haemophilia A

Management
- i.v. factor IX

Von Willebrand's disease (K&C, p. 463)
- Three types (all chromosome 12)
  — Type 1: mild disease, autosomal dominant
  — Type 2: mild disease, autosomal dominant
  — Type 3: severe disease, autosomal recessive
- Bleeding follows trauma and surgery

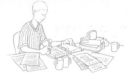

I Spontaneous epistaxis
I Defect of platelet adhesion combined with factor VIII:C deficiency

Management   I Intranasal DDAVP (vasopressin)
I Factor VIII/von Willebrand factor if required

ACQUIRED COAGULATION DEFECTS

Vitamin K deficiency (K&C, p. 463)

I Failure of synthesis of vitamin K-dependent factors
I Reduced factors II, VII, IX and X
I Reduced protein C and S

Aetiology   I Inadequate stores (newborn children)
I Malabsorption (fat-soluble vitamin)

I Oral anticoagulants, e.g. warfarin

Investigations   I Elevated prothrombin time and APTT

Management   I Intravenous vitamin K

Liver disease (K&C, p. 463)

I Vitamin K deficiency
I Reduced clotting factor synthesis
I Thrombocytopenia
I Abnormal platelet function

Disseminated intravascular coagulation (DIC) (K&C, p. 463)

I Uncontrolled fibrin production in blood vessels
— Malignancy
— Septicaemia
— Transfusion reactions
— Placental abruption
— Trauma
— Burns
— Snake bites

Investigations   I Elevated prothrombin time
I Low platelets
I Elevated FDPs

Clinical features   ▌ Haemorrhage
▌ Shock
▌ Epistaxis, bleeding gums

Management   ▌ Platelets
▌ Fresh frozen plasma (FFP)
▌ Cryoprecipitate
▌ Blood if required

Massive blood   ▌ Lack of factors VIII and V in transfusion blood
transfusion   ▌ Few platelets
▌ Citrate in transfusions lowers serum calcium
▌ If giving > 10 units check clotting and platelets
▌ Consider platelets and fresh frozen plasma
▌ Calcium i.v.

Clotting factor   ▌ 10% of haemophiliacs – antibodies against factor
autoantibodies   VIII
▌ SLE
▌ Post-childbirth

Antiphospholipid antibodies
▌ Found in 10% of those with SLE
▌ → Recurrent arterial and venous thrombosis
▌ Recurrent miscarriages
▌ Patients have elevated APTT
▌ Management
— Anticoagulation
— Aspirin

Anticoagulant drugs (*K&C*, pp. 466–469)
Warfarin   ▌ Vitamin K antagonist
▌ Increases prothrombin time

Heparin   ▌ Potentiates antithrombin III
▌ Elevates APTT

Low molecular   ▌ Can be given subcutaneously
weight heparin   ▌ Predictable anticoagulant effect

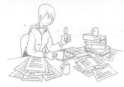

UNCONTROLLED BLEEDING DUE TO ANTICOAGULATION WITH WARFARIN

Severe bleeding
Stop warfarin immediately
i.v. access
  Give 5 mg of i.v. vitamin K by slow infusion
Fresh frozen plasma or clotting factors II, IX, X and VII
Blood transfusion if required

Less severe bleeding
e.g. Epistaxis or haematuria or INR > 8
Withhold warfarin
Consider vitamin K 0.5 mg i.v.

Fibrinolytics
- Activate plasmin
- Recombinant t-Pa
- Streptokinase

Anti-platelet drugs
- Aspirin
- Clopidogrel

THROMBOEMBOLIC DISEASE (*K&C*, p. 465)

- Thromboembolic disease is a very common cause of death; just under 50% of adult deaths result from its manifestation
  — Coronary artery thrombosis
  — Cerebral artery thrombosis
  — Pulmonary embolism (PE)

Thrombus
- Formation of solid clot in a vessel

Embolus
- Fragment of clot carried to a distant site
- → Obstruction of a vessel

Arterial thrombus
- Associated with atheroma
- → Platelet attachment
- → Propagation of thrombus

Venous thrombus
- Occurs in normal vessels
- Commonly deep leg veins
- Risk factors – Table 15.8

Table 15.8   Risk factors for deep vein thrombosis

Patient
Age
Obesity
Immobility
Smoking

Diseases
Previous DVT/PE
Malignancy
Thrombophilia
Myocardial infarction
Infection
Inflammatory bowel disease
Nephrotic syndrome
Polycythaemia
Surgery or trauma

Thrombophilia (K&C. p. 466)

- Recurrent venous thrombosis
- Venous thrombosis under the age of 40
- Often a family history

Aetiology
- Factor V Leiden syndrome
- Antithrombin deficiency
- Protein C and S deficiency
- Antiphospholipid syndrome (page 294)

Deep vein thrombosis (DVT) (K&C, p. 832)

- Formation of thrombus in
  — Deep calf vein
  — Axillary vein

Clinical features
- Pain and tenderness
- Swelling of the limb
- Redness of overlying skin
- Pulmonary embolism

Investigations
- Doppler ultrasound of the vein
- Venography (intravenous contrast)

Management
- Intravenous heparin *or*
- Low molecular weight heparin

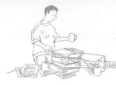

❚ Warfarin
❚ Bed rest
❚ Graduated pressure stockings

Complications ❚ Phlebitis
❚ Venous eczema

Pulmonary embolism (*K&C*, p. 718)

❚ Obstruction of a branch of the pulmonary artery by clot from a DVT

PULMONARY EMBOLUS

Patient is
In pain – pleuritic chest pain
Dyspnoeic
Shocked – hypotension and tachycardia

Give
High-flow oxygen
i.v. access

History
Risk factors for PE
Presence of a DVT
Thrombophilia
Oral contraceptive pill
Smoking
Concomitant illness/surgery/immobility

Investigations
Full blood count
Coagulation screen
D-dimer or FDPs (raised in PE)
Chest X-ray – oligaemic patch
ECG
Tachycardia
Right axis deviation and bundle branch block
S wave in lead I, Q wave and inverted T in lead III

Consider
Thrombolysis if shocked with no contraindications

Anticoagulate
Heparin bolus and i.v. infusion

Confirm diagnosis
$\dot{V}/\dot{Q}$ scan, CT angiogram

Clinical features Small or medium PE
  I Pleuritic chest pain
  I Shortness of breath
  I Haemoptysis in 30%
  I Tachypnoea
  I Pleural rub
  I Coarse crackles
  I Pleural effusion

Massive PE
  I Collapse
  I Shock
  I Cardiac arrest electromechanical dissociation
  I Elevated JVP ('a' wave)
  I Gallop rhythm

Recurrent PE
  I Breathlessness
  I Weakness
  I Syncope
  I Gradual deterioration

Investigations I Chest X-ray – oligaemic area
  I ECG
    — S wave in lead I, Q wave and inverted T in lead III
    — Right axis deviation
    — Right bundle branch block
  I D-dimers in blood are elevated
  I V̇/Q̇ scan
    — Nucleotide scan
    — Demonstrates defects in perfusion of the lung
      in areas with normal ventilation
  I Blood gases – hypoxia and low Pa_{CO_2}
  I Echocardiogram — high PA pressure
  I Pulmonary angiography/CT angiogram

Management I High-flow oxygen
  I Analgesia
  I Intravenous heparin *or*
  I Low molecular weight heparin
  I Consider thrombolysis (rtPa)

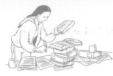

Haematological malignancy

These are malignant proliferations of

▌ Lymphocytes
 — Hodgkin's disease
 — Non-Hodgkin's lymphoma
 — Chronic lymphocytic leukaemia
 — Myeloma
▌ Immature lymphocytes
 — Acute lymphoblastic leukaemia
 — Hairy cell leukaemia
▌ Myeloid cells
 — Acute myelogenous leukaemia
 — Chronic myeloid leukaemia

LYMPHOMAS

Hodgkin's disease (Table 15.9) *(K&C, p. 496)*
▌ B or T cell lymphoma

Clinical features
▌ Lymphadenopathy
▌ Fever ⎫
▌ Drenching sweats ⎪
▌ Weight loss ⎬ B symptoms
▌ Alcohol-induced pain ⎭
▌ Hepatomegaly
▌ Splenomegaly

Investigations
▌ Blood count – anaemia
▌ ESR ↑
▌ Uric acid sometimes ↑
▌ Chest X-ray – mediastinal mass
▌ CT scan
 — Lymphadenopathy
 — Liver or spleen
▌ Lymph node biopsy and histology
▌ Bone marrow biopsy (shows Sternberg–Reed cells)

Management
▌ Depends on
 — Stage and histology
 — Site of tumour
 — Presence of B symptoms

Table 15.9 *Staging of Hodgkin's Disease (modified Ann Arbor classification)*

Stage*	Features
I	Single organ or single lymph node region
II	Two or more lymph node regions on the same side of the diaphragm One lymph node region and one other organ
III	Lymph nodes on both sides of the diaphragm Splenic involvement
IV	Extralymphatic involvement Lung Liver Bone Bone marrow

*Presence of B symptoms is denoted with a 'b' after the stage.
Bulky disease is denoted with an 'x' after the stage.
Lack of both is denoted with an 'a'.

❙ Radiotherapy
❙ Chemotherapy
❙ Myeloablation and stem cell support

Prognosis ❙ 40–70% at 20 years
❙ Depends on stage of original tumour

Non-Hodgkin's lymphoma (K&C, p. 498)

Low grade
❙ Older people
❙ Incurable
❙ Slow progression

High grade
❙ Any age
❙ Aggressive
❙ Curable

Clinical features ❙ Lymphadenopathy
❙ Symptoms due to site of tumour

Investigations ❙ Blood count
    — Anaemia
    — Thrombocytopenia

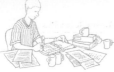

I Liver chemistry
I Chest X-ray
I CT scan of abdomen and thorax
I Bone marrow biopsy
I Lymph node biopsy

Management   I Depends on grade
I Radiotherapy
I Chemotherapy

Burkitt's   I Associated with Epstein–Barr virus
lymphoma   I Endemic in West Africa
I Jaw, abdominal and ovarian tumours
I Curable

ACUTE LEUKAEMIAS (*K&C*, p. 490)

Epidemiology   I Rare: 5 in 100 000

Aetiology   I Unknown in most cases
I T-cell leukaemia – retrovirus (HTLV-1)
I Specific genetic mutations
I Chromosome translocations, e.g. t(15; 17)
I Environmental factors
I Ionizing radiation

Clinical features   I Bone marrow failure
I → Weakness and tiredness due to anaemia
I → Bruising due to thrombocytopenia
I → Repeated infections

Investigations   I Blood count
I Blood film – leukaemic blast cells
I Bone marrow – blast cells

Management   I Correct anaemia and thrombocytopenia
I Treat any infection
I Chemotherapy to achieve remission
I Myeloablation with stem cell support to clear
marrow of malignant cells

Acute myelogenous leukaemia (AML)

I Classified by cell type (Table 15.10)
I 70% alive at 1 year → 20% alive at 5 years

I Treatment aims for complete remission
I Followed by bone marrow ablation

Acute lymphoblastic leukaemia (ALL)

I Predominantly a disease of children
I Cure rate 50–60% in children, 30% in adults
I Central nervous system involvement common
I → Prophylactic intrathecal chemotherapy

CHRONIC LEUKAEMIAS (K&C, pp. 493–495)

I Chronic leukaemias occur in older patients, most of whom die within 5 years of diagnosis
I Clinical course consists of a chronic illness lasting 3–4 years, followed by transformation into an acute leukaemia or sometimes myelofibrosis in the case of chronic myeloid leukaemia

Chronic myeloid leukaemia (CML)

Clinical features I Anaemia
I Night sweats and fever
I Weight loss
I Splenomegaly → pain

Investigations I Blood count – raised white count
I Multiple myeloid precursors

Table 15.10 Classification of acute myelogenous leukaemia (AML)

FAB (French, American, British) type	Description	Notes
M1	Myeloblastic	No maturation of blasts
M2	Myeloblastic	Maturation of blasts seen
M3	Promyelocytic	Associated with DIC *All-trans*-retinoic acid (ATRA) → remission
M4	Myelomonocytic	Skin and gum lesions, CNS involvement
M5 M6 M7	Monoblastic Erythroblastic Megakaryoblastic	} Very rare

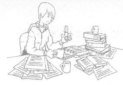
I Bone marrow biopsy
I Genetic testing for the Philadelphia chromosome
(9; 22 translocation) (positive in 90–95%)

Management I Interferons → remission in 10%
I Hydroxyurea reduces white cell count
I Myeloablation with bone marrow transplant

Chronic lymphocytic leukaemia (CLL)

Clinical features I Often an incidental finding
I Infections due to neutropenia
I Anaemia (may be due to haemolysis)
I Lymphadenopathy
I Hepatosplenomegaly

Investigations I Haemoglobin low or normal
I White count $> 15 \times 10^9/L$
I 40% lymphocytes
I Platelets low or normal
I Serum immunoglobulins may be low

Management I Nothing if asymptomatic
I Steroids for haemolysis
I Fludarabine or chlorambucil

Hairy cell leukaemia

I Rare
I Usually a B cell tumour
I Cells have filament-like projections

MYELOPROLIFERATIVE DISORDERS (K&C, pp. 440–443)

I Uncontrolled proliferation of a blood cell line
I Can transform into acute leukaemias or from one
myeloproliferation to another

Polycythaemia vera (Table 5.8)

I Red cell proliferation
I Patients usually > 60 years old

Clinical features I Tiredness
I Depression
I Tinnitus

I Vertigo
I Visual disturbance
I Itching after a hot bath
I Gout (due to increased cell turnover)
I Thrombosis or haemorrhage
I Plethora and cyanosis
I Splenomegaly

Investigations I Haemoglobin raised
I Packed cell volume (haematocrit) ↑
I 50% have ↑ platelets
I 75% have ↑ white cells
I Uric acid ↑
I Leucocyte alkaline phosphatase ↑

Management I Venesection
I Chemotherapy
I Allopurinol to avoid gout

Prognosis I 30% → myelofibrosis
I 5% → AML

Essential thrombocythaemia
I Platelet count > 1000 × 10^9/L
I → Bruising and bleeding
I Increased risk of thrombosis

Myelofibrosis I Stem cell proliferation
I Bone marrow fibrosis

Clinical features I Anaemia
I Weight loss
I Splenomegaly
I Bone pain
I Gout

Investigations I Anaemia
I High platelets
I 'Dry' bone marrow aspirate
I High uric acid

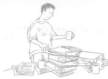

Manangement I Blood transfusion
I Folic acid
I Chemotherapy and radiotherapy
I Splenectomy may be required

Prognosis I 10–20% → AML

Myelodysplasia I Stem cell defects
I → Bone marrow failure
I Abnormal red cells, leucocytes and platelets

Management I Supportive therapy
I Low-intensity chemotherapy

MULTIPLE MYELOMA AND HYPERGLOBULINAEMIA (*K&C*, pp. 501–502)

I Clonal expansion of plasma cells resulting in very high production of a single immunoglobulin (paraprotein) or an immunoglobulin component

Myeloma I Elderly patients

Clinical features I Bone lesions → pain and fractures
I Hypercalcaemia
I Bone marrow infiltration
I → Anaemia, neutropenia
I Renal impairment
I Hyperviscosity syndrome (Table 15.11)

Investigations I Blood count (anaemia, low white cells)
I Elevated ESR
I Elevated calcium
I Protein electrophoresis – monoclonal band
I Skeletal X-ray survey – lytic lesion, e.g. skull

Table 15.11 Complications of hyperviscosity syndrome

Headaches
Visual disturbance – retinal artery and vein occlusion
Cerebrovascular accidents – indication for urgent plasmapheresis
Thrombophilia

■ 24-hour urine for light chain proteins
■ Bone marrow aspirate – plasma cells

Management ■ Supportive treatment
■ Steroids and radiotherapy for bone lesions
■ Chemotherapy

Waldenström's macroglobulinaemia
■ Older males
■ IgM paraprotein
■ → Hyperviscosity syndrome (Table 15.11)
■ Lymphadenopathy
■ Malaise and weight loss

Platelet disorders (K&C, pp. 458–460)

■ Platelets, derived from megakaryocytes, are involved in the formation of clots (see p. 105)

Thrombocytopenia
■ Low platelet count
■ Low production in bone marrow
■ High destruction in circulation
■ Causes – see Table 15.13

Autoimmune thrombocytopenic purpura
■ Follows viral infection in children (acute)
■ Idiopathic in adult women (chronic)
■ 60% have anti-platelet antibodies

Table 15.12 Causes of eosinophilia

Parasites	Lung disease
Ascaris	Asthma
Hookworm	Allergic bronchopulmonary
Strongyloides	aspergillosis
	Churg–Strauss syndrome
Allergy	
Allergic rhinitis	**Skin disorders**
Drug reactions	Urticaria
	Pemphigus
Malignancy	Eczema
Hodgkin's disease	**Others**
Carcinoma	Sarcoidosis

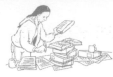

Table 15.13   Causes of thrombocytopenia

Reduced production	Immune destruction
Leukaemia	Autoimmune idiopathic
Aplastic anaemia	thrombocytopenic purpura
Megaloblastic anaemia	SLE
Myeloma	**Coagulation**
	DIC
Drugs	Haemolytic uraemic
Co-trimoxazole	syndrome
Infections	**Other**
Viral infection	Hypersplenism

- → Purpuric rash
- Epistaxis and menorrhagia
- Treat with steroids/splenectomy

Thrombocytosis

- High platelet count
- Haemorrhage
- Inflammation (any site)
- Essential thrombocythaemia (see above)

Self-assessment questions

Multiple choice questions

1. A 36-year-old woman has the following full blood count: Hb 10.1 g/dL, MCV 76 fl, MCH 24, WCC 9.4, Platelets 187. The following are possible diagnoses:
   A. Megaloblastic anaemia
   B. Sickle cell disease
   C. Menorrhagia
   D. Folate deficiency
   E. Polycythaemia rubra vera

2. The following statements about haemoglobin are correct:
   A. Adult haemoglobin comprises two α and two γ chains
   B. Each haemoglobin molecule comprises four globin chains and one haem group
   C. Deoxyhaemoglobin is insoluble
   D. β-thalassaemia is an inherited inability to synthesize β globin chains

E. Each haemoglobin molecule can carry four oxygen molecules

3. The following are true of vitamin B_{12} absorption:
   A. It requires the presence of intrinsic factor
   B. Intrinsic factor is produced by gastric parietal cells
   C. Active absorption takes place in the jejunum
   D. Chronic pancreatitis is a cause of vitamin B_{12} deficiency
   E. Oral B_{12} is useful in the treatment of pernicious anaemia

4. In autoimmune haemolytic anaemia:
   A. The direct Coombs' (globulin) test will be positive
   B. The autoantibody is always IgG class
   C. Haemoglobinuria may occur
   D. *Mycoplasma* pneumonia is a recognized cause
   E. Jaundice is a recognized symptom

5. Regarding pernicious anaemia:
   A. Anti-parietal cell or anti-intrinsic factor antibodies are detectable
   B. Chronic hyperplastic gastritis results
   C. There is an increased risk of gastric cancer
   D. Oral intrinsic factor will reverse the vitamin B_{12} deficiency
   E. Men are as commonly affected as women

6. The following are appropriate blood transfusion options:
   A. Group O donor to group A recipient
   B. Group A Rhesus-positive donor to group A Rhesus-negative recipient

C. Group AB Rhesus-negative donor to group O Rhesus-negative recipient
D. Group B Rhesus-positive donor to group A Rhesus-positive recipient
E. Group A donor to group AB recipient

7. The following are recognized complications of blood transfusions:
   A. Urticarial rash
   B. Hepatitis C infection
   C. Fever
   D. Anaphylactic shock
   E. Disseminated intravascular coagulation

OSCE questions

1. With reference to the following blood test results, answer the questions below: Hb 9.8 g/dL, WCC 7.2, Platelets 198, MCV 101 fl, Blood film: hypersegmented neutrophils.
   A. What is the haematological diagnosis?
   B. List three possible causes of your diagnosis.
   C. Name two tests that would help you in determining the diagnosis.

2. You are presented with a unit of blood, a patient with an identification label and the cross-match results. Explain the procedures involved in checking the blood against the cross-match results and against the patient in order to administer the blood safely.

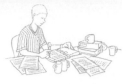

Short answer questions

1. Outline the pathological processes involved in:
   A. Sickle cell disease
   B. β-thalassaemia major
   C. Hydrops fetalis

2. Outline the causes of:
   A. Iron deficiency anaemia
   B. Megaloblastic anaemia
   C. Inherited haemolytic anaemias

3. Write short notes on the following:
   A. The structure of haemoglobin
   B. Coombs' tests
   C. Glucose-6-phosphate dehydrogenase deficiency

Essay questions

1. Outline the causes, investigation and management of iron deficiency anaemia.

2. A 23-year-old African man is admitted with severe knee and chest pain. He is known to have sickle cell disease. Briefly describe the pathological basis of the disease and outline the management of this patient.

3. Discuss the possible complications of blood transfusion and their management.

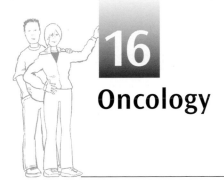

16

Oncology

(*K&C*, p. 473) Oncology studies the management of 'malignant disease', illness arising from the uncontrolled proliferation of a cell clone. The clone characteristically is able to invade adjacent tissues (local spread) and seed to distant sites via the vascular or lymphatic circulation (metastasis). Malignancy is an important cause of death worldwide, most notably in the developed world (Fig.16.1). Specific malignancies are discussed in the appropriate system chapter.

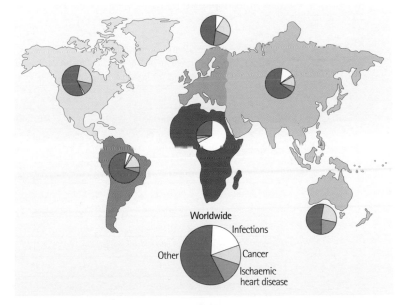

Fig. 16.1 Causes of mortality by continent demonstrating the relative importance of infection, malignancy and heart disease. Malignancy is responsible for roughly 13.5% of all male and 11.7% of all female deaths worldwide. (Data from the World Health Organization, 1999)

427

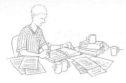

Cancer epidemiology

Sex differences (Table 16.1)
- Sex-specific tumours (e.g. prostate)
- Risk factors (e.g. alcohol intake, smoking)
- Genetic variation
- Hormonal variation

Age differences

Childhood cancers
(age 3–13 years)
- Hereditary, e.g. retinoblastoma
- Haematological, e.g. acute leukaemia

Adult cancers
- Frequency increases with age

Geographical differences (*K&C*, p. 475)
- Variation in genetics
- Variation in environmental factors, e.g.
  — Gastric cancer (Fig. 16.2)
  — Hepatocellular carcinoma secondary to chronic viral hepatitis

Table 16.1 Age-standardized mortality for the ten highest causes of malignancy-related death in the UK in 2000 (Globocan 2000, International Agency for Research on Cancer)

Rank	Male Site	Male Mortality	Female Site	Female Mortality
1	Lung	48.6	Breast	26.8
2	Colon and rectum	18.7	Lung	21.1
3	Prostate	18.5	Colon and rectum	13.8
4	Stomach	10.1	Ovarian	8.3
5	Oesophagus	8.7	Pancreas	5.3
6	Bladder	7.0	Stomach	4.8
7	Pancreas	6.6	Oesophagus	4.0
8	Lymphoma	5.8	Lymphoma	3.9
9	Leukaemia	4.9	Leukaemia	3.3
10	Brain	4.5	Brain	3.0

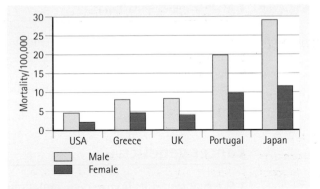

Fig. 16.2 Geographical variation in the mortality from gastric cancer. (Data from the World Health Organization, 1997)

Cancer aetiology (K&C, p. 474)

Smoking
- Associated with 30% of cancer deaths in the UK
- Implicated in several cancers
  — Lung carcinoma
  — Oral cavity cancers
  — Oesophageal carcinoma
  — Bladder (transitional cell carcinoma)

Alcohol
- Oral cavity cancers
- Oesophageal carcinoma
- Colorectal carcinoma

Environmental risks

Asbestos
- Mesothelioma
- Lung carcinoma

Hydrocarbons
- Lung carcinoma
- Skin cancers

UV light
- Melanoma
- Basal cell carcinoma
- Squamous cell carcinoma

Drugs

Oestrogens
- Vaginal carcinoma
- Endometrial carcinoma

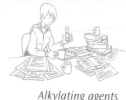

Alkylating agents ▌ Acute myeloid leukaemia

Infections ▌ Viral hepatitis – hepatocellular carcinoma
▌ *Schistosoma* – bladder cancer
▌ *Helicobacter pylori* – gastric cancer
▌ Epstein–Barr virus – Burkitt's lymphoma
▌ Papillomavirus – cervical cancer

Cancer genetics (K&C, p. 475)

▌ Malignancy results from genetic mutations that
lead to uncontrolled proliferation of a cell clone
▌ These mutations and abnormalities can arise in
several ways

Chromosome ▌ Chronic myeloid leukaemia – 9:22 translocation
abnormalities (Philadelphia chromosome) positive in 95%
▌ Acute promyelocytic leukaemia – 15:17
translocation positive in > 90%
▌ Burkitt's lymphoma 8:14 translocation
→ *myc* gene over-expressed

Failure of ▌ Mutation of DNA repair systems → hereditary
DNA repair cancer syndromes, e.g.
— Xeroderma pigmentosum
— Ataxia telangiectasia
— *BCRA1* and *2* in breast cancer
— Mismatch repair mutations in colon cancer

Tumour ▌ Mutation of tumour suppressor genes → over-
suppressors expression of mutated gene product
▌ Failure of control of cell cycle → uncontrolled
proliferation
▌ e.g. *p53* mutations in GI cancers

Inherited cancers ▌ Specific mutations increase the risk of malignancy
if inherited, e.g.
— *apc* gene: familial adenomatous polyposis
— *BCRA* genes: breast and ovarian cancer
— *Rb* gene: hereditary retinoblastoma

Oncogenes

- Genes which, if activated inappropriately by a mutation, → malignancy, e.g.
  - *C-Myc:* cervical cancer, Burkitt's lymphoma, breast cancer
  - *K-Ras:* colorectal cancer
- The gene may have a cell cycle regulatory role
  - *bcl-2* expression → resistance of apoptosis → a proliferating clone that is open to further mutations → malignant transformation

Cancer biology (K&C, pp. 475–476)

Cell proliferation

- Uncontrolled proliferation
- Often loss of cell differentiation
- → Exponential growth curve
- 'Doubling time' describes the growth rate
- → Very variable between tumour types
- As tumour enlarges, growth may slow due to:
  - Limitation of blood supply
  - Local production of growth inhibitors

Local invasion

- Penetration of malignant cells into other tissues
- Associated with loss of intercellular adhesion
- Increased production of proteolytic enzymes

Lymphatic spread

- Tumours seed to locally draining lymph nodes

Dissemination (Table 16.2)

- Invasion into blood vessels or lymphatics
- Allows seeding of cells to distant sites
- Metastases → organs with a dense vasculature, e.g.
  - Liver
  - Lungs
  - Bone marrow
- Tumour cells express ligands for endothelial receptors
- → Increased adhesion and invasion
- → Specific metastatic patterns, e.g. breast cancer → long bones

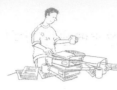

Table 16.2 Common sites of metastasis	
Site	**Origin**
Bone	Breast
	Bronchus
	Thyroid
	Prostate
	Kidney
Intracerebral	Bronchus
	Breast
	Stomach
	Prostate
	Thyroid
	Kidney
Liver	GI tract
	Breast
	Bronchus

Diagnosis of cancer (K&C, p. 477)

Clinical features
- Specific combinations of symptoms and signs can suggest particular malignancies
- e.g. Painless jaundice and weight loss → pancreatic cancer
- Characteristics of a palpable mass suggesting malignancy,
  — Fixed to deep tissues
  — Fixed to overlying skin
  — Hard/'craggy' texture
  — Overlying ulceration
  — Lymphadenopathy

Imaging
- Can be highly suggestive of malignancy
- e.g. Chest X-ray in lung cancer

Tissue diagnosis
- Vital for confirmation of diagnosis and guiding treatment
- Tumour type
- Degree of differentiation (tumour grade)

Methods
- CT- or ultrasound-guided biopsy

❙ Endoscopic biopsy
❙ Laparoscopic biopsy

Tumour staging
(Table 16.3)

❙ Assessment of distribution of tumour
❙ Classification varies with tumour
❙ Staging investigations required, e.g.
— CT scanning
— Lymph node sampling

Tumour markers

❙ Serum markers for the presence of malignancy
❙ Useful in following response to treatment
❙ Can help demonstrate relapse post-therapy
❙ Rarely useful in initial diagnosis
❙ e.g.
— Ca-125 – pancreatic/ovarian/GI cancer
— Ca-19-9 – GI and pancreatic cancers
— α-fetoprotein – hepatocellular carcinoma
— β-human chorionic gonadotrophin (HCG) –
choriocarcinomas, testicular carcinoma

Screening

❙ Investigations used to detect premalignant tissue or
malignancy in those in whom cancer has not been
diagnosed
❙ e.g.
— Mammograms for breast cancer
— Smears for cervical cancer

Surveillance

❙ Investigations to detect recurrence of malignancy
following treatment for a previous cancer
❙ e.g.
— Mammography after breast cancer
— Prostate-specific antigen (PSA) for progression of
prostatic cancer

Table 16.3   The TNM system

T		Extent of primary tumour
N	N0	No involved lymph nodes
	N1–4	Lymph nodes involved
M	M0	No metastases
	M1	Metastases present

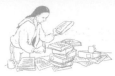

Treatment of malignancy (K&C, p. 479)

I Therapeutic efforts in oncology are aimed at
— Complete destruction of the tumour (curative therapy)
— Reduction of the tumour mass in order to improve life expectancy
— Reduction of symptoms of the cancer (palliative care)

Surgical resection I May be curative (complete tumour removal)
I May be palliative (symptomatic relief but not curative)

Radiotherapy I High-energy electromagnetic radiation
I Targeted at specific site
I Useful adjuvant therapy to reduce relapse rate

Chemotherapy I Drug therapy aimed at killing tumour cells
I Also kills normal cells
I Given in cycles to allow normal cells to recover

Antimetabolites I Block cell metabolism
— Folic acid antagonists: methotrexate
— Nucleic acid analogues: 5-fluorouracil

Plant alkaloids I Inhibit microtubule formation
I → Block cell replication
— Vincristine

Taxanes I Inhibit microtubule formation
I Useful in breast and ovarian cancers
— Docetaxel

Cytotoxic antibiotics I Block DNA replication
— Doxorubicin

Platinum analogues I Cross-link DNA strands
I → Block DNA replication
— Cisplatin

| *Alkylating agents* | ▌Block DNA synthesis |
| | — Cyclophosphamide |

| **Endocrine therapy** | ▌Hormonal manipulation of tumour cells that express hormone receptors on their surface |
| | — Tamoxifen – blocks oestrogen receptor |

| **Biological therapy** | ▌Use of immunologically active substances |
| | — e.g. α-interferon in melanoma/myeloma |

Adjuvant therapy	▌Specific therapy used in combination with another therapy modality
	▌Used to treat undetected metastases
	— Breast and colon cancers

Myeloablation with stem cell support	▌High-dose chemotherapy and radiotherapy
	▌Aims to kill all dividing cells
	▌Haemopoietic stem cells then given
	▌→ Reverses resultant bone marrow failure
	▌Stem cells may be
	— Allogenic: from a matched donor
	— Autologous: taken from patient before therapy
	▌Collection of stem cells may be via
	— Bone marrow sampling
	— Peripheral blood sampling

Complications of treatment (K&C, p. 483)

Failure of therapy	▌Incomplete surgical resection
	▌Tumour resistance to chemotherapy
	▌Failure of response to radiotherapy

Nausea and vomiting	▌Common
	▌Treat with antiemetics (Fig. 16.3)
	— Metoclopramide
	— Domperidone
	— $5HT_3$ antagonists (ondansetron)

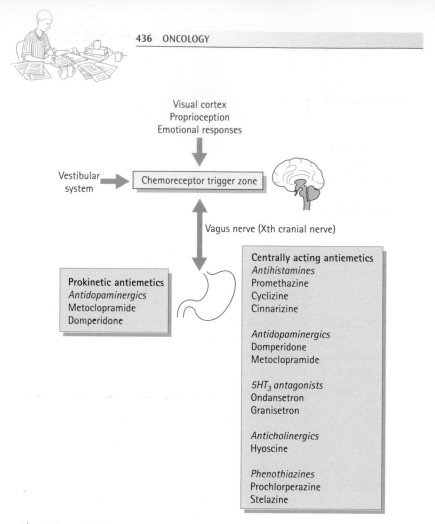

Fig. 16.3   Mechanisms of action of antiemetics.

Hair loss	▌ Difficult to avoid, but regrows after therapy
Bone marrow suppression	▌ Dose-dependent effect of therapy
Neutropenia	▌ ↑ Bacteria, viral and fungal infection ▌ Treat with antibiotics ▌ Stem cell stimulating factors, e.g. GM-CSF

Thrombocytopenia	▮ → Bleeding ▮ Treat with platelet transfusion
Anaemia	▮ Treat with blood transfusion
Cardiotoxicity	▮ Dose-dependent effect of doxorubicin
Neurotoxicity	▮ Occurs with vincristine ▮ Must never be given intrathecally
Sterility	▮ Common with alkylating agents ▮ ♂ Sperm storage prior to therapy ▮ ♀ Ovum storage (still experimental)
Mucositis	▮ Mucosal inflammation – notably of the mouth and GI tract after radiotherapy

Palliative care (*K&C*, pp. 507–509)

Therapy aimed at reducing symptoms due to the malignancy

Pain	▮ Occurs in 70% of cancers ▮ → Step up analgesia until relief obtained — Paracetamol and non-steroidal anti-inflammatory drugs (NSAIDs) — Weak opioids – codeine +/– paracetamol — Strong opioids – morphine or diamorphine
Specific analgesics	▮ Naproxen for bone pain ▮ Amitriptyline/gabapentin for pain due to nerve damage ▮ Carbamazepine/gabapentin for neuropathic pain
Continuous subcutaneous infusions	▮ Allow continuous delivery of analgesia, antiemetics and sometimes anxiolytics
Patient-controlled analgesia	▮ Continuous analgesia with the ability for the patient to give limited extra doses

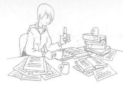

Complications of analgesics

Opioids
I Constipation, nausea vomiting
I Respiratory and CNS depression

NSAIDs
I GI ulceration
I GI bleeding
I Renal failure

Non-drug approaches
I Surgery to reduce tumour mass
I Radiotherapy
I Nerve blocks
I Steroids to reduce local inflammation

Gastrointestinal symptoms

Anorexia
I → Nasogastric feeding if appropriate

Nausea and vomiting
I → Appropriate antiemetic therapy

Bowel obstruction
I → Surgical bypass
I Antispasmodics – hyoscine
I Antiemetics
I Nasogastric tube to reduce vomiting

Psychological support
I Effective communication with the patient
I Honesty about diagnosis and prognosis
I Support for emotional crisis
I Full explanations of symptoms

Self-assessment questions

Multiple choice questions

1. Smoking has been associated with an increased risk of the following:
   A. Bronchial cancer
   B. Oesophageal cancer
   C. Transitional cell carcinoma
   D. Pharyngeal cancer
   E. Ulcerative colitis

2. Regarding malignancy:
   A. A translocation between chromosomes 9 and 22 is seen in 10% of chronic myeloid leukaemia
   B. *p53* mutations are common in gastrointestinal malignancy
   C. *Helicobacter pylori* is associated with a decreased risk of gastric cancer

D. Kaposi's sarcoma is only seen in immunocompromised patients

E. Family history is important in determining the risk of breast cancer

3. In the treatment of malignancy

A. Surgery is always carried out with the aim of a cure

B. Nausea is a rare side-effect of chemotherapy

C. Combination chemotherapy is rarely more efficacious than single therapy

D. Methotrexate is a folate metabolism antagonist

E. Vincristine can be given intrathecally

4. The following are common sites of metastasis for the named primary cancer:

A. Intracerebral: breast carcinoma

B. Long bones: osteosarcoma

C. Vertebral column: prostatic carcinoma

D. Liver: bronchial carcinoma

E. Liver: cutaneous basal cell carcinoma

5. The following are 5HT$_2$ antagonist antiemetics:

A. Metoclopramide

B. Cyclizine

C. Granisetron

D. Prochlorperazine

E. Diazepam

OSCE questions

1. Identification of a bronchial carcinoma on a plain chest X-ray.

2. Interpretation of a full blood count from a patient following chemotherapy showing neutropenia and thrombocytopenia.

Short answer questions

1. Write short notes on the following complications of chemotherapy:

A. Nausea and vomiting

B. Hair loss

C. Bone marrow suppression

2. Outline the role of the following in the aetiology of cancer:

A. Tobacco smoking

B. Electromagnetic radiation

C. Viral infections

D. Family history of malignancy

Essay questions

1. Outline the different groups of drugs that may be used in the treatment of chemotherapy-induced nausea and vomiting. Discuss their mechanisms of action.

2. A 56-year-old man presents with a 3-month history of weight loss (8 kg) and a short history of jaundice associated with dark urine and pale stools. List the differential diagnoses and discuss his management.

3. Discuss the role of screening for malignancy. Illustrate your answer with examples of screening techniques and their target patient groups.

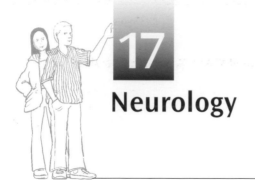

Neurology

Examining the nervous system

(*K&C*, p. 1125)

This is explained in some detail here as it is often dreaded but need not be if an organized and thoughtful approach is taken.

General rules
- Explain carefully to patients what you want them to do for each part of the examination and why
- It is often helpful to ask the patient to copy your actions, rather than trying to explain a complicated manoeuvre
- Always compare one side with the other
- Organize your examination into categories
  - Mental state
  - Cranial nerves
  - Motor function
  - Reflexes
  - Coordination and gait
  - Sensation

Equipment
- Pen torch
- Snellen eye chart or pocket vision card
- Ophthalmoscope
- Tendon hammer
- 128 and 512 Hz tuning forks
- Cotton wool
- 'Neuropins' or paper clips
- Orange stick

MINI-MENTAL STATUS EXAMINATION (see p. 500)

Ten questions give an indication of cerebral function, including orientation in time and place and long- and short-term memory; mark correct responses out of 10

I Name?
I Age?
I Address?
I Where are you now?
I Name of the monarch?
I Name of the prime minister?
I Dates of the Second World War?
I Remember the following address and repeat it when asked: 42 West Street, Edinburgh (ask the patient to recall this after asking of the rest of the questions)
I What time is it now?
I Count backwards from 20 to 10

CRANIAL NERVES

General observation
(K&C, p. 1129)

I Ptosis (III)
I Facial droop or asymmetry (VII)
I Hoarse voice (X)
I Articulation of words, dysarthria (V, VII, X, XII)
I Abnormal eye position (III, IV, VI)
I Abnormal or asymmetrical pupils (II, III)

I Olfactory

I Ask the patient about changes in or absence of sense of smell

II Optic

I Examine the optic fundi for
— Papilloedema
— Optic atrophy
— Maculopathy
— Hypertensive or diabetic retinopathy

Test visual acuity

I Allow the patient to use glasses
I Ask the patient to read a Snellen eye chart with each eye
I Record the smallest line the patient can read for each eye

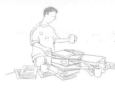

I Visual acuity is reported as a pair of numbers (20/20) where the first number represents how far the patient is from the chart and the second number is the distance from which the 'normal' eye can read a line of letters. For example, 20/40 means that at 20 feet the patient can only read letters a 'normal' person can read from twice that distance

Test visual fields

I Position yourself at eye level a metre or so in front of the patient and ask him/her to look into your eyes

I Hold your hands out to the sides halfway between you and the patient and wiggle a finger on both hands asking the patient to indicate which side he/she sees the finger move; if the patient only sees one side this indicates a lateral field defect or sensory neglect on that side

I Test the four quadrants of each eye while asking the patient to cover the opposite eye comparing with your own fields of vision for the appropriate eye

Test pupillary reactions

I Ask the patient to look into the distance

I Shine a bright light obliquely into each pupil in turn

I Look for both the direct (same eye) and consensual (other eye) reactions

I Test accommodation
— Hold your finger about 10 cm from the patient's nose
— Ask him/her to look into the distance and then at your finger
— Look for constriction of the pupil and convergence of the eyes to near vision

III Oculomotor

(*K&C*, p. 1134)

I Look for ptosis

I Test extraocular movements (superior, medial and inferior rectus and inferior oblique muscles)
— Holding your finger about 1 metre in front of the patient, ask him/her to follow your finger with the eyes without moving the head

— Check horizontal, vertical and oblique gaze using a cross or 'H' pattern
— Pause during upward and lateral gaze to check for nystagmus
❙ Test pupillary reactions to light

IV Trochlear (superior oblique muscle)
❙ Inward and downward movement of eyes (see above)

VI Abducens (lateral rectus muscle)
❙ Lateral eye movement (see above)

V Trigeminal (K&C, p. 1136)

Motor   ❙ Ask the patient to first open the mouth and then clench the teeth
❙ Palpate the temporal and masseter muscles as this is done

Sensory   ❙ On both sides, use cotton wool to test
— The forehead (olfactory division)
— The cheeks (maxillary division)
— The Jaw (mandibular division)

Corneal reflex   ❙ Ask the patient to look up and away
❙ From the other side, touch the cornea (not sclera) lightly with a fine wisp of cotton wool
❙ Look for the normal blink reaction of both eyes
❙ Repeat on the other side

VII Facial   ❙ Observe for any facial droop or asymmetry
(K&C, p. 1137)   ❙ Ask the patient to do the following, noting any weakness or asymmetry
— Raise eyebrows
— Close both eyes tightly
— Smile or show the teeth
— Puff out the cheeks
❙ Central vs peripheral
— With an upper motor neurone lesion (stroke), crossover of innervation means that function is preserved over the upper part of the face (forehead, eyebrows, eyelids)
— With a lower motor neurone lesion (Bell's palsy), the entire side of the face droops

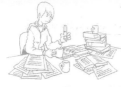

VIII Vestibulocochlear (K&C, p. 1139)

▌ Rub your fingers together next to one ear while whispering a number in the other and ask the patient to tell you the number
▌ Repeat for the other side

Weber's test
▌ Use a 512 Hz tuning fork
▌ Place the base of the vibrating tuning fork firmly on top of the patient's head
▌ Ask the patient where the sound appears to be coming from (normally in the midline)
— In sensorineural deafness there will be deafness in the affected ear
— In conductive deafness, the sound will be heard better in the deaf ear

Rinne's test
(to compare air and bone conduction)
▌ Use a 512 Hz tuning fork
▌ Place the base of the vibrating tuning fork against the mastoid bone behind the ear
▌ When the patient no longer hears the sound, hold the end of the fork near the patient's ear and ask if he or she can hear it now (air conduction is normally greater than bone conduction)
— In conductive deafness bone conduction is better than air conduction

IX and X Glossopharyngeal and vagus (tested together) (K&C, p. 1141)

▌ Ask the patient to swallow a sip of water, look for choking or dribbling
▌ Ask patient to say 'Agh', watching the movements of the soft palate and the pharynx. The uvula deviates away from the affected side
▌ Test the gag reflex (unconscious patient)
— Touch the back of the throat on the soft palate with an orange stick on each side
— It is normal to gag after each stimulus

XI Accessory

▌ From behind, look for wasting of the trapezius muscles
▌ Ask the patient to shrug the shoulders against resistance
▌ Ask the patient to turn the head against resistance. Watch and palpate the sternomastoid muscle on the opposite side

XII Hypoglossal
I Look at the tongue for wasting or fasciculation (lower motor neurone lesion)
I Ask the patient to
— Protrude the tongue
— Move the tongue from side to side
I The tongue moves towards the side of any lesion

MOTOR FUNCTION (CORTICOSPINAL OR PYRAMIDAL TRACTS) (K&C, p. 1143)

Observation
I Involuntary movements (e.g. tremor, tics, fasciculation)
I Wasting and asymmetry (pay particular attention to the hands, and shoulder and thigh girdles)

Muscle tone
I Ask the patient to relax
I Holding the patient's hand, flex and extend his/her wrist and elbow
I Place both your hands on the thigh and gently roll the leg from side to side watching for corresponding movement of the foot
I There is normally a small, continuous resistance to passive movement
I Observe for decreased (flaccid) or increased (rigid/cogwheeling/spastic) tone

Power
Pronator drift
I This is a short screening test for muscle strength
I Ask the patient to hold both arms straight out in front, palms up and eyes closed
I With an upper motor neurone lesion, the patient will not be able to maintain extension and supination (and 'drifts' into pronation and flexion)

Muscle strength
I Test strength by asking the patient move against your resistance
I Always compare one side to the other

Other tests of power
I Flexion (C5, C6, biceps) and extension (C6, C7, C8, triceps) at the elbow
I Extension at the wrist (C6, C7, C8, radial nerve)
I Squeeze two of your fingers as hard as possible ('grip', C7, C8, T1)

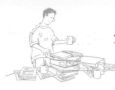

Table 17.1   Muscle strength grading scale

Grade	Description
0/5	No muscle movement
1/5	Visible muscle movement, but no movement at the joint
2/5	Movement at the joint, but not against gravity
3/5	Movement against gravity, but not against added resistance
4/5	Movement against resistance, but less than normal
5/5	Normal strength

- Finger abduction (C8, T1, ulnar nerve)
- Opposition of the thumb (C8, T1, median nerve)
- Flexion (L2, L3, L4, iliopsoas) and extension at the hip (S1, gluteus maximus)
- Adduction (L2, L3, L4, adductors) and abduction at the hips (L4, L5, S1, gluteus medius and minimus)
- Extension (L2, L3, L4, quadriceps) and flexion (L4, L5, S1, S2, hamstrings) at the knee
- Dorsiflexion (L4, L5) and plantar flexion (S1) at the ankle
- Grade strength on a scale from 0 to 5 (Table 17.1)

TENDON REFLEXES (K&C, p. 1148)

- Use a tendon hammer with as little force as needed to provoke a response
- Reinforcement
    — If the reflexes are not elicited as above then ask the patient to clench the teeth or grasp the hands together and then pull apart
    — Retest reflexes as this task is performed
- Reflexes should be graded on a 0 to 4 'plus' scale (Table 17.2)

Biceps (C5, C6)
- Position the patient with the arms relaxed across the lap and partially flexed at the elbow with the palm down

Table 17.2   Tendon reflex grading scale

Grade	Description
0	Absent
1+ or +	Hypoactive
2+ or ++	'Normal'
3+ or +++	Hyperactive without clonus
4+ or ++++	Hyperactive with clonus

I Place your thumb or finger on the biceps tendon
I Tap your finger with the reflex hammer
I Watch for flexion of the elbow

Triceps (C6, C7) I Hold the patient's hand across the chest
I Tap the triceps tendon above the elbow with the reflex hammer
I Watch for extension of the elbow

Brachioradialis I Rest the forearm on the abdomen or lap
(C5, C6) I Tap the radius about 3–5 cm above the wrist
I Watch for flexion and supination of the forearm

Knee (L2, L3, L4) I Hold your arm under the patient's flexed knees, taking the weight of the legs on your forearm
I Tap the patellar tendon just below the patella
I Note contraction of the quadriceps and extension of the knee

Ankle (S1, S2) I Dorsiflex the foot at the ankle with your hand, with the knee slightly bent and the leg rotated laterally
I Tap the Achilles tendon
I Watch and feel for plantar flexion at the ankle

Clonus I Support the knee in a partly flexed position
I With the patient relaxed, quickly pull the foot into dorsiflexion
I Observe for sustained rhythmic beats of dorsiflexion

Plantar response I Run a key or orange stick firmly along the lateral
(Babinski) aspect of the sole of each foot

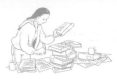

I Flexion of the big toe is normal
I Extension of the big toe with fanning of the other toes is abnormal and indicates an upper motor neurone lesion

COORDINATION AND GAIT (CEREBELLOSPINAL CONNECTIONS) (K&C, p. 1146)

Rapid alternating movements (dys-diadochokinesis)

I Ask the patient to tap the back of one hand with, alternately, the palmar and dorsal aspects of the other hand as accurately and quickly as possible

Point-to-point movements (finger–nose and heel–shin)

I Ask the patient to touch your index finger and his/her nose alternately several times. Move your finger about slowly as the patient performs this task. Holding your finger still, ask the patient to touch his/her nose and then your finger with the eyes closed. Repeat for the other side
I Ask the patient to place one heel on the opposite knee and run it down the shin to the big toe and back again. Repeat with the patient's eyes closed
I Look for past-pointing, intention tremor and clumsiness

Romberg's test (cerebellar connections and dorsal columns)

I Ask the patient to stand with the feet together and eyes closed for 5–10 seconds without support (Be prepared to catch the patient if unstable)
I The test is positive if the patient becomes unstable (indicating a vestibular or proprioceptive problem)

Gait

I Ask the patient to walk across the room, turn and come back and then walk heel-to-toe in a straight line

SENSATION (K&C, p. 1149)

General

I Compare symmetrical areas on the two sides of the body and distal and proximal areas of the extremities
I When you detect an area of sensory loss map out its boundaries in detail

I Test the following areas
— Shoulders (C4)
— Inner and outer aspects of the forearms (C6 and T1)
— Thumbs and little fingers (C6 and C8)
— Front of both thighs (L2)
— Medial and lateral aspect of both calves (L4 and L5)
— Little toes (S1)

Light touch (dorsal columns)
I Use a piece of cotton wool to touch the skin lightly
I Ask the patient to respond whenever a touch is felt

Pain (spinothalamic tracts)
I Use a suitable sharp object (e.g. Neuropin or paperclip) to test 'sharp' or 'dull' sensation

Temperature (spinothalamic tracts)
I This can be left out if pain sensation is normal
I Use a tuning fork heated or cooled by water and ask the patient to identify 'hot' or 'cold'

Vibration (dorsal columns)
I Use a low-pitched tuning fork (128 Hz)
I Place the stem of the fork over the radial head or medial malleolus, and ask the patient to tell you if he/she feels the vibration

Position sense (dorsal columns)
I Hold the patient's big toe away from the other toes with your fingers on each side of the toe
I Show the patient 'up' and 'down.'
I Ask the patient to close the eyes and to identify the direction in which you move the toe
I Test the fingers in a similar fashion

Dermatomes
I See Figure 17.1

Neurological investigations

ROUTINE (K&C, p. 1154)

I See Table 17.3

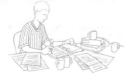

Fig. 17.1
Dermatomes of spinal roots and ophthalmic (V$_1$), maxillary (V$_2$) and mandibular (V$_3$) divisions of the trigeminal nerve.

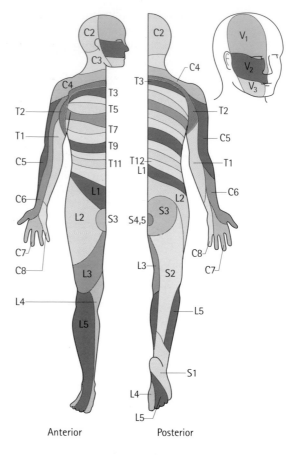

Anterior   Posterior

NEURORADIOLOGY

Skull X-ray
| Skull fracture
| Paget's disease
| Myeloma
| Intracranial calcification
| Intrasellar tumour

Pituitary fossa X-ray
| Enlargement with pituitary tumours

Spinal X-rays
| Fractures/vertebral collapse
| Metastases

Table 17.3 *Abnormalities in routine investigations and possible causes*

Test	Result	Potential cause/effect
Urinalysis	Glycosuria	Polyneuropathy
	Bence Jones protein	Cord compression
Blood film	Raised MCV	Vitamin B_{12} deficiency
ESR	Prolonged	Vasculitis
Serum electrolytes	Low potassium	Weakness
	Low sodium	Confusion/coma
Serum calcium	Low	Tetany/spasms
Serum creatine phosphokinase (CPK)	Raised	Muscle disease
Chest X-ray	Tumour	Metastases Paraneoplastic syndrome
Thyroid function	Hypothyroidism	Confusion/dementia
Vitamin B_{12}	Low	Polyneuropathy Confusion/dementia Subacute combined degeneration of the cord

I Spondylosis
I Tuberculosis

Computed tomography (CT)

Brain I Cerebral tumours
I Intracranial haemorrhage
I Infarction
I Subarachnoid haemorrhage
I Midline shift
I Hydrocephalus
I Cerebral atrophy
I Pituitary lesions

Spine I Cord/bone lesions

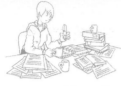

Magnetic resonance imaging (MRI)
- Greater resolution than CT for small lesions and does not require contrast injection
- Contraindicated in patients with metal implants, e.g. aneurysm clips
- Plaques (multiple sclerosis, MS)
- Nerve root compression
- Spinal cord lesions
- Blood vessel imaging

Cerebral angiography
- Intra-arterial or intravenous contrast is injected to demonstrate arterial or venous systems, e.g. berry aneurysms, arteriovenous malformations

Myelography
- Contrast is injected into lumbar subarachnoid space and imaged with CT scanning or X-ray to demonstrate spinal cord compression and lesions

Positron electron tomography (PET)
- Maps function of specific areas of brain

ELECTRICAL STUDIES (K&C, p. 1156)

Electroencephalography (EEG)
- Records electrical brain activity from scalp electrodes on 16 channels
- Used in
  — Epilepsy (spikes or spike and wave abnormalities)
  — Diffuse brain disorders (slow waves, e.g. hepatic encephalopathy)

Electromyelography (EMG)
- Demonstrates abnormal muscle innervation and myopathies

Nerve conduction studies
- Nerve entrapment
- Neuropathies

Visual evoked potentials (VEP)
- Record time for visual stimulus to reach the visual cortex
- Document previous retrobulbar neuritis

LUMBAR PUNCTURE (LP) AND CEREBROSPINAL FLUID (CSF) EXAMINATION (K&C, p. 1157)

Indications for lumbar puncture
- Diagnosis of meningitis or encephalitis
- Intrathecal injection of contrast or drugs
- Diagnosis of subarachnoid haemorrhage
- Measurement of CSF pressure (Table 17.4)
- Therapeutic removal of CSF
- Detection of miscellaneous CSF abnormalities, e.g. oligoclonal bands in MS

Contraindications for lumbar puncture
- Raised intracranial pressure
- Suspected intracranial or spinal cord mass lesion
- (Unconscious patients and those with papilloedema must have CT scan to exclude raised intracranial pressure or mass lesion before LP)
- Platelet count $< 40 \times 10^9/L$
- Abnormal coagulation

BRAIN BIOPSY

- Inflammatory and degenerative brain diseases
- CT-guided sampling of mass lesions

Table 17.4   Normal CSF

Appearance	Protein
Crystal clear, colourless	0.2–0.4 g/L
Pressure	**Glucose**
60–150 mmH$_2$0	2/3–1/2 blood glucose level
Cell count	**Microbiology**
5/mm^3	Sterile
No polymorphs	
No red blood cells	

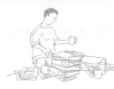

Unconsciousness and coma (K&C, p. 1159)

I Coma is a state of unrousable unresponsiveness
I Consciousness is graded using the Glasgow Coma
Scale (GCS – Table 17.5)

Aetiology of coma   I Diffuse brain dysfunction (see Table 17.6)
I Brainstem lesion
I Brainstem compression (coning)

Table 17.5   Glasgow Coma Scale

Eye opening (E)	
Spontaneous	4
To speech	3
To pain	2
None	1

Motor function (M)	
Obeys commands	6
Localizes to pain	5
Withdraws	4
Flexion	3
Extension	2
None	1

Verbal function (V)	
Orientated	5
Confused conversation	4
Inappropriate words	3
Incomprehensible sounds	2
None	1

Table 17.6   Causes of diffuse brain dysfunction

Drug overdose, alcohol	Hypothyroidism
Hypoglycaemia	Adrenal failure
Hyperglycaemia	Hyponatraemia
Hypoxia	Hypernatraemia
Hypertensive encephalopathy	Metabolic acidosis
Uraemia	Hypothermia, hyperpyrexia
Hepatic encephalopathy	Epilepsy
CO_2 retention	Encephalitis
Hypercalcaemia	Head injury
Hypocalcaemia	Subarachnoid haemorrhage

COMA

Check A B C (airways, breathing, circulation)
Immobilize cervical spine if head or spinal injury suspected
Look for warning cards/bracelets etc, e.g. diabetics, epileptics

Examination

Glasgow Coma Score
Rectal temperature
Smell breath for alcohol/ketones
Blood pressure
Pupils
    Bilateral fixed dilated – Brainstem death, barbiturates,
                              hypothermia
    Single fixed dilated – coning
    Pinpoint – pontine lesions, opiates
Fundi for papilloedema
Eye movements
    Doll's head reflex
    Fixed lateral gaze
Lateralizing signs
    Facial drooping
    Muscle tone
    Plantar responses
    Tendon reflexes

Investigations

Drug screen
Serum biochemistry
Serum glucose
Thyroid function tests
Blood cultures
ECG
CT scan or MRI of brain
LP and CSF examination (only after raised intracranial
    pressure excluded)
EEG
Serum cortisol

Immediate management

Careful observation to detect changes in vital functions or
    depth of coma
Protect airway
Ventilate if necessary

Longer-term management

Skin care
Pressure area care
Oral hygiene
Nutrition (nasogastric feeding or percutaneous endoscopic
    gastrostomy tube)
Eye care
Urinary catheter only if essential

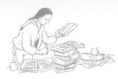

Epilepsy (K&C, p. 1173)

▌ A continuing tendency to suffer epileptic seizures, a seizure being a convulsion or transient abnormal event resulting from paroxysmal discharge of cerebral neurones

Prevalence   ▌ 2% of the population has two or more seizures

Classification   ▌ By clinical pattern of seizures (Table 17.7)

Generalized
▌ Absence (petit mal)
▌ Myoclonic

Table 17.7   *Clinical pattern of epileptic seizures*

Generalized tonic-clonic seizures
Warning – vague
Tonic phase – body becomes rigid before patient falls (often with a cry), biting the tongue and with urinary incontinence
Clonic phase – a generalized convulsion with rhythmic jerking of muscles and frothing at the mouth
Recovery – patient is drowsy or confused, or in a coma for several hours (post-ictal)

Absence seizures
Patient becomes still and staring and looks pale
Eyelids may twitch
Attack lasts a few seconds usually, during which the patient is unresponsive
No recollection of the event

Partial (focal) seizures
Aura, e.g. strange smell, tingling in a limb
Motor (Jacksonian)
　　Jerking movements begin at the angle of the mouth or in the hand, spreading to involve the limbs on the side opposite from the epileptic focus
　　Patient remains conscious
　　Paralysis of the affected limbs may follow for several hours (Todd's paralysis)
Temporal lobe epilepsy
　　May be simple or complex
　　Feeling of unreality, often déjà-vu, associated with absence attacks, vertigo or visual hallucinations

▌ Tonic-clonic (grand mal)
▌ Tonic
▌ Akinetic

Partial
▌ Simple (e.g. Jacksonian, no impairment of consciousness)
▌ Complex (impairment of consciousness)

Aetiology
▌ Genetic
▌ Developmental abnormalities
▌ Trauma
▌ Surgery
▌ Pyrexia (in children, febrile convulsions)
▌ Intracranial mass
▌ Infarction
▌ Alcohol/drug withdrawal
▌ Encephalitis
▌ Metabolic abnormalities, e.g. hyponatraemia, hypoglycaemia

Investigations
▌ EEG (abnormal during seizures, often normal in between)
▌ CT scan/MRI scan
▌ Serum biochemistry
▌ Chest X-ray

Management
During seizure
▌ Maintain airway and physical safety
▌ Rectal or i.v. diazepam 5–10 mg if seizure does not stop spontaneously

Prophylactic
▌ For recurrent seizures
▌ First-line drugs
— Sodium valproate
— Carbamezepine
— Phenytoin
— Ethosuximide (petit mal)

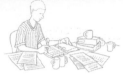

STATUS EPILEPTICUS

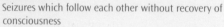

Definition
Seizures which follow each other without recovery of consciousness

Management
Nurse the patient in an area with full ventilatory support available if required and with cardiac monitoring facilities

Diazepam 10–20 mg i.v. at a rate of 2.5 mg/30 seconds until fitting stops (up to a maximum of 40 mg); beware of respiratory depression

Loading dose of i.v. phenytoin, 15 mg/kg at a rate < 50 mg/minute

Maintenance phenytoin i.v. or oral depending on patient's ability to take it

If status continues unresponsive to treatment for more than 90 minutes, the patient needs to be anaesthetized with thiopental or propofol and ventilated

❙ Second-line drugs
— Lamotrigine
— Vigabatrin
— Gabapentin
— Clobazam
— Phenobarbital

Toxic drug effects   *All drugs*
❙ Ataxia
❙ Nystagmus
❙ Dysarthria

Phenytoin
❙ Gum hypertrophy
❙ Hypertrichosis
❙ Osteomalacia
❙ Folate deficiency
❙ Polyneuropathy

Driving   ❙ It is illegal to drive if any form of seizure or unexplained loss of consciousness has occurred during the past year

❙ In the UK it is essential that a doctor inform patients of the driving regulations; it is then the patient's responsibility to inform the licensing authority

OTHER CAUSES OF DROP ATTACKS, BLACKOUTS AND EPISODES OF DISTURBED CONSCIOUSNESS
(K&C, p. 1180)

❙ Diagnosis can usually be determined from the history
❙ A witness account of an attack is especially valuable

Aetiology   ❙ Syncope, e.g. simple, micturition
❙ Transient ischaemic attack (see p. 477)
❙ Panic attack
❙ Cardiac arrhythmia, e.g. Stokes Adams attack
❙ Aortic stenosis
❙ Hypoglycaemia
❙ Hypocalcaemia
❙ Vertigo

Movement disorders (K&C, p. 1182)

Parkinson's disease

❙ Combination of tremor, rigidity and akinesia

Prevalence   ❙ Increases with age
❙ 1:200 over 70 years of age
❙ Less prevalent in smokers

Aetiology   ❙ Idiopathic
❙ Drug-induced, e.g. phenothiazines
❙ MPTP (methylphenyltetrapyridine, impurity in illegally synthesized opiates)
❙ Encephalitis lethargica

Pathology   ❙ Cell degeneration in the substantia nigra
❙ Loss of dopamine in the extrapyramidal nuclei

Clinical features   ❙ Micrographia
❙ Falls

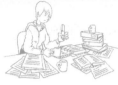
- 4–7 Hz resting tremor (pill-rolling)
- Increased tone throughout the range of movement
- Cogwheel rigidity (stuttering rigid tone combined with tremor)
- Poverty of movement
- Mask-like facies
- Reduced blinking
- Stooping, shuffling gait
- Poor arm swinging
- Monotonous speech, slurring dysarthria
- Normal power
- Brisk reflexes
- Downgoing plantars
- Cognitive function initially preserved; late dementia sometimes occurs

Investigations
- No diagnostic test; diagnosis made on clinical grounds

Management
- Levodopa plus dopa decarboxylase inhibitor e.g. Sinemet or Madopar; start gradually increasing the dose until adequate response or limiting side-effects (see below)
- Dopaminergic agonists, e.g. bromocriptine
- Neurosurgery (occasionally for intractable tremor)
- Physiotherapy
- Physical aids

Side-effects of levodopa

Short-term
- Nausea and vomiting
- Confusion
- Visual hallucinations
- Chorea

Long-term
- End-of-dose dyskinesia
- On–off syndrome
- Chorea
- Dystonic movements

Prognosis
- Variable

I Usually worsens over 10–15 years with death from bronchopneumonia

Huntington's disease (K&C, p. 1186)

I Inherited progressive chorea and dementia in middle life

Prevalence I 5:100 000

Aetiology I Autosomal dominance with full penetrance
I Children of an affected parent have a 50% chance of inheriting the mutation on chromosome 4

Pathology I Cerebral atrophy
I Loss of neurones in caudate nucleus and putamen
I Depletion of γ-aminobutyric (GABA), angiotensin-converting enzyme (ACE) and met-enkephalin in substantia nigra

Clinical features I Chorea (sudden involuntary jerky semi-purposeful movements, flitting from one part of the body to another)
I Progressive dementia

Investigations I MRI or CT shows atrophy of caudate nucleus

Management I Phenothiazines may reduce chorea

Prognosis I Death 10–20 years after onset

Screening I Mutation analysis is available for presymptomatic screening in families but no effective treatment is known to alter disease progression

Other causes of chorea I Sydenham's chorea (rheumatic fever)
I Drugs, e.g. phenytoin
I Thyrotoxicosis
I Stroke
I Systemic lupus erythematosus (SLE)

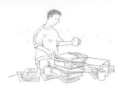

Multiple sclerosis (K&C, p. 1189)

I Multiple plaques of demyelination in the brain and spinal cord disseminated in time and place
I Clinical diagnosis: two neurological events separated in time and neurological location

Prevalence
I Increases moving north from the Equator
I 60–100/100 000 in the UK

Aetiology
I Increased concordance among monozygotic twins
I HLA haplotype A3, B7, D2 and DR2 is more common

Environmental
I ?Viral infection
I ?Dietary antigens

Pathology
I Plaques of demyelination particularly in
— Optic nerves
— Periventricular region
— Brainstem and cerebellar connections
— Cervical spinal cord
— Corticospinal tracts
— Posterior columns

Clinical patterns
I Relapsing/remitting
I Chronic progressive
I See below

Investigations
Imaging
I MRI brain and spinal cord (visualizes multiple plaques)

CSF
I Oligoclonal bands in 80%
I Raised mononuclear cell count 5–60 cells/mm^3

Visual evoked responses
I Delayed following optic neuropathy

Management ▌ No treatment has been shown to alter long-term outcome
▌ Corticosteroids – i.v. methylprednisolone or ACTH may speed recovery in acute relapses
▌ β-interferon – reduces relapse rate but not long-term outcome
▌ Physiotherapy
▌ Occupational therapy
   — Walking aids
   — Wheelchairs
   — Car/house conversions
▌ Speech therapy
▌ Counselling

Prognosis ▌ Unpredictable course ranging from grave disability to mild and benign

Optic neuropathy
Clinical features ▌ Blurred vision in one eye
▌ Mild ocular pain
▌ Recovery within 1–2 months
▌ Optic disc swelling (optic neuritis)
▌ Normal disc (retrobulbar neuritis)
▌ Optic atrophy
▌ Relative afferent pupillary defect (dilatation of the affected eye when light is transferred from the good eye to the affected eye)

Brainstem demyelination
Clinical features ▌ Double vision
▌ Vertigo
▌ Facial numbness
▌ Weakness
▌ Dysphagia
▌ Pyramidal tract signs
▌ Nystagmus
▌ Ataxia
▌ Cranial nerve defects
▌ Internuclear ophthalmoplegia

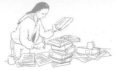

Spinal cord lesion

Clinical features
- Difficulty walking
- Sensory abnormalities
- Electric shock-like pains radiating down trunk and limbs caused by neck flexion (Lhermitte's sign)
- Urinary symptoms (incontinence, retention)
- Spastic paraparesis
- Increased tone
- Weakness
- Brisk reflexes
- Up-going plantars
- Sensory level

Other presentations of MS

- Epilepsy
- Trigeminal neuralgia
- Tonic spasms of a hand
- Organic psychosis
- Dementia

Infections and inflammatory conditions of the nervous system (K&C, p. 1191)

Meningitis

Aetiology
- See Table 17.8

Clinical features
- Headache
- Neck stiffness
- Fever
- Photophobia
- Vomiting
- Rigors
- Positive Kernig's sign
- Petechial/purpuric rash (meningococcal septicaemia)
- Drowsiness/focal signs (suggest complication, e.g. raised intracranial pressure/abscess)

Table 17.8   Causes of meningitis

Bacteria	HIV
Neisseria meningitides	Epstein–Barr virus (EBV)
Streptococcus pneumoniae	**Fungi**
Staphylococcus aureus	Cryptococcus neoformans
Listeria monocytogenes	Candida
Gram-negative bacilli	
Haemophilus influenzae	**Chronic inflammatory**
Mycobacterium tuberculosis	**conditions**
Treponema pallidum	Sarcoidosis
	Behçet's disease
Viruses	Syphilis
Enterovirus	
Echovirus	**Malignancy**
Coxsackie virus	**Blood**
Polio virus	Following subarachnoid
Herpes simplex	haemorrhage

Investigations
I CT of brain to exclude raised intracranial pressure
I Lumbar puncture (Table 17.9)
I Blood cultures
I Blood glucose
I Chest X-ray
I Skull X-ray (if trauma)
I Throat swab for *Neisseria*

Management
I Immediate parenteral antibiotics (Table 17.10); do not wait for LP/CT
I Further treatment depends on results of blood or CSF culture and sensitivities
I Viral meningitis requires no specific treatment
I i.v. steroids with first dose of antibiotics

Prophylaxis
I Meningococcus is notifiable

Table 17.9   CSF findings in meningitis

	Appearance	Mononuclear cells (per mm³)	Polymorphs (per mm³)	Protein (g/L)	Glucose (% blood glucose)
Normal	Crystal clear	< 5	Nil	0.2–0.4	> 50
Viral	Clear/turbid	10–100	Nil	0.4–0.8	> 50
Pyogenic	Turbid/purulent	< 50	200–300	0.5–2	< 50
TB	Turbid/viscous	100–300	0–200	0.5–3	< 30

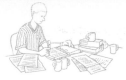

Table 17.10   Antibiotics in meningitis

Suspected organism	Antibiotic
Unknown	Ceftriaxone
Meningococcus	Benzylpenicillin Ceftriaxone
Pneumococcus	Ceftriaxone
TB	Rifampicin

▌ Family and very close contacts should be treated with ciprofloxacin or rifampicin to eradicate carriage
▌ Meningococcal vaccine to close contacts

Acute viral encephalitis (*K&C*, p. 1194)

Aetiology
▌ Herpes simplex
▌ Echovirus
▌ Coxsackie virus
▌ Mumps
▌ EBV
▌ Adenovirus
▌ Varicella zoster
▌ Influenza
▌ Measles
▌ Rabies

Clinical features
▌ Often mild and self-limiting
▌ HSV-1 infection may be more serious
▌ Headache
▌ Fever
▌ Mood change
▌ Drowsiness
▌ Seizures
▌ Focal signs
▌ Coma

Investigations
▌ CT scan (may show diffuse oedema)
▌ EEG (characteristic slow wave changes in HSV)
▌ CSF (increased mononuclear cells, slightly raised protein)

Management
▌ i.v. aciclovir for suspected HSV-1

Prognosis ❙ 20% mortality in serious cases, with many others suffering long-term severe brain damage

Herpes zoster (Shingles) (*K&C*, p. 1195)

❙ Recrudescence of varicella zoster virus infection within a dorsal root ganglion

Clinical features ❙ Typical blistering rash affecting dermatome supplied by the affected nerve root

Trigeminal nerve (ophthalmic division)
❙ Rash affects the eye and may cause corneal scarring

Facial nerve (Ramsay Hunt syndrome)
❙ Facial palsy
❙ Vesicles on ear lobe, external auditory meatus and fauces

Treatment ❙ Aciclovir

Complications ❙ Post-herpetic neuralgia

Neurosyphilis
(*K&C*, p. 1196)

Meningovascular syphilis
❙ Subacute meningitis with cranial nerve palsies or paraparesis

Tabes dorsalis
❙ Demyelination of dorsal roots
❙ Charcot's joints (neuropathic)
❙ Ataxia
❙ Stamping gait
❙ Widespread sensory loss
❙ Argyll Robertson pupils (small irregular pupil, fixed to light, constricts to accommodation)
❙ Ptosis
❙ Optic atrophy

Generalized paralysis of the insane (GPI)
❙ Dementia
❙ Weakness
❙ Tremor
❙ Brisk reflexes
❙ Extensor plantars
❙ Argyll Robertson pupils

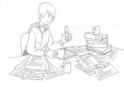

Taboparesis
▌ Congenital neurosyphilis
▌ Features of tabes dorsalis and GPI in childhood

Management ▌ Parenteral penicillin for 2–3 weeks

Sporadic Creutzfeldt–Jakob disease (CJD) *(K&C, p. 1197)*

Aetiology ▌ Prion disease
▌ Can be passed on from surgical specimens, autopsy material (e.g. corneal grafts) and human pituitary hormones

Pathology ▌ Spongiform changes in brain

Clinical features ▌ Slowly progressive dementia develops after age 50

New variant CJD ▌ First noted in Britain in 1995

Aetiology ▌ Prion disease
▌ Linked to ingestion of meat from cattle infected with bovine spongiform encephalopathy (BSE)

Clinical features ▌ Younger patients
▌ Early neuropsychiatric symptoms
▌ Ataxia
▌ Dementia
▌ Myoclonus
▌ Chorea
▌ Death

Brain abscess ▌ A focal area of bacterial infection causing an
(K&C, p. 1198) expanding mass lesion in the cerebrum or cerebellum

Aetiology ▌ *Streptococcus milleri*
▌ *Bacteroides* spp
▌ *Staphylococcus* spp
▌ Fungi
▌ Parameningeal infection, e.g. ear, nose, paranasal sinuses
▌ Skull fracture
▌ Distant infection, e.g. pneumonia, infective endocarditis
▌ Immunosuppression, e.g. HIV infection

Clinical features ▌ Headache
                     ▌ Fever
                     ▌ Focal signs
                     ▌ Seizures
                     ▌ Vomiting
                     ▌ Drowsiness
                     ▌ Papilloedema

Investigations ▌ Imaging (mass lesion on CT or MRI +/− hydrocephalus)
                  ▌ Blood cultures
                  ▌ Raised ESR
                  ▌ Raised white cell count
                  ▌ Look for a local/distant focus of infection
                  ▌ Lumbar puncture is contraindicated

Management ▌ Parenteral antibiotics
              ▌ Surgical decompression

Prognosis ▌ Mortality 25%
             ▌ Persistent epilepsy common in survivors

Intracranial tumours (Table 17.11) (*K&C*, p. 1198)

▌ Primary intracranial tumours account for about
   10% of all neoplasms

Table 17.11   Intracranial tumours

Type	Prevalence
Metastases Bronchus Breast Stomach Prostate Thyroid Kidney Lymphoma (associated with AIDS)	50%
Primary malignant Astrocytoma Oligodendroglioma	35%
Benign Meningioma Neurofibroma	15%

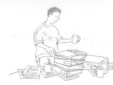
Table 17.12 Symptoms and signs of raised intracranial pressure

Headache	Bradycardia
Vomiting	Decerebrate posturing (coning)
Papilloedema	False localizing signs
Impaired consciousness	VI nerve lesion
Respiratory depression	III nerve lesion

Clinical features
- Direct mass effect on function, e.g. hemiparesis
- Raised intracranial pressure (Table 17.12)
- Seizures

Investigations
- CT or MRI scanning
- Brain biopsy

Management
- Reduce cerebral oedema using corticosteroids and/ or i.v. mannitol
- Anticonvulsants
- Surgery
- Radiotherapy

Prognosis
- 50% survival at 2 years for malignant tumours

Headache and migraine (K&C, pp. 1201–1203)

Tension headache
- The vast majority of chronic and recurrent headaches

Clinical features
- Throbbing headache
- Tight band sensation
- Pressure behind eyes

Management
- Avoid precipitating causes
- Simple analgesia

Migraine
- Recurrent headaches associated with visual and gastrointestinal disturbance

Pathology
- Vasodilatation and oedema of blood vessels
- Release of vasoactive substances

Classical migraine

Clinical features
- Prodrome
  - — Teichopsia (flashes)
  - — Jagged lines
  - — Unilateral patchy scotoma
  - — Lasts 15 minutes to 1 hour
- Headache hemicranial or generalized
- Nausea and vomiting
- Generally irritable
- Preference for the dark
- Sleeping

Other patterns
- Migraine without aura
- Hemiplegic migraine

Differential diagnosis
- Subarachnoid haemorrhage
- Transient ischaemic attack
- Partial seizures

Management
- Avoid precipitating features

During attack
- Paracetamol
- Antiemetics
- Sumatriptan (5HT agonist)
- Ergotamine

Prophylaxis
- Pizotifen, methysergide (5HT antagonists)
- Propranolol
- Amitriptyline (low-dose)

Cluster headaches
- Affect adults in third and fourth decades
- ♂ > ♀

Clinical features
- Recurrent bouts of excruciating pain centred around one eye
- Wakes patient at night
- Vomiting
- Watering and congestion of affected eye
- Transient ipsilateral Horner's syndrome

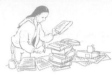

Management	▌ Usually unhelpful
	▌ No analgesia effective for headache
	▌ Lithium carbonate for prophylaxis
	▌ Oxygen during attack

Other causes of headache	▌ Subarachnoid haemorrhage
	▌ Meningitis
	▌ Sinusitis
	▌ Brain tumours
	▌ Temporal arteritis
	▌ Benign intracranial hypertension
	▌ Head injury

Cerebrovascular disease and stroke

(Table 17.13) *(K&C, p. 1163)*

▌ Stroke is the third commonest cause of death in the UK

▌ A stroke is a focal neurological deficit due to a vascular lesion lasting > than 24 hours (if the patient survives)

▌ A transient ischaemic attack (TIA) is a focal neurological deficit lasting < 24 hours

Risk factors	▌ Hypertension
	▌ Smoking
	▌ Family history
	▌ Hyperlipidaemia
	▌ Afro-Caribbean race
	▌ High-dose oral contraceptive pill

Table 17.13 Types of cerebrovascular disease

Thromboembolic infarction
Cerebral and cerebellar haemorrhages
Dissection of carotid or vertebral arteries
Subarachnoid haemorrhage
Subdural and extradural haemorrhage
Cortical venous and dural sinus thrombosis

Transient ischaemic attacks (K&C, p. 1165)

Clinical features   I Focal deficit depends on part of brain affected

Carotid system
I Amaurosis fugax
— visual loss
I Aphasia (dominant side)
I Hemiparesis
I Hemianopic visual loss

Vertebrobasilar system
I Diplopia
I Vertigo
I Vomiting
I Dysarthria, choking
I Ataxia
I Transient global amnesia

Evidence of source of embolus
I Atrial fibrillation
I Carotid bruit
I Valvular heart disease
I Subclavian artery stenosis

Cerebral infarction (K&C, p. 1166)

Clinical features   I Focal deficit depends on part of brain affected (see below)
I Initially flaccid areflexic weakness followed by spastic tone, brisk reflexes and extensor plantars
I See Figure 17.2 for arterial supply to the cerebral cortex

Dysphasia
I Dominance
— Almost all right-handed and 50% of left-handed people have language function in the left hemisphere
I Expressive dysphasia
— Lesion in Broca's area in frontal lobe
— Reduced fluency of speech
— Failure to construct sentences
— Comprehension preserved

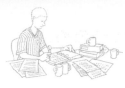

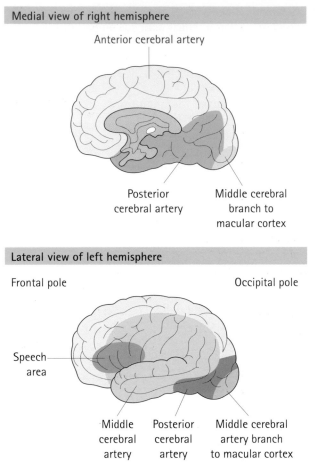

Medial view of right hemisphere

Anterior cerebral artery

Posterior cerebral artery

Middle cerebral branch to macular cortex

Lateral view of left hemisphere

Frontal pole

Occipital pole

Speech area

Middle cerebral artery

Posterior cerebral artery

Middle cerebral artery branch to macular cortex

Fig. 17.2 Arterial supply to the cerebral cortex.

❙ Receptive dysphasia
  — Lesion in Wernicke's area in temporo-parietal region
  — Fluent speech with incorrect words
  — Use of jargon
  — Sounds like nonsense
  — Failure of comprehension

Middle cerebral/internal carotid artery (internal capsule stroke)
▌ Hemiparesis (limbs and face)
▌ Aphasia (dominant side)
▌ Hemianopic visual loss
▌ Dysarthria

Posterior inferior cerebellar artery (brainstem stroke)
▌ Coma, altered consciousness
▌ Vertigo
▌ Vomiting
▌ Dysphagia, choking
▌ Ataxia
▌ Contralateral loss of pain on face

Important parts of examination of patients with cerebrovascular disease
▌ Neurological signs
▌ Source of embolus (e.g. carotid bruit, atrial fibrillation)
▌ Blood pressure (in both arms)
▌ Optic fundi (hypertensive retinopathy, papilloedema)

Investigations
▌ CT/MRI imaging of brain (Chapter 5)
  — Demonstrates site
  — Distinguishes between infarct or haemorrhage
▌ Carotid Doppler scanning
▌ Magnetic resonance angiography (for possible surgery)
▌ Blood count
▌ ESR
▌ Blood glucose, lipids
▌ Syphilis serology
▌ Chest X-ray
▌ ECG
▌ Echocardiogram

Management
▌ Identify and treat risk factors where possible
▌ Antihypertensive therapy
▌ Aspirin 75 mg per day or other antiplatelet therapy
▌ Anticoagulation (for atrial fibrillation)
▌ Surgery (internal carotid endarterectomy)
▌ Fibrinolytics in acute stroke

Rehabilitation
▌ Physiotherapy
▌ Speech therapy
▌ Occupational therapy

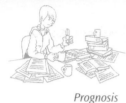

Prognosis
- 30–40% survival at 3 years (among initial survivors)
- 10% chance of further stroke within a year

Intracerebral haemorrhage (K&C, p. 1171)
- Accounts for 30% of strokes

Aetiology
- Rupture of microaneurysms

Risk factors
- Hypertension

Clinical features
- Difficult to distinguish between haemorrhage and infarction
- Haemorrhage may be accompanied by headache and coma

Investigations
- CT head (Chapter 5)

Management
- As for infarction except avoid antiplatelet and anticoagulant drugs

Subarachnoid haemorrhage (K&C, p. 1171)
- Spontaneous arterial bleeding into subarachnoid space

Prevalence
- 6:100 000/year
- Accounts for 10% of cerebrovascular events

Aetiology
- Saccular 'berry' aneurysms (70%)
- Arteriovenous malformation (AVM) (10%)
- No lesion (20%)

Clinical features
- Sudden onset of severe occipital headache
- Vomiting
- Loss of consciousness
- Neck stiffness
- Positive Kernig's sign
- Papilloedema and retinal haemorrhages

Investigations
- CT scan
- Lumbar puncture (if CT undiagnostic) – red cells and/or xanthochromia in CSF
- Carotid and vertebral angiography

Management	*Immediate*

Management   *Immediate*
I Bed rest
I Treat hypertension
I Dexamethasone
I Nimodipine

Later
I Neurosurgical aneurysm clipping or coil insertion

Prognosis   I 50% mortality at presentation
I 10–20% more die in early weeks

Chronic subdural   I Accumulation of blood in subdural space following
haematoma   rupture of a vein after head injury (sometimes
(*K&C*, p. 1173)   trivial)

Clinical features   I May be delayed
I Headache
I Drowsiness
I Confusion
I Focal deficits

Management   I Often conservative
I Usually resolve spontaneously without surgical
drainage

Degenerative disorders

Motor neurone   I Progressive degeneration of lower motor neurones
disease   and upper motor neurones of the cortex, cranial
(*K&C*, p. 1208)   nerve nuclei and spinal cord

Prevalence   I 6:100 000
I Slight male predominance

Clinical features   I Progressive muscular atrophy – progressive
weakness and wasting of arm and hand muscles
I Amyotrophic lateral sclerosis – progressive spastic
tetraparesis or paraparesis with wasting and
fasciculation

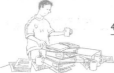

I Progressive bulbar palsy – degeneration of lower cranial nerve nuclei

Clinical features
I Muscle wasting
I Fasciculation
I Reflexes absent or exaggerated
I Dysarthria
I Dysphagia
I Nasal regurgitation of fluids
I Choking
I Bulbar and pseudobulbar palsy (see p. 488)
I Ocular movements are not affected
I Cerebellar or extrapyramidal signs do not occur
I Dementia is unusual
I Sphincter function is usually preserved
I No sensory signs

Investigations
I Diagnosis made on clinical grounds
I EMG – denervation of muscles with preserved motor conduction velocity

Prognosis
I Relentlessly progressive course
I Death within 3 years

Management
I No effective treatment

Friedreich's ataxia
(*K&C*, p. 1211)
I Progressive degeneration of dorsal root ganglia, spinocerebellar tracts and corticospinal tracts

Aetiology
I Abnormal gene for fraxitin (unknown function)

Clinical features
I Difficulty walking from about 12 years of age
I Ataxia of gait and trunk
I Nystagmus
I Dysarthria
I Absent reflexes in legs
I Optic atrophy
I Pes cavus
I Cardiomyopathy

Neuropathy

▌ A pathological process affecting peripheral nerves

Pathology
▌ Demyelination
▌ Axonal degeneration
▌ Wallerian degeneration (after nerve section)
▌ Compression
▌ Infarction
▌ Infiltration

MONONEUROPATHIES

▌ Caused by peripheral nerve compression

Carpal tunnel syndrome (*K&C*, pp. 522 and 1213)
▌ Median nerve compression in carpal tunnel (at wrist)

Aetiology
▌ Idiopathic
▌ Hypothyroidism
▌ Diabetes mellitus
▌ Pregnancy
▌ Rheumatoid arthritis
▌ Obesity
▌ Acromegaly

Clinical features
▌ Tingling in fingers (especially at night)
▌ Weakness of thenar muscles
▌ Wasting of thenar eminence
▌ Weakness of abductor pollicis brevis (raising thumb away from palm)
▌ Weakness of opposition of thumb and little finger
▌ Tinel's sign (reproduction of tingling by tapping over carpal tunnel)
▌ Sensory loss of palm and radial three and a half fingers

Management
▌ Splint wrist
▌ Surgical decompression

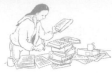

Ulnar nerve compression

I Usually occurs after trauma at elbow

Clinical features

I Wasting and weakness of interossei and hypothenar muscles
I Sensory loss in the ulnar one and a half fingers

Radial nerve compression ('Saturday night palsy')

I Occurs after nerve is compressed against humerus when arm is draped over a hard chair for several hours

Clinical features

I Wrist drop
I Weakness of finger extension

Mononeuritis multiplex

I Multiple mononeuropathies

Aetiology

I Diabetes mellitus
I Leprosy
I Vasculitis
I Sarcoidosis
I Amyloidosis
I Malignancy
I Neurofibromatosis
I HIV infection

POLYNEUROPATHIES

Guillain–Barré syndrome
(*K&C*, p. 1214)

I Acute inflammatory post-infective polyneuropathy
I Follows 1–3 weeks after infection (often trivial, or *Campylobacter* infection)

Clinical features

I Weakness of distal limb muscles +/– numbness
I Weakness ascends over days for up to 3 weeks
I Can affect respiratory and facial muscles in 30%

Variants
I Autonomic neuropathy
I Miller–Fisher syndrome (affecting ocular muscles, and with ataxia)

Investigations ▌ Diagnosis is made on clinical grounds
▌ Nerve conduction studies (demyelinating neuropathy)
▌ CSF (cell count normal, protein raised 1–3 g/L)

Management ▌ Measurement of respiratory function (arterial blood gases, vital capacity, FEV_1)
▌ Assisted ventilation if necessary
▌ High-dose i.v. γ-globulin
▌ Plasmapheresis
▌ Subcutaneous heparin for prevention of thromboembolism

Prognosis ▌ Spontaneous gradual recovery

OTHER POLYNEUROPATHIES (Table 17.14)
(*K&C*, pp. 1216–1217)

Thiamin deficiency (Wernicke–Korsakoff syndrome)
Clinical features ▌ Ocular signs
— Nystagmus
— Bilateral rectal palsies
— Fixed pupils
▌ Ataxia
▌ Confusion (amnestic syndrome, with loss of short-term memory)

Investigations ▌ Reduced red cell transketolase

Management ▌ Parenteral thiamine

Table 17.14 Other polyneuropathies

Metabolic	Thalidomide
Diabetes mellitus	Vincristine
Uraemia	Cisplatin
Porphyria	**Vitamin deficiencies**
Amyloidosis	Thiamin (B_1)
Toxic	Pyridoxine (B_6)
Alcohol	Vitamin B_{12}
Drugs	Nicotinic acid
Phenytoin	**Non-metastatic manifestation**
Isoniazid	**of malignancy**
Metronidazole	

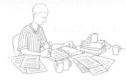
Vitamin B$_{12}$ deficiency (subacute combined degeneration of the cord)

Aetiology ▌ See page 394

Clinical features ▌ Distal sensory loss
— Light touch
— Vibration sense
— Joint position sense
▌ Absent ankle jerks
▌ Extensor plantars
▌ Optic atrophy
▌ Dementia

Investigations ▌ Reduced serum B$_{12}$
▌ Macrocytosis
▌ Megaloblastic bone marrow

Management ▌ Parenteral B$_{12}$

Peroneal muscular atrophy (Charcot–Marie–Tooth disease)

▌ Inherited sensorimotor neuropathy
▌ Several types: autosomal dominant and recessive

Clinical features ▌ Distal limb wasting and weakness
▌ Inverted 'champagne bottle' legs
▌ Pes cavus
▌ Clawing of toes
▌ Loss of sensation
▌ Loss of reflexes

Autonomic neuropathy

Aetiology ▌ Diabetes mellitus
▌ Guillain–Barré syndrome
▌ Amyloidosis

Clinical features ▌ Postural hypotension
▌ Retention of urine
▌ Impotence
▌ Diarrhoea
▌ Diminished sweating
▌ Cardiac arrhythmias

Muscle disease (K&C, pp. 1222–1224)

Aetiology	∎ See Table 17.15
Myasthenia gravis	∎ Disorder of the neuromuscular junction
Prevalence	∎ 4:100 000 ∎ ♀ > ♂ (2:1) ∎ Age of onset about 30 years

Aetiopathogenesis	∎ Unknown aetiology
	∎ IgG antibodies to acetylcholine receptor
	∎ Immune complex deposits on postsynaptic membrane
	∎ Destruction of acetylcholine receptor
	∎ Thymic hyperplasia in 70%
	∎ Associated with
	  — Thyroid disease
	  — Rheumatoid arthritis
	  — Pernicious anaemia
	  — SLE

Clinical features	∎ Weakness and fatigability of muscles
	  — Proximal limb
	  — Extraocular
	  — Speech
	  — Facial expression
	  — Mastication
	∎ Ptosis
	∎ Reflexes preserved but fatigable

Table 17.15   Causes of myopathies

Type	Example
Inflammatory	Polymyositis
Metabolic	Cushing's syndrome
Myasthenic	Myasthenia gravis
Hereditary	Duchenne muscular dystrophy
Myotonias	Myotonic dystrophy
Channelopathies	Periodic paralysis

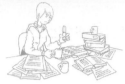

> ### TENSILON TEST
>
> An i.v. bolus of 10 mg edrophonium (anticholinesterase) is given
>
> Simple exercises are performed
>
> Weakness improves immediately after drug, lasting 2–3 minutes before fatigability begins

Investigations
I Tensilon test
I Serum acetylcholine receptor antibodies (positive in 90%)
I Mediastinal imaging for thymoma (chest X-ray, CT, MRI)

Management
I Oral anticholinesterases, e.g. pyridostigmine
I Thymectomy (improves prognosis)
I Corticosteroids
I Azathioprine
I Plasmapheresis

Lambert–Eaton myasthenic-myopathic syndrome

I Non-metastatic manifestation of small cell carcinoma of the bronchus due to defective acetyl-choline release at the neuromuscular junction

Clinical features
I Muscle weakness and absent reflexes which improve with contraction

Dystrophia myotonica

I Autosomal dominant inheritance

Clinical features
I Cataracts
I Frontal baldness
I Ptosis
I Facial weakness
I Progressive distal muscle weakness
I Mild intellectual impairment
I Cardiomyopathy
I Hypogonadism
I Glucose intolerance

Cranial nerve defects

▌ See Table 17.16

Table 17.16 Cranial nerve defects

Nerve	Causes	Features
I	Head injury	Loss of smell (anosmia)
II	Optic neuritis Optic nerve compression Visual pathway lesion	See MS Tunnel vision (if at chiasma) See Figure 17.3
III	Coning Aneurysm of posterior inferior carotid artery Diabetes	Ptosis Eye points down and out Fixed dilated pupil
IV	Rare	Diplopia looking away and down
V	Brainstem lesion Acoustic neuroma Cavernous sinus thrombosis	Sensory loss (face and tongue) Loss of corneal reflex Deviation of jaw towards lesion
VI	MS Glioma Raised intracranial pressure	Convergent squint Diplopia looking towards lesion
VII	Upper motor neurone lesion (infarction) Lower motor neurone lesion (Bell's palsy, Ramsay Hunt syndrome, parotid gland disease)	Facial muscle weakness Loss of taste on anterior two-thirds of tongue
VIII	Acoustic neuroma Meningitis Head injury Drugs – gentamicin	Sensorineural deafness Vertigo Nystagmus
IX and X	Brainstem infarct Motor neurone disease Carcinoma of nasopharynx	Weakness of elevation of pharynx Loss of gag reflex Hoarseness Dysphagia Bulbar or pseudobulbar palsy
XI	Syringobulbia Motor neurone disease Carcinoma of nasopharynx	Weakness of sternomastoid and trapezius
XII	Brainstem infarct Motor neurone disease Carcinoma of nasopharynx	LMN lesion; unilateral wasting, weakness and fasciculation of tongue UMN lesion; stiff, spastic tongue

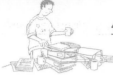

SPECIFIC CRANIAL NERVE AND BRAINSTEM DEFECTS

Optic pathway (*K&C*, p. 1130)

I See Figure 17.3

Bell's palsy (*K&C*, p. 1138)

I Common acute, isolated facial nerve palsy

Aetiology I Viral infection (often herpes simplex) causes swelling of nerve within petrous temporal bone

Clinical features I Unilateral lower motor neurone facial weakness and droop
I Loss of taste on anterior two-thirds of tongue

Investigations I Diagnosis made on clinical grounds

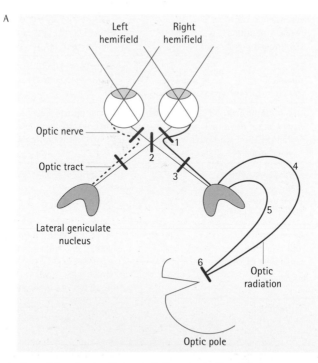

Fig. 17.3 Lesions of the visual pathway. **A.** Optic nerve tracts and lesions.

B

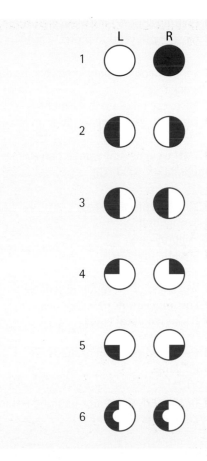

Fig. 17.3 *(continued)* **B.** Visual field defects caused by lesions in the optic pathway. *Lesion 1:* This is analogous to losing an eye. One eye is completely blacked out. *Lesion 2:* Here only inputs from the nasal retinas are cut, so peripheral vision is lost on both sides. This can be caused by a pituitary tumour. (The pituitary lies just under the optic chiasm.) C *Lesion 3:* Homonymous hemianopia: loss of the left hemifield. Both eyes are blind to anything on the left side of the world (assuming the eyes are pointed straight ahead). *Lesion 4:* The lower optic radiations are carrying information from the upper visual world so vision is lost in the upper quadrants of the left hemifield. *Lesion 5:* Here the parietal portion of the optic radiations are cut, so the lower visual world is affected on one side. *Lesion 6:* When the cortex itself is lesioned, vision at the fovea is spared, perhaps because there is such a large representation of the fovea in the cortex, or perhaps due to overlapping blood supply. The loss of vision is not a complete hemifield, then, but a notched hemifield. This is called macular sparing.

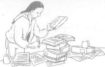
Management	**I** Prednisolone 60 mg reducing to zero over 10 days
	I Closure of eyelid to protect cornea

Prognosis	**I** Spontaneous improvement begins during second week
	I Recovery takes up to 12 months
	I Less than 10% have residual severe weakness

Bulbar palsy
(*K&C*, p. 1142)

I LMN weakness of cranial nerve nuclei within medulla (IX, X, XI, XII)

Aetiology

I Motor neurone disease
I Syringobulbia
I Poliomyelitis
I Myasthenia gravis

Clinical features

I Weakness of elevation of palate
I Loss of gag reflex
I Paralysed vocal cords
I Dysphagia
I Nasal regurgitation of fluids
I Choking

Pseudobulbar palsy (*K&C*, p. 1143)

I Bilateral upper motor neurone lesion of lower cranial nerve nuclei

Aetiology

I Motor neurone disease
I Multiple sclerosis
I Multi-infarct dementia
I Severe head injury

Clinical features

I Stiff, slow, spastic tongue (not wasted)
I Dysarthria
I Dry gravelly voice
I Preserved gag reflex
I Exaggerated jaw jerk
I Emotional lability

Horner's syndrome (*K&C*, p. 1133)

I Lesion of the cervical sympathetic pathway

Aetiology
- Brainstem stroke
- Coning
- Syringomyelia
- Apical lung cancer (Pancoast's tumour)
- Cervical rib
- Brachial plexus trauma

Clinical features
- Ptosis
- Myosis (constricted pupil)
- Enophthalmus
- Loss of sweating on side of face

Spinal cord disease

Spinal cord compression (K&C, p. 1206)

Aetiology
- See Table 17.17

Clinical features
- Radicular pain
- Spastic paraparesis or tetraparesis
- Sensory loss to level of compression
- Sphincter disturbance (retention of urine and incontinence)

Investigations
- Plain spinal X-rays
- Chest X-ray

Table 17.17   Causes of spinal cord compression

Within the cord
Spinal cord neoplasms
Transverse myelitis

In the meninges
Epidural abscess
Epidural haemorrhage
Ependymoma
Meningioma

Outside the cord
Vertebral neoplasms (metastases, myeloma)
Disc lesions
Vertebral collapse

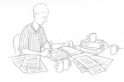
I MRI
I Myelography

Management   **I** Surgical decompression if possible

Syringomyelia and syringobulbia (K&C, p. 1206)

I A fluid-filled cavity (syrinx) within the cervical spinal cord (syringomyelia) or extending up into the brainstem (syringobulbia)

Aetiology   **I** Arnold–Chiari malformation
I Spina bifida
I Hydrocephalus
I Intrinsic cord tumours

Pathology   **I** The expanding cavity within the cord destroys spinothalamic neurones, anterior horn cells, lateral corticospinal tracts, sympathetic trunk, trigeminal, IX, X XI and XII nuclei

Clinical features   **I** Loss of pain and temperature sensation in upper limbs
I Painless burns
I Trophic changes
I Normal light touch sensation
I Loss of upper limb reflexes
I Wasting of small muscles of hands
I Spastic paraparesis
I Neuropathic joints
I Brainstem signs, e.g. bulbar palsy, Horner's syndrome

Investigations   **I** MRI

Management   **I** No effective treatment or surgery

Self-assessment questions

Multiple choice questions

1. The following are true in epilepsy:
   A. Generalized convulsions are characterized by loss of consciousness
   B. Absence seizures are generalized
   C. Absence seizures are commonest in adults
   D. Temporal lobe seizures may be partial or generalized
   F. Todd's paralysis follows temporal lobe seizure

2. In epilepsy:
   A. The EEG is usually diagnostic between fits
   B. Generalized seizures should be treated immediately with intravenous diazepam
   C. It is the doctor's responsibility to inform the driving authorities when a patient is diagnosed with epilepsy
   D. Ataxia usually signifies drug toxicity
   E. Phenytoin causes alopecia

3. In Parkinson's disease the following statements are true:
   A. Smoking predisposes to Parkinson's disease
   B. Males are more commonly affected
   C. There is dopamine loss in the extrapyramidal nuclei
   D. Incidence is 1:200 over 70 years of age
   E. It may be caused by alcohol abuse

4. Parkinson's disease
   A. Is characterized by an intention tremor
   B. Causes cogwheel rigidity
   C. May progress to dementia
   D. Is diagnosed by characteristic findings on CT brain scan
   E. Is characterized by extensor plantar reflexes

5. Huntington's disease:
   A. Is inherited in an autosomal dominant manner
   B. Is caused by a mutation on chromosome 4
   C. Is associated with rheumatic fever
   D. Is characterized by involuntary movements
   E. Causes dementia

6. Multiple sclerosis:
   A. May cause afferent pupillary defect
   B. Is characterized by increased concordance between monozygotic twins
   C. Has a pathology characterized by neurofibrillary tangles
   D. Invariably leads to severe disability
   E. Is associated with recent *Campylobacter* infection

7. The following are symptoms of motor neurone disease:
   A. Muscle wasting
   B. Ophthalmoplegia
   C. Frontal balding
   D. Cerebellar ataxia
   E. Bulbar palsy

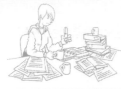

8. Causes of mononeuritis multiplex include:
   A. Diabetes mellitus
   B. Sarcoidosis
   C. Vitamin B_{12} deficiency
   D. HIV infection
   E. Thiamine deficiency

9. Causes of polyneuropathy include:
   A. Porphyria
   B. Thalidomide
   C. Thyrotoxicosis
   D. Guillain–Barré syndrome
   E. Malignancy

10. The clinical features of autonomic neuropathy are:
    A. Hypertension
    B. Impotence
    C. Polydipsia
    D. Diarrhoea
    E. Infertility

11. The following statements about cerebrospinal fluid (CSF) are correct:
    A. It normally contains no red cells
    B. In bacterial meningitis the lymphocyte count is raised
    C. In viral meningitis glucose is lower than one-third of blood glucose
    D. In subarachnoid haemorrhage, xanthochromia occurs after 18 hours
    E. In Guillain–Barré syndrome protein is raised with a normal cell count

12. The following statements about CNS infections are true:
    A. Herpes zoster causes a symmetrical rash
    B. Prion diseases are transferred by droplet spread
    C. Acute viral encephalitis is commonly caused by rotavirus
    D. Meningococcal septicaemia causes a purpuric rash
    E. Tuberculous meningitis is associated with high CSF protein

13. The following statements about Creutzfeldt–Jakob disease (CJD) are true:
    A. It is caused by a herpes virus infection
    B. It can be passed on in corneal grafts
    C. New variant CJD is less common in vegetarians
    D. It causes spongiform changes in the brain
    E. It is treatable with antiretroviral drugs

14. The following are aetiologically linked with brain abscess:
    A. Middle ear infection
    B. Lumbar puncture
    C. Skull fracture
    D. HIV
    E. Multiple sclerosis

15. The following are symptoms and signs of raised intracranial pressure:
    A. Headache
    B. Vomiting
    C. Tachycardia
    D. Facial nerve palsy
    E. Papilloedema

16. Risk factors for cerebrovascular disease include:
    A. Diabetes mellitus
    B. Hypertension
    C. Asian race
    D. Family history
    E. Hypothyroidism

17. Aetiological factors in transient ischaemic attacks include:
   A. Atrial fibrillation
   B. Deep venous thrombosis
   C. Coronary artery disease
   D. Warfarin therapy
   E. Polycystic kidney disease

18. Chronic subdural haematoma:

A. Is due to arteriovenous malformation in 10% of cases
B. Is usually precipitated by severe head injury
C. Is characterized by a classical 'lucid period'
D. Most often requires surgical drainage
E. May be asymptomatic

Extended matching questions

Question 1 *Theme: difficulty walking/limb weakness*

A. Embolic stroke
B. Spinal cord compression
C. Guillain–Barré syndrome
D. Foot drop
E. Phenytoin toxicity
F. Motor neurone disease
G. Multiple sclerosis
H. Parkinson's disease
I. Huntington's disease
J. Friedreich's ataxia
K. Hysteria

For each of the following questions, select the best answer from the list above:

I. A 34-year-old housewife presents with difficulty walking due to weakness in her legs, 2 weeks after recovering from a bout of food poisoning. Examination shows absent tendon reflexes and 4/5 power in both legs.
What is the most likely diagnosis?

II. A 70-year-old right-handed hypertensive smoker presents with sudden onset of weakness in the left leg and difficulty speaking.
What is the most likely diagnosis?

III. A 61-year-old solicitor presents with a 1-year history of increasing difficulty walking. His wife has noticed his hands shaking and his secretary finds his handwriting has become too small to read.
What is the most likely diagnosis?

Question 2 *Theme: headache*

A. Migraine
B. Temporal arteritis
C. Primary brain tumour
D. Hypertension
E. Subarachnoid haemorrhage
F. Meningitis
G. Encephalitis
H. Tension headache
I. Trigeminal neuralgia

For each of the following questions select the best answer from the list above:

I. A 24-year-old student presents with recent onset of flu-like symptoms, headache, vomiting, photophobia and neck stiffness. He is pyrexial (38.7°C), with a purpuric rash on the trunk.
What is the most likely diagnosis?

II. A 32-year-old female legal secretary has a 6-month history of episodic throbbing right-sided headaches associated with nausea, often on Saturday mornings.
What is the most likely diagnosis?

III. A 51-year-old Afro-Caribbean female with chronic renal failure and diabetes presents with a 3-week history of headache and blurred vision.

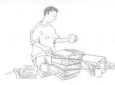
Fundoscopy reveals retinal haemorrhages and papilloedema. What is the most likely diagnosis?

Question 3 *Theme: loss of consciousness/coma*

A. Grand mal epilepsy
B. Vasovagal faint
C. Hyperglycaemia
D. Hysteria
E. Hypothermia
F. Head injury
G. Drug overdose
H. Meningoencephalitis
I. Septicaemia
J. Stroke
K. Alcohol excess
L. Hypoglycaemia

For each of the following questions select the best answer from the list above:

I. A 48-year-old female diabetic is found unconscious in bed. Her husband died recently and she was last seen arguing with her son the previous day. She visited her GP complaining of insomnia a week ago.
What is the most likely diagnosis?

II. A 75-year-old female is found unconscious in bed and smells of urine. She is pyrexial (38.5°C) and a urine dipstick shows positive nitrites. What is the most likely diagnosis?

III. An 88-year-old female not seen for several days is found unrousable in her front room on New Year's Day. On examination her pulse is 58 and regular, her BP is 90/60, there are no focal neurological signs but tendon reflexes are depressed. The ECG shows J waves. What is the most likely diagnosis?

Short answer questions

1. Write short notes on pseudobulbar and bulbar palsy.

2. Write short notes on visual evoked responses.

3. Write notes on the causes of chorea.

4. Write notes on Guillain–Barré syndrome.

5. Write notes on the neurological manifestations of vitamin B_{12} deficiency.

6. Describe the inheritance and clinical features of dystrophia myotonica.

7. Describe the procedure and interpretation of the Tensilon test.

8. Write brief notes on Charcot–Marie–Tooth disease.

9. Describe the causes and clinical features of Bell's palsy.

10. Write notes on Horner's syndrome.

11. Write short notes on the lateral medullary syndrome.

12. Write notes on subarachnoid haemorrhage.

13. Make notes on the Glasgow Coma Scale.

14. What are the risks for cerebrovascular disease?

15. Write notes on dysphasia.

16. Write short notes on the differential diagnosis of meningism.

17. Write short notes on Creutzfeldt–Jakob disease (CJD).

18. Write notes on the management of status epilepticus.

19. Write short notes on the side-effects and toxicity of phenytoin.

20. Describe the features of temporal lobe epilepsy.

21. Describe the principles and uses of the EEG in clinical practice.

Essay questions

1. Outline the major causes of polyneuropathy.

2. Describe the pathogenesis and clinical features of motor neurone disease.

3. Outline the causes, clinical features and diagnosis of paraparesis.

4. Describe the principles of treatment in epilepsy.

5. Explain how you would distinguish between different causes of transient loss of consciousness.

6. Describe the non-pharmacological management of stroke.

7. Describe the clinical features of a dominant hemisphere stroke.

8. Describe the causes, clinical features and emergency treatment of suspected meningitis.

9. Write an essay on brain tumours.

10. Describe the clinical features and essential aspects of management in Parkinson's disease.

11. Describe the pathogenesis and clinical patterns in multiple sclerosis.

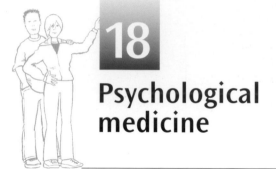

Psychological medicine

- Patients with psychiatric problems can present with physical manifestations such as depression manifesting as irritable bowel syndrome
- Chronic/severe physical ill health can result in psychological disease such as depression after a stroke
- Psychiatric symptoms can be part of a physical disease such as depression in hypothyroidism
- Patients with psychiatric disease can develop physical problems

The psychiatric history (K&C, p. 1226)

The psychiatric history is different in some ways from standard history taking. Corroboration and additional details should be sought from a relative or friend. The history should include the following:

Reason for referral	I Why and how the patient came to the attention of the doctor
Complaints	I As reported by the patient
Present illness	I Detailed account of the illness from its beginning to the present day I Include the degree of insight on the patient's part

Family history	I Family atmosphere in childhood
	I Early stresses (death or separation)
	I Mental illness in family members

Family history
I Family atmosphere in childhood
I Early stresses (death or separation)
I Mental illness in family members

Personal history
I Short biography of childhood, school, jobs, marriage/divorce and children
I Present housing, social and financial situation

Personality
I Attitudes, beliefs, moral values and standards
I Leisure activities and interests
I Usual reaction to stress and setback

Medical history
I Health in childhood
I Menstrual and sexual history
I Previous mental health
I Use of alcohol, drugs and tobacco

Examining the mental state

(*K&C*, pp. 1227–1229)

APPEARANCE/GENERAL BEHAVIOUR

I Can give information about mood
I Facial appearance
I Posture
I Movement

SPEECH

I Disorders of thinking are recognized from speech

Disorders of stream (amount and speed) of thought

Pressure of thought
I Varied ideas arise in abundance
I Characteristic of mania
I Occurs in schizophrenia

Poverty of thought
I Patient reports lack/absence of thoughts
I Characteristic of depression
I Occurs in schizophrenia

Thought blocking
I Abrupt and complete interruption of stream
I Strongly suggests schizophrenia

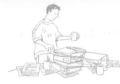

Disorders of form of thought

Flight of ideas
- Quickly moving from topic to topic
- Distracted by clues in the immediate environment
- Clang associations (using words with similar sounds)
- Punning
- Rhyming

Perseveration
- Persistent and inappropriate repetition
- Occurs in dementia and other conditions

Loosening of associations
- Lack of clarity
- 'Knight's move' thinking
- 'Word salad'

MOOD

- Affect/feeling/emotion

Changes in nature of mood
- Depression
- Anxiety
- Elation
- Phobia

Changes in fluctuation of mood
- Loss of emotion (apathy)
- Reduced variation in mood (blunted)
- Rapidly and excessively changeable mood (labile)

Inappropriate mood
- Incongruous mood such as laughing when describing death of close relative

THOUGHT CONTENT (WORRIES AND PREOCCUPATIONS)

Obsession
- Recurrent persistent thoughts

Compulsion
- Repetitive, seemingly purposeful action
- Must be carried out
- Urge to resist

Insight
- Degree to which patient recognizes own illness

ABNORMAL BELIEFS AND INTERPRETATION OF EVENTS (DELUSIONS)

I Delusions are abnormal beliefs arising from distorted judgements
I They are
— False
— Held with absolute conviction
— Not modifiable by reason/experience
I Persecutory delusions – paranoid thoughts
I Delusions of worthlessness/grandeur
I Nihilism
I Thought insertion – the belief that thoughts are implanted from outside
I Thought withdrawal
I Thought broadcasting – the belief that unspoken thoughts are known to others

ABNORMAL EXPERIENCE REFERRED TO THE ENVIRONMENT, BODY OR SELF

I Illusions
I Hallucinations
I Depersonalization – the patient feels 'unreal'/detached/remote
I Derealization – the external environment feels unreal/remote

COGNITIVE STATE/MEMORY

I Assessed using mental test score ('Folstein score') (page 500)

Organic mental disorders (K&C, pp. 1263–1265)

Delirium/toxic confusional state
I Impairment of consciousness associated with abnormalities of perception and mood

Aetiology
I See Table 18.1

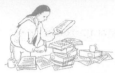

THE MINI-MENTAL STATE EXAMINATION

'What day of the week is it?' [1 point]

'What is the date today?' day:month:year [1 point each]

'What season is it?' [1 point]

'What country are we in?' [1 point]

'What is the name of this town?' [1 point]

'What are two main streets nearby?' [1 point]

'What floor of the building are we on?' [1 point]

'What is the name of this place?' [1 point]

Say the following then give the patient a piece of paper: 'I am going to give you a piece of paper. When I do, take it in your right hand. Fold the paper in half with both hands and put the paper down on your lap.' [1 point for each of three actions]

Show a pencil and ask what it is called [1 point]

Show a wristwatch and ask what it is called [1 point]

Say the following: 'I am going to say something and I would like you to repeat it after me: No ifs and buts' [1 point]

Say: 'Please read what is written here and do what it says them show a card with 'Close your eyes' written on it [1 point if correct action carried out]

Say: 'Write a complete sentence on this sheet of paper' [1 point if sentence contains a verb and makes sense]

Say: 'Copy this drawing'

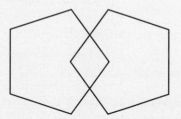

[1 point if angles are preserved and if the two figures intersect to form a four-sided figure]

Say: 'I am going to name three objects. After I have finished saying all three

I want you to repeat them, e.g. apple, table, penny' [1 point each for first try]

Say: 'Now I would like you to take 7 away from 100. Now take 7 away from the number you get and repeat until I tell you to stop' [Score 1 point each time the difference is 7 – continue until five subtractions done]

Say: 'Now name those three objects I told you earlier' [1 point each]

A score < 25 suggests dementia but consider depression or acute confusional state

Table 18.1   Causes of delirium

Infection
Any infection, particularly if high fever

Metabolic disturbance
Electrolyte upset
Hepatic/renal failure
Hypoxia

Endocrine
Hypoglycaemia
Cushing's syndrome

Intracranial
Trauma
Tumour
Abscess
Subarachnoid haemorrhage
Epilepsy

Drug intoxication
Anticonvulsants
Anxiolytics/hypnotics
Opiates

Drug/alcohol withdrawal

Vitamin deficiency
Thiamine (Wernicke–Korsakoff syndrome)
Nicotinic acid (pellagra)
Vitamin B_{12}

Clinical features
❚ Acute – clears within days
❚ Fluctuant with lucid periods
❚ Worse at night
❚ Visual hallucinations may occur
❚ Patient is frightened, suspicious, restless and uncooperative
❚ More common in elderly patients

Investigations
❚ To determine underlying cause
❚ Bloods
   — Full blood count (FBC)
   — Urea and electrolytes (U&E)
   — Glucose
   — Liver function tests (LFTs)
   — Calcium

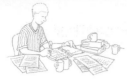

— B$_{12}$
— T$_4$
I Blood, urine cultures
I ECG
I Chest X-ray
I CT of brain

Management
I Treat underlying cause
I Nurse carefully in a well-lit area
I Communicate clearly and concisely
I Give repeated information to orientate (family/carers can be useful for this)
I Ensure adequate hydration
I Sedate if necessary, e.g. haloperidol i.m.
I Paracetamol if febrile
I Review all drugs and stop all but essential ones

Dementia
I Disturbance of higher cortical functions in the absence of clouded consciousness

Aetiology
I See Table 18.2

Differential diagnosis
I Depression

Investigations
I Blood
— FBC
— U&E
— Glucose
— LFTs
— Calcium
— B$_{12}$
— T$_4$
— Syphilis serology
— HIV antibodies if indicated and patient counselled
I Chest X-ray
I CT/MRI

Alzheimer's disease

Neuropathology
I Neuronal loss
I Neurofibrillary tangles
I Senile plaques
I Amyloid deposition

Table 18.2   Causes of Dementia

Degenerative	**Toxic**
Alzheimer's disease	Alcohol
Pick's disease	Occupational
Huntington's disease	**Traumatic**
Parkinson's disease	Post-head injury
Normal pressure	Boxing (punch drunk
hydrocephalus	syndrome)
Vascular	**Anoxic**
Cerebrovascular disease	Cardiac arrest
Cranial arteritis	Respiratory failure
Metabolic	Carbon monoxide poisoning
Uraemia	**Vitamin deficiency**
Renal dialysis	Thiamine
Hepatic failure	Vitamin B_{12}
Remote effects of carcinoma	**Infections**
Endocrine	Encephalitis
Hypothyroidism	Creutzfeldt–Jakob disease
Hypocalcaemia	HIV
Intracranial	Syphilis
Subdural haematoma	
Tumour	

Aetiology
▌ Early onset – autosomal dominant, chromosome 14; 21 mutation
▌ Familial – ?apolipoprotein E gene

Clinical features
▌ Inability to learn new information or recall previously learnt information
▌ Decline in language, particularly names
▌ Apraxia – unable to carry out motor functions
▌ Agnosia – unable to identify/recognize objects
▌ Impairment of organizing/sequencing
▌ Behavioural change – wandering, agitation, aggression
▌ Paranoia

Management
▌ Cholinesterase inhibitors may benefit selected patients

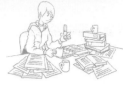

Vascular dementia/multi-infarct dementia

Clinical features
- Second commonest cause of dementia
- History of transient ischaemic events/ cerebrovascular accident

Management
- Aspirin to prevent further events

Schizophrenia (K&C, p. 1261)

- Abnormal integration of emotional and cognitive functions

Epidemiology
- 2–4/1000 annual incidence
- 1% lifetime risk

Aetiology
- Genetic – lifetime risk in patients with first-degree relative affected is 12%
- Altered neurotransmitters
  — ↑ Dopamine activity
  — Altered serotonin metabolism
- environmental triggers
  — High expressed emotion
  — More common in patients born in winter/spring

Clinical features
- Peak onset late adolescence
- ♀ = ♂

Diagnosis
- Based on presence of first-rank symptoms:
- Auditory hallucinations
- Thought withdrawal
- Thought insertion
- Thought interruption
- Thought broadcasting
- Delusions
- External controlled emotions
- Somatic passivity and feelings (feeling that thoughts and acts are due to the influence of others)

Subtypes   *Paranoid schizophrenia*
I Most common presentation
I Insidious onset
I Later age of onset
I Persecutory delusions dominate
I Threatening auditory hallucinations
I Appearance and behaviour well preserved

Simple schizophrenia
I Insidious deterioration in personality
I Starts in early adolescence
I Delusions and hallucinations absent
I Increasing eccentricity
I Slow withdrawal from society

Hebephrenic schizophrenia
I Shallow and inappropriate mood
I Disturbed and disorganized thought processes
I Speech rambling and incoherent
I Aimless, purposeless behaviour
I Hypochondriasis

Catatonic schizophrenia
I Rare in developed world
I Marked psychomotor disturbance
I Episodes of hyperkinesis and stupor
I Delusions and hallucinations

Chronic schizophrenia
I Thought disorder
I Negative symptoms (lack of drive/social withdrawal)

Management   I Combination of drug and social treatment
delivered by multidisciplinary team

Drugs
I Antipsychotics/neuroleptics
— Dopamine antagonists (chlorpromazine,
haloperidol, sulpiride); unwanted side-effects
are shown in Table 18.3

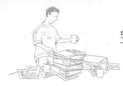

Table 18.3 Unwanted effects of neuroleptic drugs

Common effects
Extrapyramidal
Acute dystonia
Parkinsonism
Akathisia (restless, repetitive and irresistible need to move)
Tardive dyskinesia (mouthing and smacking of the lips,
    grimaces and contortions of the face/neck)

Autonomic
Hypotension
Failure of ejaculation

Anticholinergic
Dry mouth
Urinary retention
Constipation
Blurred vision

Metabolic
Weight gain

Rare effects
Hypersensitivity
Cholestatic jaundice
Leucopenia
Skin reactions

Others
Precipitation of glaucoma
Galactorrhoea
Amenorrhoea
Cardiac arrhythmias
Seizures
Retinal degeneration (high-dose thioridazine)

Neuroleptic malignant syndrome
  Hyperthermia
  Muscle rigidity
  Tachycardia
  Labile BP
  Pallor
  Elevated white cell count, creatine kinase, liver function tests
  Treatment: lower temperature, bromocriptine, dantrolene

— Other agents (clozapine, risperidone,
  olanzapine)

Psychological treatment
▌ Reassurance and support

MANAGEMENT OF THE AGITATED PATIENT

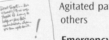

Suggested by
Agitated patient who is likely to harm him/herself or
others

Emergency treatment
Talk calmly to patient: if this fails, get help to restrain
him/her
Check blood sugar, oximetry, coma scale and for focal
neurological deficit
If not hypoglycaemic or hypoxic and has good coma scale
with no focal neurology, then consider sedation with 5 mg
i.m. haloperidol (repeat up to 20 mg if needed)
If alcohol or benzodiazepine withdrawal likely, then use
lorazepam 2 mg

Initial investigations
Bloods – FBC, U&E, glucose, calcium, LFTs
Blood and urine cultures if sepsis suggested
Measure arterial blood gases
ECG
Chest X-ray

Social treatment
❚ Structured work and social programme

Mood (affective) disorders (K&C, p. 1241)

❚ Spectrum of disorders ranging from depression
through to mania
❚ Patients who suffer attacks of both have bipolar
disorder (Fig. 18.1)

Aetiology   *Physical*
❚ Genetic – 10–15% of first-degree relatives affected

Fig. 18.1
Bipolar disorder.

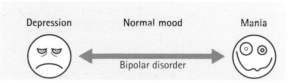

Depression   Normal mood   Mania

Bipolar disorder

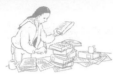

I Neurotransmitter imbalance – reduced in
depression/increased in mania
I Hormonal
  — Loss of diurnal variation of cortisol
  — Oral contraceptives/pregnancy/premenstrual

Psychological
I Maternal deprivation
I Learned helplessness

Social
I Stressful life events
I Sexual abuse in childhood

Clinical features   I See Table 18.4
I Range of severity (Fig. 18.2)
  — Severe life-threatening disease
  — Minor forms

DIFFERENTIAL DIAGNOSIS

Mania   I Drug-induced psychosis
  — Amphetamines
  — Cannabis
  — Steroids
I Acute schizophrenia
I Dementia
I Hyperthyroidism

Fig. 18.2   Depressive psychosis   Mania
Mood disorders.

Moderate depressive   Hypomania

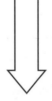

Mild depressive   Mild euphoria

Table 18.4   Clinical features of depression and mania

Characteristic	Depression	Mania
Mood	Depressed Miserable Unhappy	Elevated Labile Infectious
Talk	Slow Impoverished Monotonous Incomplete	Fast Pressurized Punning/rhyming Flight of ideas
Energy	Lacking Retarded or agitated Apathetic	Excessive Restless Distractible

Ideation	Feelings of
	  Futility
	  Guilt
	  Self-reproach
	  Unworthiness
	Hypochondriasis
	Worrying
	Suicidal thoughts
	Delusions of guilt
	Nihilism
	Persecution
		Grandiose
		Self confident
		Delusions of
		  Wealth
		  Power
		  Influence
		  Religious significance
		Persecutory delusions

Cognition	Verbal memory impaired Pseudodementia if elderly	Disturbance of memory retrieval
Physical	Early waking Poor appetite Weight loss Constipation Loss of libido Impotence Fatigue Bodily aches and pains	Insomnia Weight loss
Behaviour	Poverty of movement/expression Retardation/agitation	Disinhibition Increased sexual interest Excessive drinking/spending

Hallucinations	Auditory
	  Abusive
	  Hostile
	  Critical
		Fleeting auditory
		Occasionally visual

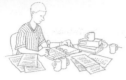
Depression
- Malignancy
- Hypothyroidism/hyperparathyroidism
- Cushing's syndrome
- Infection
- Neurological diseases (multiple sclerosis, Parkinson's)
- Collagen disorders
- Cerebral ischaemia
- Heart failure
- Porphyria
- Drugs
  — Steroids
  — Oestrogen/progesterone
  — Hypotensive agents
  — Anti-parkinsonian agents
  — Anticancer drugs
- Psychiatric disorders
  — Schizophrenia
  — Alcohol/drug abuse
  — Anxiety
  — Dementia
- Normal bereavement reaction (Table 18.5)

MANAGEMENT (K&C, pp. 1244–1246)

Depression
- Drugs
  — Tricyclic antidepressants (TCAs), e.g. amytriptyline; see Table 18.6 for unwanted effects
  — Serotonin reuptake inhibitors, e.g. fluoxetine
  — Noradrenaline reuptake inhibitors, e.g. reboxetine
  — Monoamine oxidase inhibitors, e.g. phenelzine
- Electroconvulsive therapy (ECT)
  — Rapid action
  — Used in life-threatening depression

Mania
- Acute attacks
  — Neuroleptic drugs, e.g. haloperidol
- Prophylaxis
  — Lithium – Table 18.6 lists unwanted effects
  — Regular check on drug levels (narrow therapeutic window)

Table 18.5 Clinical features of normal grief reaction and depressive illness after bereavement (morbid grief reaction)

Characteristic	Normal bereavement	Morbid grief reaction
Onset	Immediately after loss	Delayed for weeks/months
Duration	Weeks	Months/years
Pattern	Slow acceptance and adjustment	Denial loss and refusal to accept implications
Grief	Expressed openly	Expressed with difficulty
Guilt	Mild regret in early stage	Marked guilt often present

Table 18.6 Unwanted effects of drugs used in affective disorders

Tricyclic antidepressants	Lithium
Anticholinergic effects	GI symptoms
Dry mouth	Hypothyroidism
Constipation	Fine tremor
Tremor	Weight gain (increased
Blurred vision	appetite)
Urinary retention	Polyuria/polydipsia
Postural hypotension	Toxic symptoms
Cardiac effects	Drowsiness
ECG changes	Blurred vision
Arrhythmias	Tremor
Lowered seizure threshold	Ataxia
Weight gain	Dysarthria
Sedation	Convulsions
Mania	Coma and death
Agranulocytosis (mianserin)	

— Regular check on renal function (renal excretion)
— Regular check on thyroid function
— Carbamazepine
— Valproate

Psychological I Psychotherapy
I Cognitive/behavioural therapy

Social I Assistance with social problems
I Group support
I Stress management
I Family/carer support

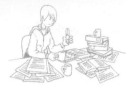

Puerperal affective disorders (K&C, p. 1243)

I Childbirth has a higher relative risk of depression than life events or physical illness
I Treatment of these disorders is as for any other affective disorder

Maternity blues

Clinical features I Brief episodes of emotional lability, irritability and tearfulness
I Occurs in 50% of women 2–3 days post-partum
I Resolves spontaneously

Postpartum psychosis

Clinical features I 1 in 500–1000 births
I Onset usually within 2 weeks of birth
I Classical features of affective psychosis plus confusion and disorientation
I If severe, patient may have delusions that child is deformed, evil or affected in another way which can lead to suicide or infanticide
I Responds well to treatment
I 15–20% recur in next puerperium

Postnatal depression

Clinical features I Depression occurs in 10–20% of mothers in first post-partum year
I Clinically similar to other depressive illness
I Recovery after a few months

Suicide and deliberate self-harm

(K&C, p. 1249)

Suicide

Risk factors I Living alone
I Immigrant status
I Recent bereavement/separation/divorce
I Unemployment/retirement
I Male sex
I Older age

❚ Family or previous history of
  — Affective disorder
  — Suicide
  — Alcohol abuse
❚ Previous suicide attempt
❚ Drug/alcohol addiction
❚ Severe depression/early dementia
❚ Incapacitating, painful physical illness

Deliberate self-harm (DSH)

❚ ♀ > ♂
❚ Most patients < 35 years
❚ 90% involve self-poisoning
❚ Formal psychiatric disorder is unusual
❚ 1–2% kill themselves in the following year
❚ Assessment procedure – see Table 18.7
  Indications for referral to psychiatric team – see Table 18.8

Table 18.7   Deliberate self-harm

Establish the following in all DSH patients:

Reason for attempted suicide
Method of suicide attempt and how discovered
Suicidal intent
Risk factors for suicide (see text)
Evidence of current psychiatric disease
Evidence of drug/alcohol abuse

Table 18.8   Indications for referral to psychiatrist

Absolute indications
Clinical depression
Psychosis
Clearly pre-planned suicide attempts
Persistent suicidal intent
Violent method used

Relative indications
Alcohol/drug abuse
Patients with risk factors for suicide (see above)
Persistent suicide attempts
Any patient giving concern

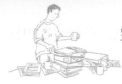

Neuroses and stress-related/somatoform disorders (K&C, pp. 1250–1254)

Anxiety disorder

Clinical features ▌ See Table 18.9

Differential diagnosis *Psychiatric disorders*
▌ Depression
▌ Schizophrenia
▌ Dementia
▌ Drug/alcohol dependence
▌ Benzodiazepine withdrawal

Physical disorders
▌ Hyperthyroidism
▌ Hypoglycaemia
▌ Phaeochromocytoma

Management *Psychological*
▌ Reassurance about physical symptoms
▌ Relaxation training
▌ Psychotherapy

Table 18.9 Clinical features of anxiety

Physical	Lack of libido
Gastrointestinal	
Dry mouth	*Nervous system*
Dysphagia	Tinnitus
Epigastric pain	Blurred vision
Flatulence	Dizziness
Diarrhoea	Headache
	Sleep disturbance
Respiratory	
Sensation of chest	**Psychological**
constriction	Apprehension and fear
Difficulty inhaling	Irritability
Over-breathing	Difficulty concentrating
	Distractibility
Cardiovascular	Restlessness
Palpitations	Sensitivity to noise
Chest pain	Depression
	Depersonalization
Genitourinary	Obsessional symptoms
Frequency	
Failure of erection	

Drugs
I β-blockers for physical symptoms
I Short courses of benzodiazepines

Obsessive compulsive disorder

I Characterized by obsessional thinking and compulsive behaviour with varying degrees of anxiety/depression and depersonalization

Clinical features
I Persistent and intrusive obsessions/compulsions
I Functioning impeded
I Constant need to check
I Repetitive/superstitious actions

Management
I Behaviour therapy
— Response prevention
— Modelling
I Serotonin reuptake inhibitors (may need higher doses than those used in depression)

Dissociative (conversion) disorder (previously known as hysteria)

I Characterized by
— Absence of physical pathology
— Unconscious production
— Absence of sympathetic overactivity

Clinical features
I ♀ > ♂
I Rarely occurs in those > 40 years
I See Table 18.10

Table 18.10   Common dissociative/conversion symptoms

Mental	Tremor
Amnesia	Aphonia
Fugue	Mutism
Pseudodementia	Sensory symptoms
Sleep-walking	Repeated vomiting
Multiple personality	Globus hystericus
Psychosis	Hysterical fits
Physical	Dermatitis artefacta
Paralysis	Blindness
Gait disorder	Deafness

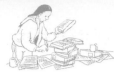

I May confer advantage (secondary gain)
I Patients' emotional distress is less than expected

Management I Psychotherapy

Somatoform disorders I Patients
— Repeatedly present with physical problems
— Have repeatedly negative findings on clinical investigation
— Have no demonstrable physical cause

Clinical features *Hypochondriasis*
I Preoccupation with ill health
I Disproportionate and unjustified concern

Somatization disorder (Münchausen's disorder)
I Repeatedly present with a variety of medical symptoms
I Undergo repeated investigations/operations
I May have medical connections

Management I Reassure
I Explore psychological/social problems
I Avoid repeated investigations
I Graded exercise programmes
I Trial of an antidepressant

Acute stress reaction and post-traumatic stress disorder
I Occur in individuals in response to exceptional physical or psychological stress

Acute stress reaction I Lasts a few hours/days
I Initial state of 'daze'
I Then a phase of either
— Withdrawal/stupor *or*
— Agitation/over-activity
I Commonly associated with autonomic signs of anxiety

Post-traumatic stress disorder I Delayed/protracted response to a stressful event
I 'Flashbacks'

I Intense distress in/avoidance of situations resembling the event (including anniversaries)
I Emotional blunting/numbness
I Detachment from others
I Hypervigilance
I Insomnia
I Anxiety and depression
I Occasionally suicide

Management I Counselling

Drug and alcohol abuse and dependence (K&C, pp 1256–1260)

I Current evidence suggests that drinking up to 28 units a week (for men) or 21 units a week for women carries no long-term health risk

Alcohol dependence syndrome
Clinical features I Compulsive need to drink
I Altered alcohol tolerance
I Stereotyped pattern of drinking
I Drinking takes primacy over other activities
I Repeated withdrawal symptoms (see Ch.10)
I Relief drinking to avoid withdrawal, e.g. early morning drinking
I Rapid relapse if patient drinks again following a period of abstinence

Management *Psychosocial support and group therapy*
I e.g. Alcoholics anonymous

Drugs
I Disulfiram (Antabuse) reacts with alcohol to form acetaldehyde which produces unpleasant symptoms to discourage drinking
I Acamprosate alters neurotransmitters and is said to reduce cravings

Drug abuse I For commonly used illicit drugs the desired and adverse effects are shown in Table 18.11

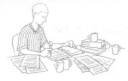
Table 18.11   Desired and adverse effects of commonly used 'illicit' drugs

Drug	Desired effects	Adverse effects
Solvents ('glue sniffing')	Euphoria Floating sensation	Amnesia Visual hallucinations Inhalation of vomit Bone marrow/brain/liver/kidney toxicity Aggressive/impulsive behaviour Tolerance
Amphetamines	Stimulant Euphoria	Psychological dependence Restlessness Over-activity Paranoid psychosis
Cocaine	Stimulant Hyperarousal	Dependence Paranoid ideation Fits Coronary artery spasm Perforation of nasal septum if inhaled
Cannabis	Exaggeration of pre-existing mood	No definite withdrawal syndrome or tolerance
MDMA ('Ecstasy')	Psychodelic effects	Hyperpyrexia Acute hepatic/renal failure Possible chronic brain damage
Hypnotics (e.g. Benzodiazepines)	Relaxation Sleep induction	Dependence Withdrawal syndrome Respiratory depression
Narcotics (Morphine, Heroin, Codeine, Methadone, Pethidine	Calm Slight euphoria Analgesia Flattening of emotions	Marked and rapid tolerance Withdrawal syndrome Respiratory depression Complications of injecting Infection (e.g. HIV/hepatitis B and C/ endocarditis) Vein thrombosis

Management   ▍ Withdrawal programmes, e.g. using methadone
▍ Psychosocial support to help the addict live without
drugs

Eating disorders (K&C, pp. 1266–1267)

Anorexia nervosa
Aetiology   ▍ Genetic
▍ Childhood sexual abuse

I Dietary problems in early life
I Family factors
— Over-protective
— Rigid
— Unresolved conflict
I Social factors
— Higher social class
— Occupation – ballet dancers/nurses

Clinical features
I BMI (body mass index) < 17.5
I Intense wish to be thin
I Morbid fear of fatness
I Amenorrhoea in women
I ♀ ≫ ♂
I Onset in adolescence, rare > 30 years
I Previous history of chubbiness/fatness
I Relentless pursuit of low body weight
I Distorted image of own body
I Eats little
I Avoids carbohydrates
I Vomiting/excess exercise/purging
I Loss of sexual interest
I Lanugo hair

Management
I Behaviour therapy – Goal setting/reward for weight/dietary intake
I Psychotherapy
I Family therapy

Bulimia nervosa

Clinical features
I Binge eating
I Self-induced vomiting
I Laxative abuse
I Misuse of drugs, e.g. diuretics, thyroxine, anorectics
I ♀ ≫ ♂
I Often associated with anorexia nervosa
I Premorbid personality – neurotic traits
I May be associated with
— Depression
— Alcohol dependence
I Fluctuation in body weight
I Periods irregular

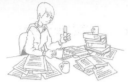
Consequences of vomiting
I Cardiac arryhthmias
I Renal impairment secondary to low K^+
I Muscular paralysis
I Tetany – hypokalaemic alkalosis
I Swollen salivary glands
I Eroded dental enamel

Management   I Behaviour therapy
— 'Eating diary'
— Identify and avoid stimuli to bingeing

Psychiatry and the law (K&C, p. 1269)

Compulsory section under the Mental Health Act

Conditions   I For a patient to be held against his/her will under the Mental Health Act he/she must be
— Suffering from a defined mental disorder
— A risk to his/her and/or other people's health or safety
— Unwilling to accept hospitalization voluntarily

Sections   I See Table 18.12 for details

Table 18.12   Important sections of the Mental Health Act 1983

Section	Duration	Signatures required	Purpose
2	28 days	2 doctors (1 approved) plus nearest relative or social worker	Assessment and treatment
3	6 months	2 doctors (1 approved) plus nearest relative or social worker	Treatment
4	72 hours	1 doctor plus relative or social worker	Emergency admission
5(2)	72 hours	Doctor in charge of patient's care	Emergency detention of a patient already in hospital
5(4)	6 hours	Nurse (RMN)	Emergency detention of a patient already in hospital
136	72 hours	Police officer	Psychiatric assessment of patients in public places

Self-assessment questions

Multiple choice questions

1. The following are first-rank symptoms of schizophrenia:
   A. Thought broadcasting
   B. Thought withdrawal
   C. Apraxia
   D. Auditory hallucinations
   E. Persecutory delusions

2. In dementia the following are correct:
   A. Consciousness is clouded
   B. Multi-infarct dementia is the commonest cause
   C. Dementia can be genetically inherited
   D. Dementia can result from repeated head trauma
   E. A CT scan is indicated

3. In toxic confusional state:
   A. Elderly patients are more commonly affected
   B. Patients should be nursed in a darkened room
   C. Patients may require intravenous fluids
   D. There is usually resolution after a few days
   E. Antibiotics may be indicated

4. Patients with depression:
   A. Sleep well
   B. Have increased sexual interest
   C. May have auditory hallucinations if disease is severe
   D. Have a family history of depression in 50% of cases
   E. Can be treated with psychotherapy

5. The following are features of mania:
   A. Delusions of wealth
   B. Weight loss
   C. Excessive drinking
   D. Flight of ideas
   E. Critical hallucinations

6. Lithium:
   A. Is used to prevent depression
   B. Undergoes renal excretion
   C. Causes hyperthyroidism
   D. Needs therapeutic drug level monitoring
   E. Is used to treat acute attacks of mania

7. Suicide is more common in:
   A. Men
   B. Young people
   C. Mild depression
   D. Stroke patients
   E. Patients with a family history of suicide

8. In deliberate self-harm:
   A. 75% is by self poisoning
   B. There is often an associated psychiatric disorder
   C. Patients with depression should be referred to a psychiatrist
   D. A violent method makes suicide more likely
   E. Patients who planned to be discovered are at higher risk of suicide

9. Anxiety disorder may present as:
   A. Chest pain
   B. Diarrhoea
   C. Impotence
   D. Amenorrhoea
   E. Jaundice

10. Anorexia nervosa:
    A. Patients often have uncaring family circumstances
    B. Occurs in young people
    C. Is more common in higher social classes
    D. Patients have amenorrhoea
    E. Patients think they are thin

11. Regarding the sections of the Mental Health Act:
    A. Section 2 allows patients to be held for 6 months
    B. Section 3 is for psychiatric assessment
    C. Section 5(2) relates to patients already in hospital
    D. Section 5(2) allows the patient to be detained for 72 hours
    E. Section 2 requires the signatures of two doctors and a social worker/relative

12. The following statements are correct:
    A. Obsessive compulsive disorder responds to low-dose serotonin reuptake inhibitors
    B. Paralysis is a common symptom of a conversion disorder
    C. Conversion disorder is produced unconsciously
    D. Post-traumatic stress disorder occurs immediately after a stressful event
    E. In acute stress reaction bradycardia is usual

Extended matching questions

Question 1 *Theme: agitation*

A. Acute confusional state
B. Acute mania
C. Puerperal psychosis
D. Schizophrenia
E. Obsessive-compulsive disorder
F. Alzheimer's disease
G. Anxiety disorder
H. Alcohol withdrawal syndrome
I. Cocaine abuse
J. Somatization disorder

For each of the following questions, select the best answer from the list above:

I. A 59-year-old female smoker who lives with her husband presents with agitation. On direct questioning she cannot remember details of the distant past although her short-term memory seems intact. She has lost weight but there are no other physical signs or symptoms.
What is the most likely diagnosis?

II. A 23-year-old female who was born in Jamaica but has lived in the UK since the age of 8 attends the accident and emergency department alone; she is agitated. She appears to have threatening auditory hallucinations. She also says that she is having difficulty sleeping. The casualty records show a previous attendance at a psychiatric outpatient clinic 2 years ago. The limited physical examination she allows is normal.
What is the most likely diagnosis?

III. A 48-year-old male presents with agitation. On direct questioning he admits to visual hallucinations. He has a previous history of gastrointestinal bleeding. On examination he is sweaty and the pulse rate is 110/min. Blood tests reveal the following: Hb 14.4, MCV 101. What is the most likely diagnosis?

Short answer questions

1. Write short notes on the following:
   A. Paranoid schizophrenia
   B. Causes of dementia
   C. Neuroleptic malignant syndrome

2. Write short notes on the following:
   A. Treatment of anxiety disorder
   B. Risk factors for suicide

3. Write short notes on the following:
   A. Obsessive compulsive disorder
   B. Physical consequences of bulimia nervosa
   C. Physical consequences of cocaine addiction

4. Write short notes on the following:
   A. Side-effects of antidepressants
   B. Morbid grief reaction

C. Treatment of mania
D. Puerperal psychosis

Essay questions

1. Outline the investigation and management of a patient in a toxic confusional state.

2. Discuss the side-effects of antipsychotic drugs.

3. Describe how you would psychologically assess a patient who has taken an overdose.

4. Describe the clinical features associated with anxiety disorder.

5. Describe the features of alcohol dependence syndrome and its treatment.

6. Outline the aetiological factors and clinical features of anorexia nervosa.

7. Describe the treatment options for depression.

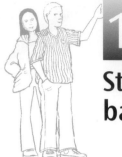

19

Statistics and evidence-based medicine

The epidemiology of a disease is a description of the demographics of the affected population and the environment from which they originate. Statistical analysis is the manipulation of data about a patient group designed to reveal similarities or differences between groups of differing patients or between treatment types. Statistical analysis is also used to describe details about a population.

Types of data

Nominal
I Mutually exclusive groups
— Male or female

Ordinal
I Ranked exclusive groups
— mild/moderate/severe

Continuous
I Numerical values that may be anywhere along a continuum
— Age

DESCRIPTIONAL STATISTICS

I A method of describing a population or a sample from that population

Mean
I The mathematical average of a set of numerical data

Mode
I The most commonly occurring value

Median	▌ The middle number when the data set is arranged in numerical order
	▌ If there is an even number of values it is the mean of the middle two

Sample mean	▌ The mathematical average of a variable measured in a sample

Population mean	▌ The mean calculated if the entire population under study were measured
	▌ Note: this is rarely achievable

Distribution	▌ The pattern of spread of values
	▌ Many biological values fit a 'normal' or Gaussian distribution, a bell-shaped curve

Normal distribution	▌ A symmetrical 'bell-shaped' curve distribution where the mean, mode and median are the same (Fig. 19.1)

Skewed distribution	▌ Very high or low values may result in an asymmetrical distribution leading to a positive (high value) or negative (low value) skew (Fig. 19.2)

Fig. 19.1 Gaussian or normal distribution. This is symmetrical about the mean. Sixty-eight per cent of all values in the data set fall within ± 1 standard deviation (SD), 95% between ± 2 SD and 99% between ± 3 SD. This is often described as the bell-shaped curve.

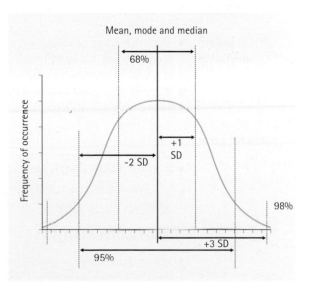

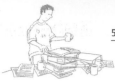
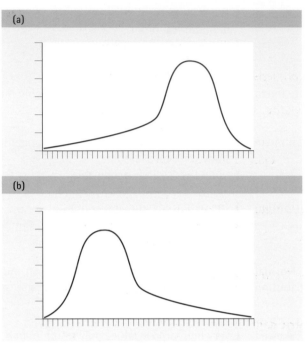

Fig. 19.2   Distributions. A. Negative skew. B. Positive skew.

Variance	❙ Describes the spread of values either side of a mean
Standard deviation	❙ Gives the range of values within which a certain proportion of the sample will lie ❙ 68% will lie ± 1 SD from the mean ❙ 95% will lie ± 2 SD from the mean ❙ 99% will lie ± 3 SD from the mean
Standard error	❙ The range within which the population mean will lie based on the sample mean ❙ It allows an estimation of the range in which the true population mean will lie when a representative sample from that population is analysed

COMPARATIVE STATISTICS

❙ Allows data from two groups to be compared, with the aim of determining whether they originated from the same population or not, or, in the context of a trial, whether the differences between them are due to luck or really exist

Hypothesis ▮ The concept being tested

Null hypothesis ▮ That no difference exists between the two samples being analysed

Bias ▮ Inequalities between the groups being compared that lead to incorrect conclusions being reached

Type 1 error ▮ A false positive result
▮ A difference is found between two groups where one does not exist

Type 2 error ▮ A false negative result
▮ No difference is detected although one does exist

Parametric data ▮ Data values fit a normal distribution

Statistical tests ▮ Tests that provide a probability value
▮ This value (the 'p' value) is the probability that the two sets of data being compared are from the same population or that no difference exists between them
▮ Statistical significance is stated to be a probability of 1 in 20 or lower that the two groups are the same ($p \leq 0.05$)

Parametric tests ▮ Used on data following a normal distribution, e.g.
— Student t test
— Paired t test

Non-parametric tests ▮ Unpaired Mann–Whitney
▮ Paired Wilcoxon

Nominal tests ▮ If data can be placed in a 2 × 2 square for example, the response to a treatment or placebo (see Fig. 19.3) – then a Chi squared test can be used

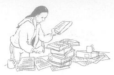

	Disease present	Disease absent	Totals
Treatment given	9	41	50
Placebo given	39	11	50
Totals	50	50	100

Fig. 19.3   The 2 × 2 table and Chi squared tests. If you consider a disease for which a treatment is given, 100 patients enter a study and are randomized to receive the treatment or a placebo. Each of the groups is mutually exclusive. An individual cannot be in more than one group. A 2 × 2 table can then be drawn up of the outcomes. In this example, 50 patients received the treatment and 41 were cured, as were 11 of those who received the placebo. Analysis of this data can be carried out using a Chi squared test in order to determine whether the treatment is statistically better than the placebo.

95% confidence intervals
- The 95% confidence interval is the range of values around the mean within which the true population mean will lie in 95% of cases
- It is calculated from the standard error. We can state that in 95% of cases, the population mean will lie ± 2 standard errors from our sample mean
- Data can therefore be expressed as a mean and 95% confidence interval, the values being the range provided by the mean ± 2 standard errors

CORRELATION AND REGRESSION (Fig. 19.4)

Correlation coefficient
- Reports on the relationship between two variables
- A value of 1 suggests a completely linear relationship
- 0 suggests that no relationship exists between them

Regression
- Allows calculation of the equation of a line drawn when two variables are plotted against each other
- Once this equation is defined, the value of one variable can be calculated when the other is known

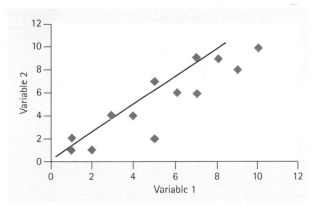

Fig. 19.4 Correlation and regression. When two variables are plotted against each other, a scatter plot results. A line of best fit can then be drawn through these points and the accuracy of the relationship between the two variables can be calculated based on the variance between each data point and the best fit line. This is the correlation coefficient.

ACCURACY OF TEST VALUES

Normal range
- For any variable there is usually a range of normal values, usually defined as the mean value $\pm$ 2 or 3 standard deviations

Sensitivity
- The ability of a test to report an abnormal result when the disease is present
- It reports on what proportion of patients with a disease will have a positive test

Specificity
- The ability of a test to return a normal result when the disease is absent
- It reports on what proportion of patients without the disease will have a negative test

Positive predictive value (PPV)
- The proportion of positive tests where the disease is actually present
- A high PPV suggests that if the test is positive, then the disease is present, i.e. there are few false positives

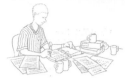

Clinical trials

I Designed to compare the effect of a therapy with either a placebo (i.e. an inactive substance) or another therapy

Randomization I Each patient entered into the trial has an equal chance of being in each of the therapy groups in the trial

Controlled trial I Comparison of one therapy against another or a placebo

Blinded I Patients do not know which therapy they are receiving

Double blind I Neither the doctor nor the patient knows which therapy is being received

Bias I Inequalities between the two groups other than the difference in therapy that they are receiving

Publication bias I Failure of negative trials to be published, so only positive data about a therapy reaches the public domain

Intention to treat I The analysis of the trial data includes all patients entered, irrespective of whether they completed the treatment course

Crossover trials I Each subject undergoes both types of therapy, one after the other
I A comparison can then be made for each individual patient

Evidence-based medicine

Definition | The conscientious, explicit and judicious use of current best evidence in making decisions about the care of individual patients

Role | EBM leads to patient care guided by the best available data on therapies available, but it is specific to the patient; in other words it aims to take into account differences between individual patients
— If a trial on hypertension were carried out in male Caucasians, its results may not be true of African women.

Resources

Cochrane Collaboration | A collection of critical appraisals of trials on specific therapies

Medline/Pubmed/ Index Medicus | Databases of biomedical studies published worldwide

Critical appraisal | The analysis of all the trials that have studied the same therapy in the same disease with a conclusion about the overall role of that therapy
| In general, only randomized controlled, preferably blinded trials are included and an intention to treat analysis is carried out

Relative risk | The percentage change in the probability of an event occurring due to the therapy given
— If the chance of a stroke on aspirin is 2% and the chance off aspirin is 4%, the relative risk of a stroke on aspirin is 50% (the proportion of strokes that would have been avoided)
| A relative risk of 100% ($\equiv 1$) suggests that the risk in each group is identical

Absolute risk | The proportion of all patients who would benefit from the therapy

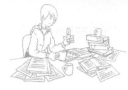

I In the above example, the chance of a stroke off aspirin is 4% while on aspirin it is 2%; therefore the absolute reduction in risk from taking aspirin is 4%–2% = 2%

Number needed to treat
I An estimation of the number of patients who would need to receive a therapy in order for a defined event to be avoided.
I In the example, 2 in every 100 patients taking aspirin will be prevented from having a stroke; to avoid 1 stroke, therefore, 50 patients have to be given aspirin

Screening and surveillance

Screening
I The investigation of a population in order to identify those who have a specific disease

Surveillance
I The investigation of an individual in order to detect recurrence of a disease

Ransom's criteria
I Criteria for an appropriate screening test
I That there is a safe and sensitive test for the disease with a high positive predictive value; the test should not have a high complication rate
I The yield of the test needs to be high enough to merit the cost of the test and the inconvenience and discomfort for both those in whom the disease is detected and those in whom it is not
I Earlier treatment of the disease has to have a benefit to the patient compared with late treatment; in other words, an effective therapy has to be available

Number needed to screen
I The number of individuals who have to be screened in order to prevent one death due to the disease

Lead time
I The time difference between detection of a disease by screening and the point at which it would have presented by causing symptoms

Epidemiology

The study of disease and the way it is distributed within the population

❚ The risk of developing a specific disease can depend on a wide variety of factors

Genetic predisposition
❚ Genetic variation between individuals alters their susceptibility to a disease
— HLA-B8 DR3 increases the risk of autoimmune disease

Exposure to causative agent
❚ Increased exposure to an infectious agent, carcinogen or other agent may be a function of geographical location, immediate personal contacts, work environment or personal habits such as diet, alcohol or smoking

Availability of healthcare
❚ Availability and utilization of healthcare resources impacts upon prevention of disease (e.g. vaccination) and the stage at which a disease presents; this may have a large impact on outcome

Social and cultural beliefs
❚ The response to disease is modified by an individual's perceptions of illness and his or her society's approach to disease management

DEFINITIONS IN EPIDEMIOLOGY

Incidence
❚ Number of new cases arising during a defined period of time
— 300 per year

Incidence rate
❚ Number of new cases per unit of population per year
— 3 per 1000 per year

Prevalence
❚ Total number of cases in a population per unit time

Prevalence rate
❚ Prevalence per unit population

Mortality
❚ Death rate per unit time

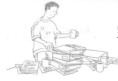

Mortality rate ❙ Death rate per unit population per unit time

Age-standardized mortality ❙ Correction of the mortality rate for a disease for age

Standardized mortality ratio
❙ Ratio of deaths observed in a cohort to the number expected across the whole population.
❙ e.g. The mortality in any specific age range in smokers is higher than that for the population as a whole

Audit and governance

❙ Audit is a method of monitoring performance and standards in healthcare
❙ Governance is the mechanism by which standards are maintained

Stages of audit
❙ Describe the variable to be audited
❙ Choose an appropriate standard to be used as a benchmark for performance
❙ Collect the data on local performance
❙ Compare local results with the standard
❙ Identify ways of improving local performance
❙ Repeat audit after implementation of the new protocols in order to assess their effect

Rules
❙ Audit should be non-confrontational and non-judgemental
❙ Individuals should not be openly targeted
❙ However, an individual doctor who is under-performing should be encouraged to improve practice and supported in doing so

Governance
❙ The means by which organizations ensure the provision of quality clinical care by making individuals accountable for setting, maintaining and monitoring performance standards
❙ Involves individuals and groups of healthcare workers in identifying best practice and how it may be achieved

Self-assessment questions

Multiple choice questions

1. Considering the following dataset: 3 4 5 5 7 9 11 12 13 15 48 186:
   A. The mode is 11
   B. The median is 10
   C. The distribution is Gaussian
   D. There is a positive skew
   E. The mean is 5

2. The following are appropriate tests for parametric data:
   A. Chi squared
   B. Paired t
   C. Mann–Whitney
   D. Student t
   E. Wilcoxon

Short answer questions

1. Discuss the role of the following in designing clinical trials:
   A. Blinding
   B. Randomization
   C. Placebo control groups

2. Define the following, giving examples of their use:
   A. Incidence
   B. Prevalence
   C. Standardized mortality ratio

Essay questions

1. What is bias? Describe the types of bias that may occur in clinical trials and the methods used to avoid it.

2. Discuss the importance of evidence-based medicine in modern healthcare. Outline the key points in deciding on the best type of therapy for a patient.

3. Define audit and its role in maintaining standards in health provision. Illustrate your answer with examples.

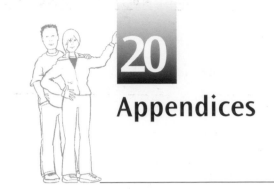

20

Appendices

A. Completion of death certificates

I Completing death certificates has been used as a station in the OSCE
I Doctors attending during the last illness of a person who dies have a statutory duty to issue a medical certificate of the cause of death
I The cause(s) of death must be stated to the best of your knowledge and belief
I Data from death certificates is used for the legal registration of death and to collect mortality statistics which are used for:
— Public health surveillance
— Research
— NHS resource allocation
I Death certificates are not to be completed by the attending doctor for cases referred to the coroner/procurator fiscal for investigation. Table 20.1 lists cases which should be referred to the coroner/procurator fiscal
I Deaths of neonates and still births have specific death certificates

NOTES FOR COMPLETION OF THE CERTIFICATE

Personal details of the deceased

Name

Age I In completed years or, if less than 1 year, in completed months

Table 20.1   A death should be referred to the coroner/procurator fiscal for investigation if:

▌ The cause of death is **unknown**
▌ The deceased was **not seen** by the certifying doctor either after death or within 14 days before death
▌ The death was **violent or unnatural or suspicious**
▌ The death may be due to an **accident**
▌ The death may be due to **self-neglect or neglect by others**
▌ The death may be due to **industrial disease or related to the deceased's employment**
▌ The death may be due to an **abortion**
▌ The death occurred during an **operation or before recovery from the effects of an anaesthetic**
▌ The death may be a **suicide**
▌ The death occurred during or shortly after **detention in police or prison custody**

Place of death   ▌ For hospital patients this is the name of the hospital
▌ For patients at home it is the private address
▌ For deaths elsewhere the locality is recorded

Circumstances of certification

Last seen alive by me   ▌ Record the date that you last saw the patient alive

Information from post-mortem   ▌ You should indicate here if the information you give takes account of a post-mortem
▌ Ring option 1 if a post mortem has been done
▌ Ring option 2 if information from the post-mortem may be available later
▌ Ring option 3 if a post-mortem is not being held

Seen after death   ▌ Ring one option (a, b or c) only to indicate whether you or another medical practitioner saw the deceased after death

Cases reported to the coroner   ▌ Some cases are discussed with the coroner/ procurator fiscal and a certificate is completed by the attending doctor after agreement with the coroner/procurator fiscal, e.g. patients dying within

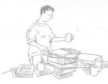

24 hours of arrival at hospital but for whom the cause of death is known
❙ If this is the case, then ring option 4 and tick box A on the back of the certificate
❙ Remember for cases referred to the coroner for investigation a certificate is not completed by the attending doctor

Cause of death statement
❙ Remember, always avoid abbreviations
❙ This section of the certificate is divided into two parts

Part I
❙ Here the immediate cause of death and any underlying cause(s) are recorded
❙ It is vital that this section is completed accurately and fully with as specific details as possible, e.g. histological cell types for malignancies if known

Example
❙ A patient died from an intracerebral haemorrhage caused by cerebral metastases from a primary malignant neoplasm of the left main bronchus
❙ This should be entered as follows:

Disease or condition that led directly to death	I (a) Intracerebral haemorrhage

Intermediate cause of death	(b) Cerebral metastases

Underlying cause of death	(c) Squamous cell carcinoma of the left main bronchus

❙ Occasionally there are apparently two distinct conditions leading to death. If there is no way of choosing between them they should be entered on the same line and it should be indicated that they are joint causes of death
❙ Do not use terms that imply a mode of dying rather than a cause of death (Table 20.2)

Table 20.2   Terms implying a mode of death rather than a cause of death

Asphyxia	Debility	Respiratory arrest
Asthenia	Exhaustion	Shock
Brain failure	Heart failure	Syncope
Cachexia	Hepatic failure	Uraemia
Cardiac arrest	Hepatorenal failure	Vagal inhibition
Cardiac failure	Kidney failure	Vasovagal attack
Coma	Renal failure	Ventricular failure
		Liver failure

Part II   ▌Any significant condition/disease that contributed to the death but which is not part of the sequence leading directly to death is recorded
▌Do not list all conditions present at the time of death
▌Do list any that may have hastened the death

Example
▌A diabetic patient died from an intracerebral haemorrhage caused by cerebral metastases from a primary malignant neoplasm of the left main bronchus
▌This should be entered as follows:

Disease or condition that led directly to death	I (a) Intracerebral haemorrhage

Intermediate cause of death	(b) Cerebral metastases

Underlying cause of death	(c) Squamous cell carcinoma of the left main bronchus

Other conditions contributing to death	II Diabetes mellitus

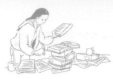

Employment-related death

- If you believe that the death may have been due to (or contributed to by) the employment followed at any time by the deceased, you should indicate this by ticking the appropriate box on the front of the certificate and report the death to the coroner/procurator fiscal

Signature of certifying doctor and name of consultant

- Sign the certificate and add your qualifications, your address and the date
- Print your name in block capitals also
- If the death occurred in hospital, the name of the consultant responsible for the care of the patient must also be recorded

Final points

- Complete the *Notice to Informant* section and the counterfoil of the certificate

B. Normal reference ranges

Normal values for laboratory tests:
These may vary from hospital to
hospital

Test	Abbreviation	Normal Range	Units
Full blood count			
Haemoglobin	Hb	Males 13.5–17.7	g/dL
		Females 11.5–16.5	g/dL
Mean corpuscular volume	MCV	80–96	fL
Mean corpuscular haemoglobin	MCH	27–33	pg
Mean corpuscular haemoglobin concentration	MCHC	32–36	g/dL
Reticulocyte count	retics	0.5–2.5%	of red cell count
Red cell count	RCC	males: 4.5–6	$\times 10^{12}$/L
		females: 3.9–5.0	$\times 10^{12}$/L
White cell count	WCC	4–11	$\times 10^9$/L
Basophils		0.01–0.1	$\times 10^9$/L
Eosinophils		0.04–0.4	$\times 10^9$/L
Lymphocytes		1.5–4.0	$\times 10^9$/L
Monocytes		0.2–0.8	$\times 10^9$/L
Neutrophils		2.0–7.5	$\times 10^9$/L
Platelets		150–400	$\times 10^9$/L

Test	Abbreviation	Normal Range	Units
Haematinics			
Serum B_{12}	B_{12}	160–925	ng/L
Serum folate		2.9–18	µg/l
Ferritin		male: 20–260	µg/L
		female: 6–110	µg/L
Iron	Fe	13–32	µmol/L
Total iron binding capacity	TIBC	42–80	µmol/L

Test	Abbreviation	Normal Range	Units
Other Haematology			
Erythrocyte sedimentation rate	ESR	< 20	mm/hour

Test	Abbreviation	Normal Range	Units
Coagulation			
Bleeding time		3–9	minutes
Active partial thromboplastin time	APTT	23–31	seconds

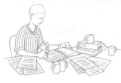
Test	Abbreviation	Normal Range	Units
Prothrombin time	PTPT	12–16	seconds
International normalized ratio	INR	1.0–1.3	

Urea and Electrolytes

Sodium	Na^+	135–146	mmol/L
Potassium	K^+	3.5–5.0	mmol/L
Chloride	Cl^-	95–106	mmol/L
Urea		2.5–6.7	mmol/L
Creatinine		79–118	µmol/L

Liver function tests

Alanine aminotransferase	ALT	5–40	IU/L
Aspartate aminotransferase	AST	12–40	IU/L
Gamma glutaryl transpeptidase	γT	10–40	IU/L
Alkaline phosphatase	ALP	39–117	IU/L
Bilirubin	Bili	<17	µmol/L

Other biochemistry

Glucose (fasting)		4.5–5.5	mmol/L
Glycosylated haemoglobin	Hb A_{1c}	3.7–5.1	
Calcium	Ca^{2+}	2.20–2.67	mmol/L
Phosphate	$PO4^{3-}$	0.8–1.5	mmol/L
C reactive protein	CRP	<10	mg/L
Urate		0.18–0.42	mmol/L

Lipids

Cholesterol	Chol	3.5–6.5	mmol/L
HDL cholesterol	HDL	male: 0.8–1.8	mmol/L
		female: 1.0–2.3	mmol/L
Triglycerides	Trig	male: 0.7–2.1	mmol/L
		female: 0.5–1.7	mmol/L

Arterial blood gases

Arterial partial oxygen pressure	Pao_2	10–13.3	kPa
Arterial partial carbon dioxide pressure	$Paco_2$	4.8–6.1	kPa
pH	pH	7.35–7.45	
Bicarbonate	HCO_3	24–28	mmol/L

C. Answers to self-assessment questions
MULTIPLE CHOICE QUESTIONS

3. Basic medical sciences

1. A. F
   B. T
   C. T
   D. F
   E. T

2. A. F
   B. T
   C. T
   D. F
   E. F

3. A. F
   B. F
   C. F
   D. T
   E. T

4. A. F
   B. T
   C. F
   D. F
   E. F

5. A. F
   B. T
   C. T
   D. F
   E. F

6. A. F
   B. F
   C. T
   D. T
   E. F

7. A. T
   B. F
   C. F
   D. T
   E. T

8. A. F
   B. T
   C. T
   D. T
   E. F

9. A. T
   B. T
   C. F
   D. T
   E. F

10. A. F
    B. T
    C. F
    D. T
    E. T

4. Clinical pharmacology

1. A. F
   B. T
   C. F
   D. T
   E. F

2. A. T
   B. F
   C. T
   D. T
   E. F

3. A. T
   B. T
   C. T
   D. T
   E. F

4. A. T
   B. T
   C. F
   D. F
   E. T

5. A. T
   B. T
   C. F
   D. T
   E. T

6. A. T
   B. T
   C. F
   D. T
   E. F

5. Radiology

1. A. T
   B. T
   C. F
   D. F
   E. F

2. A. T
   B. F
   C. F
   D. T
   E. T

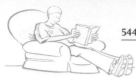

6. Clinical Chemistry

1. A. T
   B. F
   C. T
   D. T
   E. T

2. A. T
   B. T
   C. F
   D. F
   E. T

3. A. F
   B. F
   C. T
   D. F
   E. F

4. A. T
   B. T
   C. T
   D. T
   E. F

5. A. F
   B. T
   C. T
   D. T
   E. T

6. A. T
   B. T
   C. F
   D. T
   E. F

7. A. F
   B. T
   C. T
   D. T
   E. T

8. A. T
   B. T
   C. F
   D. T
   E. T

9. A. F
   B. T
   C. F
   D. T
   E. T

7. Infectious diseases

1. A. T
   B. F
   C. T
   D. T
   E. T

2. A. T
   B. F
   C. T
   D. F
   E. F

3. A. T
   B. F
   C. T
   D. F
   E. F

4. A. T
   B. T
   C. F
   D. T
   E. F

5. A. T
   B. T
   C. T
   D. T
   E. F

6. A. T
   B. F
   C. F
   D. F
   E. F

7. A. T
   B. F
   C. T
   D. T
   E. T

8. A. T
   B. F
   C. T
   D. T
   E. T

9. A. T
   B. F
   C. T
   D. F
   E. F

10. A. T
    B. T
    C. F
    D. T
    E. F

11. A. T
    B. F
    C. F
    D. F
    E. F

12. A. T
    B. F
    C. T
    D. T
    E. F

13. A. T
    B. F
    C. T
    D. F
    E. F

14. A. T
    B. T
    C. T
    D. T
    E. T

15. A. T
    B. F
    C. F
    D. F
    E. F

16. A. T
    B. F
    C. T
    D. T
    E. T

17. A. T
    B. T
    C. F
    D. F
    E. T

18. A. T
    D. T
    C. T
    D. F
    E. T

19. A. F
    B. F
    C. T
    D. T
    E. F

20. A. T
    B. T
    C. T

    D. T
    E. T

21. A. F
    B. T
    C. T
    D. F
    E. F

22. A. T
    B. F
    C. F
    D. T
    E. F

23. A. F
    B. F
    C. F
    D. T
    E. F

24. A. T
    B. T
    C. T
    D. F
    E. F

8. Respiratory medicine

1. A. T
   B. F
   C. T
   D. F
   E. T

2. A. F
   B. T
   C. T
   D. F
   E. T

3. A. T
   B. T
   C. F

   D. T
   E. F

4. A. T
   B. F
   C. F
   D. T
   E. T

5. A. T
   B. F
   C. T
   D. F
   E. T

6. A. T
   B. T
   C. F
   D. F
   E. F

7. A. T
   B. F
   C. T
   D. T
   E. T

8. A. T
   B. T
   C. F
   D. T
   E. T

9. A. T
   B. T
   C. T
   D. F
   E. T

10. A. T
    B. T
    C. F
    D. T
    E. T

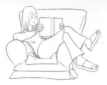

11. A. F
    B. T
    C. T
    D. T
    E. F

12. A. F
    B. T
    C. T
    D. F
    E. T

13. A. T
    B. T
    C. T
    D. F
    E. F

14. A. F
    B. T
    C. F
    D. T
    E. T

15. A. T
    B. T
    C. F
    D. T
    E. F

9. Cardiology

1. A. F
   B. T
   C. T
   D. F
   E. F

2. A. T
   B. T
   C. F
   D. T
   E. T

3. A. F
   B. T
   C. F
   D. F
   E. T

4. A. F
   B. T
   C. T
   D. T
   E. F

5. A. T
   B. F
   C. F
   D. F
   E. T

6. A. T
   B. T
   C. F
   D. F
   E. F

7. A. F
   B. T
   C. T
   D. F
   E. F

8. A. F
   B. T
   C. T
   D. T
   E. F

9. A. T
   B. F
   C. T
   D. F
   E. T

10. A. T
    B. F
    C. F

    D. T
    E. F

11. A. F
    B. T
    C. F
    D. T
    E. F

12. A. F
    B. T
    C. T
    D. T
    E. T

13. A. T
    B. F
    C. F
    D. F
    E. T

14. A. T
    B. T
    C. F
    D. F
    E. T

15. A. T
    B. T
    C. T
    D. F
    E. T

10. Gastroenterology and hepatology

1. A. T
   B. T
   C. T
   D. F
   E. T

2. A. T
   B. T
   C. F
   D. T
   E. T

3. A. F
   B. T
   C. T
   D. T
   E. T

4. A. T
   B. F
   C. T
   D. T
   E. F

5. A. I
   B. F
   C. T
   D. F
   E. T

6. A. F
   B. T
   C. T
   D. T
   E. F

7. A. T
   B. F
   C. F
   D. T
   E. T

8. A. T
   B. F
   C. T
   D. T
   E. T

9. A. T
   B. T
   C. F
   D. T
   E. T

10. A. T
    B. F

C. T
D. T
E. T

11. A. T
    B. T
    C. F
    D. T
    E. F

12. A. F
    B. T
    C. T
    D. F
    E. T

13. A. T
    B. F
    C. F
    D. F
    E. F

14. A. T
    B. F
    C. T
    D. T
    E. F

15. A. T
    B. T
    C. F
    D. T
    E. F

16. A. F
    B. F
    C. T
    D. F
    E. T

17. A. F
    B. T
    C. F
    D. T
    E. F

18. A. F
    B. T
    C. F
    D. F
    E. F

19. A. T
    B. F
    C. T
    D. T
    E. T

20. A. F
    B. T
    C. T
    D. T
    E. F

21. A. T
    B. F
    C. T
    D. T
    E. F

22. A. F
    B. F
    C. T
    D. T
    E. T

23. A. T
    B. F
    C. T
    D. F
    E. F

24. A. T
    B. T
    C. T
    D. F
    E. F

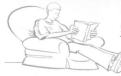

25. D

26. A. F
    B. T
    C. T
    D. F
    E. F

27. A. F
    B. F
    C. T
    D. T
    E. T

28. A. T
    B. T
    C. T
    D. T
    E. T

29. A. F
    B. T
    C. T
    D. F
    E. T

30. A. T
    B. T
    C. T
    D. F
    E. T

31. A. T
    B. T
    C. T
    D. F
    E. F

32. A. F
    B. T
    C. T
    D. F
    E. F

33. A. T
    B. T
    C. F
    D. F
    E. T

34. A. T
    B. T
    C. T
    D. F
    E. T

35. A. T
    B. T
    C. F
    D. T
    E. T

36. A. T
    B. F
    C. T
    D. F
    E. F

37. A. T
    B. T
    C. F
    D. T
    E. T

38. D

39. A. T
    B. F
    C. F
    D. T
    E. T

40. A

11. Rheumatology

1. A. T
   B. F
   C. T
   D. F
   E. T

2. A. F
   B. T
   C. T
   D. T
   E. F

3. A. F
   B. F
   C. T
   D. F
   E. F

4. A. F
   B. T
   C. F
   D. T
   E. T

5. A. T
   B. T
   C. T
   D. T
   E. F

6. A. F
   B. F
   C. T
   D. F
   E. F

7. A. F
   B. F
   C. T
   D. F
   E. F

8. A. F
   B. T
   C. F
   D. T
   E. F

9. A. F
   B. F
   C. T
   D. T
   E. T

10. A. T
    B. T
    C. F
    D. T
    E. F

11. A. T
    B. T
    C. F
    D. T
    E. F

12. A. T
    B. T
    C. T
    D. T
    E. T

12. Dermatology

1. A. T
   B. T
   C. T
   D. T
   E. T

2. A. T
   B. F
   C. T
   D. F
   E. T

3. A. F
   B. T
   C. T
   D. F
   E. T

4. A. F
   B. T
   C. T
   D. F
   E. T

5. A. F
   B. T
   C. F
   D. F
   E. F

6. A. T
   B. T
   C. T
   D. T
   E. F

7. A. T
   B. T
   C. T
   D. T
   E. T

8. A. F
   B. T
   C. T
   D. T
   E. F

9. A. F
   B. F
   C. T
   D. T
   E. F

13. Endocrinology

1. A. F
   B. F
   C. T
   D. F
   E. T

2. A. T
   B. T
   C. F
   D. F
   E. T

3. A. F
   B. F
   C. T
   D. T
   E. T

4. A. T
   B. T
   C. T
   D. F
   E. F

5. A. T
   B. T
   C. T
   D. F
   E. T

6. A. F
   B. T
   C. T
   D. F
   E. F

7. A. F
   B. T
   C. T
   D. T
   E. T

8. A. F
   B. F
   C. T
   D. T
   E. T

9. A. T
   B. T
   C. T
   D. F
   E. T

10. A. T
    B. T
    C. F
    D. T
    E. F

11. A. F
    B. F
    C. F
    D. T
    E. T

12. A. F
    B. F
    C. F
    D. T
    E. T

13. A. F
    B. F
    C. T
    D. T
    E. F

14. A. F
    B. T
    C. F
    D. F
    E. T

15. A. F
    B. T
    C. F
    D. T
    E. T

16. A. F
    B. F
    C. T
    D. F
    E. F

17. A. F
    B. T

    C. F
    D. T
    E. F

18. A. F
    B. T
    C. T
    D. F
    E. T

19. A. F
    B. T
    C. T
    D. F
    E. F

14. Renal medicine

1. A. F
   B. F
   C. F
   D. F
   E. F

2. A. T
   B. F
   C. T
   D. T
   E. F

1. A. T
   B. F
   C. T
   D. T
   E. F

4. A. T
   B. F
   C. T
   D. T
   E. F

5. A. T
   B. F

   C. F
   D. T
   E. T

6. A. T
   B. T
   C. T
   D. T
   E. T

7. A. F
   B. T
   C. F
   D. F
   E. F

8. A. T
   B. T
   C. T
   D. F
   E. T

9. A. T
   B. T
   C. T
   D. F
   E. F

10. A. T
    B. T
    C. T
    D. T
    E. T

11. A. T
    B. T
    C. T
    D. F
    E. F

12. A. T
    B. T
    C. F
    D. T
    E. F

13.
A. T
B. T
C. F
D. F
E. T

14.
A. T
B. T
C. F
D. T
E. T

15. Haematology

1.
A. F
B. T
C. T
D. F
E. F

2.
A. F
B. T
C. T
D. T
E. T

3.
A. T
B. T
C. F
D. T
E. F

4.
A. T
B. F
C. T
D. T
E. T

5.
A. T
B. F
C. T
D. T
E. F

6.
A. T
B. F
C. F
D. F
E. T

7.
A. T
B. T
C. T
D. T
E. T

16. Oncology

1.
A. T
B. T
C. T
D. T
E. F

2.
A. F
B. T
C. F
D. F
E. T

3.
A. F
B. F
C. F
D. T
E. F

4.
A. T
B. F
C. T
D. T
E. F

5.
A. F
B. F
C. T
D. F
E. F

17. Neurology

1.
A. T
B. T
C. F
D. T
E. F

2.
A. F
B. T
C. F
D. T
E. F

3.
A. F
B. F
C. T
D. T
E. F

4.
A. F
B. T
C. T
D. F
E. F

5.
A. T
B. T
C. F
D. T
E. T

6.
A. T
B. T
C. F
D. F
E. F

7.
A. T
B. F
C. F
D. F
E. T

8. A. T
   B. T
   C. F
   D. T
   E. F

9. A. T
   B. T
   C. F
   D. T
   E. T

10. A. F
    B. F
    C. F
    D. T
    E. F

11. A. T
    B. T
    C. F
    D. F
    E. T

12. A. F
    B. F
    C. F
    D. T
    E. T

13. A. F
    B. T
    C. T
    D. T
    E. F

14. A. T
    B. F
    C. T
    D. T
    E. F

15. A. T
    B. T
    C. F
    D. F
    E. T

16. A. T
    B. T
    C. F
    D. T
    E. F

17. A. T
    B. F
    C. T
    D. F
    E. F

18. A. F
    B. F
    C. T
    D. F
    E. T

18. Psychological Medicine

1. A. T
   B. T
   C. F
   D. T
   E. T

2. A. F
   B. F
   C. T
   D. T
   E. T

3. A. T
   B. F
   C. T
   D. T
   E. T

4. A. F
   B. F
   C. T
   D. F
   E. T

5. A. T
   B. T
   C. T
   D. T
   E. F

6. A. F
   B. T
   C. F
   D. T
   E. T

7. A. T
   B. F
   C. F
   D. T
   E. T

8. A. F
   B. F
   C. T
   D. T
   E. F

9. A. T
   B. T
   C. T
   D. F
   E. F

10. A. F
    B. T
    C. T
    D. T
    E. F

11.	A.	F		D.	F		C.	F
	B.	F		E.	F		D.	T
	C.	T					E.	F
	D.	T	**19. Statistics and**			
	E.	T	**evidence-based**		2.	A.	F
			medicine			B.	T
12.	A.	F					C.	F
	B.	T	1.	A.	F		D.	T
	C.	T		B.	T		E.	F

HINTS FOR ANSWERS TO EXTENDED MATCHING QUESTIONS AND OSCES

5. Radiology

OSCE 1. A. A circular lesion with an air fluid level in the right lower lung field
   B. Pulmonary abscess
      Pulmonary metastasis
      Primary bronchial carcinoma
   C. CT scan of the chest
      Blood cultures

OSCE 2. B. Radionucleotide bone scan

OSCE 3. Haemorrhage
   Pain
   Perforation of a viscus (gallbladder)

OSCE 4 A. Calcified mass in the area of the right kidney
   B. Renal cell carcinoma
      Renal calcinosis
   C. CT scan of the abdomen
      Renal ultrasound

6. Clinical chemistry

1. I. C. Confusion is non-specific. Oedema suggests right heart failure. Hypokalaemia is an unwanted effect of loop diuretics. Renal failure could be secondary to heart failure or unwanted effect of diuretics.
   II. I. Hypokalaemia, hypomagnesaemia, dehydration and normal anion gap metabolic acidosis all result from electrolyte and water losses from high ileostomy outputs.

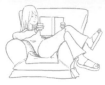

III. D. Hypoxia and low P_{CO_2} suggests respiratory problem, fever suggests infection. Low sodium is a result of syndrome of inappropriate ADH (SIADH) and is associated with pneumonia.

2. I. H. Hypercapnia and hypoxia suggest type II respiratory failure.

II. F. Metabolic acidosis with respiratory compensation (low P_{CO_2}) in a patient with diabetes who is unwell and vomiting is very suggestive of diabetic ketoacidosis.

III. C. Metabolic acidosis with high anion gap is compatible with aspirin overdose.

7. Infectious diseases

1. I. E. There is evidence of immunocompromise and/or reactivated TB (chest X-ray, lymphadenopathy, fever).

II. J. Rust-coloured sputum and peri-oral HSV are associated with *Strep. pneumoniae*.

III. F. Hepatosplenomegaly, jaundice, a fever and low platelets are all characteristic of malaria.

2. I. L. Liver ultrasound would demonstrate cholecystitis (thickened inflamed gallbadder) and cholangitis (gas in biliary tree, stones or an obstructed biliary tree). CT would be the second choice.

II. B. The clinical picture is that of malaria.

III. G. The data suggest infective endocarditis. Multiple sets of blood cultures are needed to detect the organism and derive the antibiotic sensitivities.

8. Respiratory medicine

1. I. B. Eczema suggests atopy in a young woman. Spirometry results suggest an obstructive defect. These, together with history, make asthma very likely.

II. A. Breathlessness with clubbing and weight loss strongly suggest lung cancer, especially with progressive symptoms.

III. H. Normal chest X-ray and pulmonary function tests exclude many of the answers. NSAIDs (e.g. ibuprofen) cause GI ulceration and iron deficiency particularly in elderly patients.

2. I. A. *Streptococcus pneumoniae* is the commonest cause of community-acquired pneumonia and can be associated with rust-coloured sputum.

II. E. Patient has a low CD4 count and so is at risk of opportunistic infection. Pneumocystis pneumonia can present with severe hypoxia without abnormality on examination or chest X-ray.

III. F. *Staphylococcus aureus* pneumonia can follow flu outbreaks and can cause cavitating lesions.

9. Cardiology

1. I. D. The presence of different blood pressures in each arm, interscapular pain and Marfans point to a dissected thoracic aorta.

II. B. This is exercise-induced angina in a patient with risk factors (diabetes mellitus and smoking).

III. A. The age and the relationship to food is suggestive of a gastrointestinal rather than cardiac cause.

2. I. B. The right heart failure and cardiomegaly in a drinker suggest alcoholic cardiomyopathy.

II. C. Deep vein thrombosis with a pulmonary embolus — recent travel with a swollen leg and breathlessness.

III. C. The history of diabetes and the presence of an ulcerated area could be cellulites or vascular insufficiency. The history favours the former.

3. I. B. The rate of 160 bpm and no 'p' waves in a smoker suggest AF.

II. I. The tachycardia is due to the β-agonist (it also causes tremor). If the patient was not on inhalers consider thyrotoxicosis.

III. D. The symptoms are all due to anxiety-related hyperventilation — shortness of breath and tingling of the fingers and mouth.

10. Gastroenterology

1. I. D. Autonomic neuropathy due to diabetes mellitus links the symptoms.

II. H. The mucus and low potassium suggest a tubulo-villous adenoma. The mucus is very potassium rich and can be profuse.

III. G. Ulcerative colitis (anaemia, fever and diarrhoea) all point to severe disease.

2. I. E. The risk factors of diabetes and heart disease, combined with pain and diarrhoea after food, suggest mesenteric ischaemia.

II. G. Ulcers, weight loss and anaemia, plus erythema nodosum, all point to inflammatory bowel disease and therefore Crohn's in this question.

III. H. Irritable bowel — the alternating bowel habit, bloating and left iliac fossa pain are suggestive and the weight gain discounts other pathologies.

3. I. B. Growth failure with GI symptoms points towards coeliac disease, Crohn's or cystic fibrosis. The latter is unlikely to present as late as this.

II. A. Pernicious anaemia — the low vitamin B_{12} and the history of autoimmune thyroid disease point to this.

III. E. The history suggests chronic pancreatitis — steatorrhoa and chronic alcoholism.

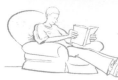

11. Rheumatology

1. I. D. Syndesmophytes are suggestive of ankylosing spondilytis and the ESR and HLA status support this.

 II. B. Osteoarthritis is a common cause of backpain. Normal bloods and no erosions on X-ray make the other diagnoses unlikely.

 III. A. Recent wrist fracture in a post-menopausal woman with normal bloods is highly suggestive of osteoporosis. She may have had steroids for her asthma, making osteoporosis more likely.

2. I. D. Elevated urate suggests gout. The distribution of the joint symptoms is compatible with gout.

 II. F. Rash, joint pains and raised inflammatory markers with a positive ANA is strongly suggestive of SLE.

 III. B. Heberden's nodes with normal ESR suggests osteoarthritis.

12. Dermatology

1. I. I. Raised, purple, painful red areas on the legs suggest erythema nodosum which is associated with Crohn's disease.

 II. A. History of atopy. Distribution suggests eczema (flexoral).

 III. F. Yellow crusts strongly suggests *Staph. aureus* infection.

2. I. F. An ulcer which is rapidly increasing in size in a patient with Crohn's disease is highly suggestive of pyoderma gangrenosum.

 II. A. The pigmentation and brown colour suggest venous ulceration.

 III. B. Being a gardener suggests UV exposure. The appearance and hard node suggests SCC rather than malignant melanoma.

13. Endocrinology

1. I. D. She has multiple endocrine neoplasia type I (a parathyroid adenoma causing hyperparathyroidism, associated with a pancreatic tumour). The high calcium resulting from this is causing the constipation and polyuria.

 II. B. She has Sheehan's syndrome — a pituitary infarction following a post-partum haemorrhage — leading to diabetes insipidus. This is rare.

 III. A. There is a metabolic acidosis (low bicarbonate), thirst, polyuria and weight loss — classical early onset diabetes mellitus.

2. I. A. She has autoimmune disease already so her risk of a further autoimmune disease is increased. Anxiety, palpitations, diarrhoea and weight loss are all pointing towards thyrotoxicosis.

II. E.   The palmar pigmentation, abdominal pain and postural hypotension suggest Addison's disease (in this case due to adrenal tuberculosis suggested by sweats, weight loss and foreign travel).

III. B.   50% of coeliac disease presents with iron deficiency. Weight loss and abdominal pain support this. The southern Irish origins increase the risk of coeliac.

14. Renal medicine

1. I. C.   The history of gout increases the risk of renal stones. The colicky pain and sudden onset in the absence of indicators of infection support this.

II. H.   The chest signs point to a pneumonia. The urinary abnormalities may be due to an atypical pneumonia (e.g. mycoplasma or legionella).

III. E.   There is an association between polycystic kidney disease and berry aneurysms that result in subarachnoid haemorrhage. The pain is probably due to bleeding into one of the renal cysts.

2. I. A.   The presence of liver cirrhosis with new acute renal failure favours hepatorenal syndrome as the cause.

II. F.   Haemolytic-uraemic syndrome results from *E. coli* O157 and occurs after food poisoning with this organism. The anaemia and thrombocytopenia are as a result of the haemolysis.

III. I.   The mass in his pelvis is his bladder. This is a classical presentation of acute retention due to prostatic enlargement.

15. Haematology

OSCE 1   A.   Macrocytic anaemia
  B.   Hypothyroidism, Vitamin B_{12} deficiency, folate deficiency
  C.   Thyroid function, Schilling test, serum B_{12} and folate

17. Neurology

1. I. C.   The distal progressive weakness and areflexia are typical of Guillain–Barré. The history of a recent GI infection supports this.

II. A.   The smoking and hypertension are key risk factors for ischaemic stroke. This is a non-dominant side event with dysphasia.

III. H.   The shuffling gait, micrographia and resting tremor all point to Parkinsons.

2. I. F.   The rash, photophobia and fever all suggest meningitis (probably meningococcal).

II. A.   The combination of abdominal symptoms and unilateral headache, probably initiated by alcohol, points to migraine.

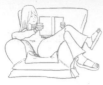

III. D. The retinal changes suggest malignant hypertension, and are not features of diabetic retinopathy.

3. I. G. All the elements are here for a benzodiazepine overdose, using drugs prescribed by the GP. She could be either ketoacidotic or hypoglycaemic but the history points to deliberate self-harm due to reactive depression.
  II. I. Scepticaemia due to urinary sepsis.
  III. E. Hypotension, bradycardia and, in particular, J waves on the ECG all point to hypothermia.

18. Psychological medicine

1. I. F. The pattern of memory loss is compatible with early dementia.
  II. D. She has first rank symptoms of schizophrenia. Her ethnicity increases the risk of this disease.
  III. H. High MCV suggests alcohol excess. Visual hallucinations, sweating and tachycardia occur in alcohol withdrawal syndrome.

D. Bibliography and further reading

Kumar P, Clark M (eds) (2002) *Clinical Medicine*, 5th edn. Edinburgh: W.B. Saunders.

Warrell D, Cox T, Firth JD, Benz EJ (eds) (2003) *Oxford Textbook of Medicine*, 4th edn. Oxford: Oxford University Press.

Hampton J (2003) *The ECG Made Easy*, 6th edn. Edinburgh: Churchill Livingstone.

Corne J, Carroll M, Delany D, Brown I (2002) *Chest X ray Made Easy* 2nd edn. Edinburgh: Churchill Livingstone.

Marshall, WJ (2000) *Clinical Chemistry* 4th edn. London: Mosby

Sackett D, Strauss S, Richardson WS, Rosenberg W, Hayes RB (2000) *Evidence Based Medicine* 2nd edn. Edinburgh: Chruchill Livingstone.

WEBSITES

www.kumarandclark.com — *Clinical Medicine* on line.

www.fleshandbones.com — A general site for medical students and instructors.

www.ncbi.nih.gov/entrez/query fcgi — Pubmed, a search engine for biomedical research.

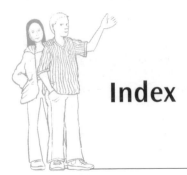

Index

Note: Question and Answer Sections are indicated in the form 14(Q),16(A) with Hints being indicated by (H). Entries in **bold** indicate tables, those in *italics* indicate figures.

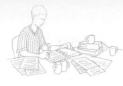

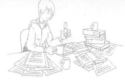

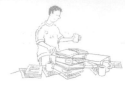

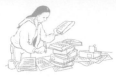

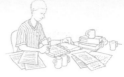

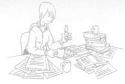

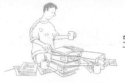

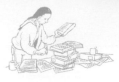

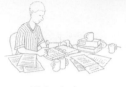

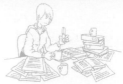

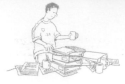

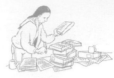

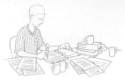

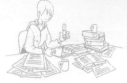